GENOTOXIC IMPURITIES

GENOTOXIC IMPURITIES
Strategies for Identification and Control

Edited by

ANDREW TEASDALE

AstraZeneca
Leicestershire, United Kingdom

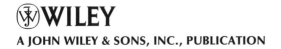

A JOHN WILEY & SONS, INC., PUBLICATION

Published by John Wiley & Sons, Inc., Hoboken, New Jersey
Published simultaneously in Canada

For general information on our other products and services or for technical support, please contact our Customer Care Department within the United States at (800) 762-2974, outside the United States at (317) 572-3993 or fax (317) 572-4002.

Wiley also publishes its books in a variety of electronic formats. Some content that appears in print may not be available in electronic formats. For more information about Wiley products, visit our web site at www.wiley.com.

Library of Congress Cataloging-in-Publication Data:

Genotoxic impurities: strategies for identification and control / edited by Andrew Teasdale.
    p. ; cm.
Includes bibliographical references and index.
ISBN 978-0-470-49919-1 (cloth)
1. Genetic toxicology.   2. Drugs–Toxicology.   I. Teasdale, Andrew.
[DNLM: 1. Mutagenicity Tests–methods.   2. Drug Toxicity–prevention & control.
3. Mutagens–adverse effects.   4. Mutagens–analysis.   5. Toxicogenetics–methods.
QU 450 G3353 2011]
RA1224.3.G463 2011
616'.042–dc22

                                    2010025374

Printed in Singapore

10 9 8 7 6 5 4 3 2 1

CONTENTS

FOREWORD

Since the turn of the millennium, the issue of genotoxic impurities (GIs) has perhaps been one of the most emotive issues facing the industry. Certainly, in advance of the formal publication of the finalized guideline, the impact was significant, resulting in, for example clinical holds, while issues were addressed. Even when the finalized guideline was published, there remained considerable concern and uncertainty. These focused on both the context of the guideline (e.g. is it appropriate to look to apply very tight controls to pharmaceuticals when the overall genotoxic burden is vast in comparison?) and its implementation (i.e. how should it be interpreted and/ or applied?).

As well as the controversy and uncertainty surrounding the guideline, it is clear that GIs occupy an almost unique position of having equal significance in terms of safety and quality. Thus, to address the challenges posed in implementing the guideline, it is necessary to adopt a multidisciplinary strategy that draws in expertise from many functions. Primary within these are the safety and chemistry functions.

Given both the level of concern and the complexity of the issue, it is timely that this book has been developed, especially as we potentially move into a new phase, with this being a proposed International Conference on Harmonization (ICH) topic.

It is hoped that this book will provide to the reader an objective commentary on the guideline as a whole, addressing both the fundamental principals and the practical implementation of the guideline. In doing so, it should provide a holistic overview of all aspects, both safety and quality, appropriately linking them together in a coherent way to provide specific, practical advice.

It is my hope that this book could in some way serve to help both industry and regulators alike, and by doing so, enable them to work together to address GI-related issues. Through this process, it is also my own hope that such a dialogue will eventually allow emerging data (e.g. evidence for the existence of thresholds) to be examined in a scientifically sound manner.

Dr. Peter Moldeus, VP Global Safety Assessment, AstraZeneca

PREFACE

When I was asked to develop a book focused on genotoxic impurities (GIs), I was both excited and at the same time slightly daunted by the prospect. I quickly realized the very significant challenge that lay ahead, given the almost unique position held by GIs. As anyone involved in this area will realize, addressing GIs is a complex issue that requires the consideration of both quality and safety matters, and the resolution of any associated problems needs a holistic approach based on the effective combination of skills from both these areas. It was therefore critical that the book address both aspects in a comprehensive manner, and to do this, I realized, would require the contribution of experts in both fields. That I feel I have been able to achieve this in the book is due to the excellent response I got from key individuals in the fields concerned. I am indebted to them for contributing to this work.

Given the complexity of the issue of GIs, it was also important that the book provide advice on the practical interpretation of regulatory guidelines covering GIs, and that this should be objective, making it useful for both industry and regulators alike. That the guideline has been controversial is clear; however, I have endeavored to present the information provided in the book in a way that deliberately avoids turning it into simplistic and emotive criticism of the regulatory position.

The book is divided into specific parts, each focused on a specific aspect of GIs. Part I focuses on the development of the guideline and the derivation of the threshold of toxicological concern (TTC). This provides an understanding of the history behind the development of regulatory guidance and of the key concept of a TTC. I believe this is critical in understanding the current position of the regulatory guidelines.

Part II is focused on safety aspects. It examines how an impurity might be evaluated using structure activity relationship (SAR) data to assess the potential for mutagenicity. Within this part, there is also an examination of the safety tests, both *in vitro* and *in vivo*, used in the experimental evaluation of the genotoxic potential of impurities. Each test is examined in terms of the end point of the test, what it specifically indicates in terms of genetic toxicity, and the strengths and weaknesses of the test. This also examines how such tests might be combined to define a strategic approach to testing.

The next chapter in Part II looks at how other safety data, including carcinogenicity data (i.e. other than simple *in vitro* Ames test data) might be utilized to define alternative limits to those defined by the TTC. In doing so, it also examines the challenges faced in the application of such data. Part II concludes with an evaluation of the challenges faced when addressing a GI that is also a metabolite, examining both the practical challenges faced when identifying such metabolites and how to assess risk when such a metabolite is discovered. This in particular examines how data derived from adsorption, distribution, metabolism, and elimination (ADME) animal studies can be used to assess the risk posed.

Part III contains two chapters that provide a perspective on the risk posed by GIs. The first chapter within this part examines the risk in context with exposure to genotoxic material from other sources. The second examines the relatively new but increasing evidence of thresholds even for mutagens that act directly on DNA, examining the implications of these discoveries, in particular how this might be developed further to improve our general understanding of the concept, beyond the limited number of GIs for which at present such data exist.

Part IV examines GIs from a quality perspective. This focuses on two critical aspects: the analysis of GIs and the evaluation of the likelihood of their presence at levels of concern.

Chapter 9 covers how the potential risk posed by GIs in terms of carryover might be practically assessed, examining the critical factors associated with such an assessment through a series of case studies. Chapters 10–13 focus specifically on the analysis of GIs, examining both the practical and strategic aspects of such analysis, again providing practical examples wherever possible.

The final chapters of Part IV look at the specific issue of sulfonate esters and their effective control and the issue of GIs formed as a result of the degradation of drug substance and/or drug product, in both cases outlining how this might be practically evaluated.

I would finally like to pay tribute to all the authors who have contributed to this work, for their dedication throughout the writing process and for the quality of their input. Without their contribution, there would be no book. I hope that as a reader you are able to share this sentiment, and that ultimately, the book is of value to you within this subject area.

The final word, though, must go to my family, my wife, and my son for their support and understanding over the time I have worked on this book. One day, perhaps, my son will understand why I have written a book about "genie-toxic" imps, as he calls it!

Andrew Teasdale

CONTRIBUTORS

Andrew Baker, AstraZeneca, Leicester, United Kingdom

Alessandro Brigo, F. Hoffman-La Roche AG, Basel, Switzerland

Frank David, Research Institute for Chromatography, Kortrijik, Belgium

Shareen Doak, Swansea University, Wales, United Kingdom

Krista Dobo, Pfizer, Groton, CT, USA

David Elder, GlaxoSmithKline, Hertfordshire, United Kingdom

Simon Fenner, AstraZeneca, Bristol, United Kingdom

Susanne Glowienke, Novartis, Basel, Switzerland

James Harvey, GlaxoSmithKline, Hertfordshire, United Kingdom

Catrin Hasselgren, AstraZeneca, Mölndal, Sweden

Charles Humfrey, AstraZeneca, Alderley Park, United Kingdom

Karine Jacq, Research Institute for Chromatography, Kortrijk, Belgium

Gareth Jenkins, Swansea University, Wales, United Kingdom

George Johnson, Swansea University, Wales, United Kingdom

Alan P. McKeown, Pfizer, Kent, United Kingdom

Lutz Müller, F. Hoffman-La Roche AG, Basel, Switzerland

Mike O'Donovan, AstraZeneca, Alderley Park, United Kingdom

Ron Oglivie, Pfizer, Kent, United Kingdom

James Parry, Swansea University, Wales, United Kingdom

Andrew Phillips, AstraZeneca, Cheshire, United Kingdom

Pat Sandra, Research Institute for Chromatography, Kortrijk, Belgium

Andrew Teasdale, AstraZeneca, Leicester, United Kingdom

Gerd Vanhoenacker, Research Institute for Chromatography, Kortrijk, Belgium

Don Walker, ex. Pfizer, Sandwich, Kent, United Kingdom

DEVELOPMENT OF GENOTOXIC IMPURITIES GUIDELINES AND THE THRESHOLD OF TOXICOLOGICAL CONCERN CONCEPT

HISTORICAL OVERVIEW OF THE DEVELOPMENT OF GENOTOXIC IMPURITIES GUIDELINES AND THEIR IMPACT

Ron Ogilvie
Andrew Teasdale

1.1 INTRODUCTION

To enable a thorough understanding of the current regulatory position relating to genotoxic impurities (GIs), it is first important to consider the history behind the events that led up to this point and their context. Like many events, the exact point at which concerns relating to the potential presence of GIs in pharmaceuticals first emerged is difficult to determine. At the time that ICH Q3 guidelines were constructed, only passing reference was made to compounds of "unusual toxicity" and the potential need for limits tighter than those defined by the guidelines. Although the term "genotoxic" is not specifically mentioned, many have taken this to refer to impurities that are genotoxic.

The first public evidence of specific regulatory concern relating to GIs was an article published within PharmEuropa in 2000,[1] which drew attention to the potential risk of formation of sulfonate esters as a result of a combination of sulfonic acids in alcoholic solution as part of a salt formation process. At this point, this publication was merely a call for "further information"; it being part of an attempt to better understand the extent of any risk involved. The publication is now seen as a landmark event, signaling a new era of focus on genotoxic impurity risk assessment and control.

In 2002, a position paper relating to GIs was published by the Committee for Proprietary Medicinal Products (CPMP[*]) on behalf of the European Medicines Evaluation Agency (EMEA) Safety Working Party (SWP) for comments in December

[*] Now Committee for Human Medicinal Products (CHMP).

Genotoxic Impurities: Strategies for Identification and Control, Edited by Andrew Teasdale
Copyright © 2010 by John Wiley & Sons, Inc.

2002.[2] Outlined below is an evaluation of this first draft position paper, and an assessment of its later significance in the context of the finalized EU guideline.

1.2 CPMP—POSITION PAPER ON THE LIMITS OF GIs—2002

1.2.1 Scope/Introduction

Within the introduction to the position paper, it was made clear that the need for such guidance was due to the fact that control over levels of genotoxic residues was not adequately addressed through existing ICH guidance.

The format of the position paper was similar to that of the final guideline, it being set out in a series of sections, which addressed the issue of GIs from both a toxicological and quality perspective. The key points from those sections are described below.

1.2.2 Toxicological Background

Within the position paper, genotoxic compounds were split into two categories:

1. Genotoxic compounds, for which sufficient evidence existed to support a thresholded mechanism.

(A thresholded mechanism is one for which a clearly discernable limit exists, below which no significant toxicological effect is observed. Several examples were given within the paper of mechanisms of genotoxicity for which a thresholded mechanism may exist, including, for example, topoisomerase inhibition, inhibition of DNA synthesis, and overload of defense mechanisms.)

2. Genotoxic compounds without sufficient evidence for a thresholded mechanism.

The position paper stated that such thresholds were either unlikely to exist, or would be difficult to prove for DNA-reactive chemicals.

This categorization of GIs, on the basis of a mechanistic understanding of toxicological action, has remained in place in the finalized guideline, and the belief that DNA reactive compounds have no threshold remains widely held.

1.2.3 Pharmaceutical (Quality) Assessment

The assumption that some "*in vivo*" genotoxins can damage DNA at any exposure level, and therefore that any level can represent a risk, led to a conservative stance being proposed in terms of quality assessment. It was stipulated that a justification must be provided in relation to the manufacturing process that clearly explained why, for that specific process, the presence of GIs was "unavoidable." The position paper also stated that wherever possible, alternative routes that avoid genotoxic residues should be used, and that an applicant was obliged to update the manufacturing process should a safer alternative process be available. If, after these steps had been taken, a risk remained, it was suggested that residual levels should be reduced to the level that was "as low as technically feasible."

1.2.4   Toxicological Assessment

The position paper made it clear that only after the use of a genotoxic reagent had been justified and every effort had been made to reduce levels should a toxicological assessment be made. Different options were provided by which risk assessments could be carried out, these being through either:

1. *Quantitative risk assessments:* This being essentially based on the linear extrapolation of the dose-response curve from rodent cancer bioassays from a high dose to low dose region. In this case, the low dose considered acceptable being one associated with a 1 in 100,000 risk. (One excess cancer death per 100,000 people exposed to the agent concerned over a lifetime [70 years].)

2. *Uncertainty factor approach:* This approach, which involves the determination of a no effect level (NOEL) from preclinical studies, along with the subsequent application of uncertainty factors, is only appropriate where a threshold-mediated mechanism has been established. Such an approach is consistent with that described within ICH Q3C—residual solvents.

The position paper in this format was a cause of significant concern. The main concern perhaps related to the safety testing requirements. For many reagents, the only safety data available often relates to limited *in vitro* studies, for example an Ames test. Such data are generally considered unsuitable for establishing a NOEL or for performing a quantitative risk assessment. Thus, to generate data to support the determination of a NOEL, or to carry out a quantitative risk assessment as prescribed in the concept paper would require the conduct of further significant *in vivo* studies. This could have resulted in a significant increase in animal studies. Thus, ultimately, alternatives to this were sought. An alternative approach, previously adopted within other spheres, such as the food arena, was the concept of a "virtual safe dose." This had been developed to deal with low-level contaminants within food. This concept itself was based on the principal of establishing a level at which any new impurity, even it was subsequently shown to be carcinogenic, would not constitute a significant risk. This paved the way ultimately for the employment within subsequent versions of the guideline of the threshold of toxicological concern (TTC for short) concept.

1.3   GUIDELINE ON THE LIMITS OF GIs—DRAFT, JUNE 2004

Significant revisions were made to the original position paper before its rerelease as a draft guideline in June 2004.[3] The revised guideline struck a more balanced note. For example, the "*as low as technically feasible*" terminology used previously was replaced with the ALARP ("as low as reasonably practical") principle, a small but in many ways significant shift in emphasis. Another important change was the removal of the requirement to introduce an alternative route/process should a safer one be identified. The need to provide justification of the route selected did, however, remain.

The most significant change was the tacit acceptance that the concept of elimination of risk in its entirety (zero risk) was going to be unachievable and therefore an alternative to this principle was required. This led to the adoption of the concept of an acceptable risk level. This acceptable risk was defined as a level sufficiently low that, even if the compound in question was ultimately shown to be carcinogenic, it would pose a negligible risk to human health. This took the form of the *TTC*. This concept obviates the need to generate extensive *in vivo* data to establish limits.

The most critical aspect of the TTC concept (the origin of its development and its derivation are described in detail in Chapter 2) is the derivation of a single numerical limit of 1.5 µg/day based on a lifetime (70 years) exposure resulting in a worst-case excess cancer risk of 1 in 100,000. Within other areas (e.g. food), a 1 in 1,000,000 figure had been applied; this was increased by a factor of ten in relation to pharmaceuticals to recognize the benefit derived from pharmaceutical treatment. This concept allows an adequate basis of safety and control limits to be established in the absence of any *in vivo* data.

The guideline, having established this TTC limit, also stated that under certain circumstances, higher limits could be established. Such circumstances included short-term exposure, treatment of a life-threatening condition for which no safer alternatives existed, where life-expectancy was less than 5 years or where the impurity was a known substance for which exposure from other sources (e.g. food) was significantly greater than that associated with exposure from pharmaceuticals. Notably, no fixed alternative limits were provided that could be applied in such instances, perhaps, as there are a myriad of potential circumstances where such considerations could apply, and thus it was considered that this topic was best left to the assessment of a specific product and a specific risk benefit analysis to agree acceptable limits. It is reasonable that product-specific risk/benefit considerations are applied, and this in many ways supports not establishing fixed acceptable limits in the guideline. This concept remains in place in the final guideline. There might, however, still be value in more specific statements in the guidance regarding necessary limits in some "extreme" circumstances (e.g. where oncology candidates are being used that themselves have known genotoxicity, it would be useful for the guidance to state that specific low-level control of potentially GIs in this instance is not required).

Since the time that the TTC concept was first introduced through this draft guideline, the TTC has come under scrutiny, principally because of its conservative nature. The guideline itself explicitly recognizes this conservatism. For this reason, the necessity of this limit has been questioned. To examine the reasons why the TTC concept was initially at least so readily accepted, it is imperative to look at it in the context of the initial concept paper. Before the TTC concept was introduced, the primary objective was elimination of risk and only where this proved impossible could limits be established. However, setting limits would, as already described, require extensive *in vivo* studies. Set in this context, the concept of an agreed baseline limit, even if conservative, was unsurprisingly seen as an attractive proposition.

One addition at this point was the widening of the scope to include excipients. This was perhaps surprising, although concerns do exist in relation to some excipients, for example modified cyclodextrins (concern over residues of alkylating agents used to modify the cyclodextrin). In many ways, excipients are very similar to existing products in that their safety has been well established through use over an extended period in multiple formulations. In addition, many are used in other areas, including the food industry, and thus any exposure related to intake of pharmaceuticals is likely to be small compared with other sources.

A major issue at this point in time was the lack of any guidance relating to permissible doses during short-term clinical trials. This led, in some instances, to the imposition of the 1.5 µg/day lifetime exposure limit, even for very short duration studies. This prompted the development from an industry perspective of a position paper, outlining a "staged" TTC concept. This is described below.

1.4 PHRMA (MUELLER) WHITE PAPER

A Pharmaceutical Research and Manufacturers of America (PhRMA) expert group, led by Lutz Mueller, sought to establish acceptable limits for GIs in APIs linked to duration of exposure. This was referred to as a "staged TTC" approach, and was based on the established principle that exposure risk was defined in terms of cumulative dose.[4] Inherent to this principle is that the risk associated with an overall cumulative dose will be equivalent in terms of risk, irrespective of dose rate and duration. Thus, short-term exposure limits could be based on linear extrapolation from accepted long-term exposure limits.

The group published the outcome of their deliberations in January 2006.[5] The key aspect of this paper, the proposed "staged TTC" limits, are displayed below in tabular form (Table 1.1).

TABLE 1.1   Proposed Allowable Daily Intakes (µg/day) for GIs during Clinical Development, a Staged TTC Approach Depending on Duration of Exposure

	Duration of exposure				
	≤1 month	>1–3 months	>3–6 months	>6–12 months	>12 months
Allowable daily intake (µg/ day) for different duration of exposure (as normally used in clinical development)	120[a] or 0.5%[c] Whichever is lower	40[a] or 0.5%[c] Whichever is lower	20[a] or 0.5%[c] Whichever is lower	10[a] or 0.5%[c] Whichever is lower	1.5[b,c]

[a] Probability of not exceeding a 10^{-6} risk is 93%.

[b] Probability of not exceeding a 10^{-5} risk is 93%, which considers a 70-year exposure.

[c] Other limits (higher or lower) may be appropriate and the approaches used to identify, qualify, and control ordinary impurities during developed should be applied.

A critical aspect of this is the application of a 1 in 1,000,000 risk factor when calculating limits for durations <12 months, as opposed to the 1 in 100,000 applied in relation to the standard TTC based on lifetime exposure. This precautionary approach was taken in recognition of the fact that during the clinical phase, studies are often performed on healthy human volunteers, and also that even for patients at this stage, the therapeutic benefit has often yet to be determined.

As well as the staged TTC principal, the paper also defined a classification system for impurities, defining five separate classes:

- Class 1: genotoxic carcinogens.
- Class 2: genotoxic—carcinogenicity unknown.
- Class 3: alerting structure—unrelated to parent.
- Class 4: alert related to parent.
- Class 5: no alerts.

Based on this classification system, the paper defined a strategy for impurity assessment based on the use of structure activity relationships (SAR). SAR evaluation is used as the first stage in order to give a preliminary evaluation of risk. Thereafter, this can be augmented by the use of safety testing, specifically the Ames test, to determine whether or not the impurity is actually genotoxic. This is particularly true where the impurity is classified as class 3. Alternatively, one can simply assume the compound in question to be genotoxic on the basis of the prediction and control in line with the appropriate TTC level.

Such a strategy, often augmented by a science-based risk assessment (incorporating factors such as reactivity of the impurity and downstream process conditions), has become the foundation of most, if not all, evaluation processes used within the industry (see Chapter 9 for a detailed evaluation of such strategies).

1.5 FINALIZED GUIDELINE ON THE LIMITS OF GIs—JUNE 2006

The finalized version of the guideline was issued June 28, 2006, with an effective date of January 1, 2007.[6] In terms of the final guideline, some key points were addressed and it is appropriate to recognize this and welcome the significant progress made from the original position paper. Outlined below are the key areas that had been addressed.

The published guidance attempted to clarify how the concepts of the guidance were to be applied to existing substances and products. A concern had been that existing medicines would be required to comply with all aspects of the new guidance. This could have led to there being a perceived shortfall in control strategies or quality for a significant number of medicinal products that had been developed in the years prior to the development of this guidance, and, furthermore, that had proved to be adequately safe across this period. The published guideline included the following specific statement.

> It also relates to new applications for existing products, where assessment
> of the route of synthesis, process control and impurity profile does not provide

reasonable assurance that no new or higher levels of genotoxic impurities are introduced as compared to products currently authorised in the EU concerning the same active substance. The same also applies to variations to existing Marketing Authorisations pertaining to the synthesis. This guideline does, however, not need to be applied retrospectively to authorised products unless there is specific cause for concern.

In practice, this has proved difficult to interpret consistently, particularly in relation to the potential "catch all" phrase "cause for concern." The impact of this uncertainty is explored in detail in the following section.

Another addition within the Recommendations section was advice over the scope of investigations in terms of what impurities should be considered as part of an assessment. The guideline stating:

As stated in the Q3a guideline, actual and potential impurities most likely to arise during synthesis, purification and storage of the new drug substance should be identified, based on a sound scientific appraisal of the chemical reactions involved in the synthesis, impurities associated with raw materials that could contribute to the impurity profile of the new drug substance and possible degradation products. This discussion can be limited to those impurities that might reasonably be expected based on the knowledge of the chemical reactions and conditions involved.

Although entirely sensible and reasonable on the face of it, in practice, this is difficult to interpret consistently. After all, what is "reasonable"? This subjective term may mean a very different thing to one person than it does to another. The impact of this difficulty in interpretation is explored in full within the next section.

Another change was the exclusion of excipients from the finalized guideline, this having present in the 2004 draft version. A separate specific position paper addressing excipients has subsequently been issued jointly by the Quality Working Party (QWP) and Safety Working Party (SWP)[7] within EMEA (and will be discussed later in this chapter).

1.6   ISSUES ASSOCIATED WITH IMPLEMENTATION

It should be recognized that many of the concepts and principles outlined in the finalized guideline were of real significance in achieving a useful guidance. However, many of the concepts outlined in the guideline also require careful implementation and leave certain concerns unaddressed.

1.6.1   The Relevance of the TTC Concept for Short Durational Exposure

The utility of the TTC concept is undeniable, but many experts were concerned, and remain concerned, that the maximum daily exposure of 1.5 µg was overly conservative (being based on the combination of several "worst case" assumptions in its derivation), and especially conservative if applied to short duration usage and acute use therapies. Importantly, the guideline as published did not provide clear guidance on what standards would be expected of investigational medicinal products during the clinical development phases, when controlled and often short duration clinical trials are conducted. It should be unnecessary to apply a control standard applicable to lifetime exposure in such short duration clinical studies, but the guideline gave no specific guidance on what standard would be expected, leaving the implementation of the guideline to be potentially inconsistent. Of primary concern was the lack of any indication as to whether or not the staged TTC concept, as outlined in the Mueller paper,[5] was acceptable or not. This led to considerable confusion and uncertainty, which was ultimately resolved with the publication, some 18 months later, of the EMEA staged TTC limits through the SWP Q&A Document.[8]

1.6.2   Lack of Clarity Regarding Drivers for Application to Existing Products

Similarly, despite the useful focusing of the scope of the applicability of the guideline on "causes for concern" and "significant change" of existing medicinal products, it left unclear what was considered to constitute a "significant cause for concern" or a "significant change."

Did a "cause for concern" exist if an existing impurity in an existing medicine had known genotoxicity (but the medicine concerned had been safely used for many years)? Did a "cause for concern" exist if an existing impurity in an existing medicine had a structural alert for potential genotoxicity but there was no known toxicological findings associated with the impurity?

Did a manufacturing change bring significant new risks if the same route of manufacture was scaled up or conducted at a different site? Did a manufacturing change bring significant cause for concern if process changes were conducted to optimize manufacture that instituted a change in manufacturing chemistry but not a change in the specification of the active substance? What about a change in manufacture of a starting material for active substance manufacture?

Such topics and a lack of clear, specific guidance in the published text left the guideline open to considerable degrees of interpretation and with it the possibility for inconsistent implementation. Indeed, there has been a considerable increase in queries linked to existing products, many asking for a full evaluation of the genotoxic risk, sometimes triggered by variations not linked to the manufacturing process.

So, one can see that even with elements of the guideline that were viewed as "positive," like the TTC concept and the risk-based application to existing products, there were elements of detail that seemed to bring a need for further clarity to support consistent implementation. And of course, there were other aspects of the published guideline that were less well received, or were simply not considered in the guideline as it was first published. These too are worthy of consideration.

1.6.3   Standards Required of Investigational Products

The lack of clear standards that would be expected of investigational products was quickly identified as a gap in the guideline. It could be considered that the original intent of the guideline had been to provide guidance on the management of potentially GIs for marketing applications, not for investigational materials, and thus to make good the "gap" in the ICH impurity guidelines. These ICH guidelines, which provide potential registration requirements for marketing applications, point to a potential need for more rigorous control for some impurity classes (e.g. GIs), but do not provide guidance on how to manage such impurities. Given this ICH-driven provenance, one might consider that the CHMP guideline as published was not intended to apply to investigational materials, but like ICH guidelines, to provide potential registration requirements for commercial products. However, the guideline's applicability was ambiguous, and, of course, with no further specific guidance for investigational materials, it was most likely that the same standards might begin to be applied to investigational materials, even if this was not the initial intent of the expert authors of the original guidance.

1.6.4 Circumstances that Support Modification of the TTC Limit

As already described, the published guideline also contained guidance to the effect that the general TTC limit (1.5 µg/day) could be modified in certain circumstances (e.g. for short duration treatments, particular indications, or patient groups) to provide for modified control of potential GIs in these products. Unfortunately, while this is potentially a very useful aspect of the guidance, the published guideline provides no further specific advice, again leaving considerable opportunity for inconsistent implementation. Similarly, and importantly, there could be some medicines, indications, or patients groups where it might be unnecessary to implement *any* rigorous, "low-level" control of potential GIs. For example, if an oncology treatment is itself known to be genotoxic, it would seem unnecessary to control potentially GIs in such an active substance to exquisite levels. Furthermore, many oncology treatments are used either post- or in tandem with cytotoxics during the clinical phase, particularly in advanced stages of the disease. The cytotoxic agent itself poses a significant but accepted risk of secondary cancer. This again challenges the value in patient safety terms, of controlling GIs to exquisitely low values, especially when the patient prognosis is also taken into account.

1.6.5 Control Requirements When Multiple GIs May Be Present

It also became clear that it was possible for a product to contain more than one potentially genotoxic impurity. However, the published guidance was not clear on what control expectations would exist when more than one potential genotoxic impurity was equally likely to be present in the active substance or product. Would each be simply controlled on the basis of individual TTC limits? This would seem reasonable given the conservative nature of the derivation of the general 1.5 µg/day TTC limit. Or would there be an expectation that the total genotoxic impurity load would be controlled to a total level of 1.5 µg/day? There might be some scientific basis for implementing such a cumulative control if the impurities were known to be (or likely to be) toxicologically similar, but far less need to do so if the impurities were known to be (or likely to be) toxicologically distinct. These are all interesting and potentially important considerations, but the published guideline provided no detailed guidance on these questions. An almost inevitable consequence of this uncertainty has been the potential for variance in interpretation by regulators and industry.

1.6.6 Application to New MAA Applications Relating to Existing Products

Of course, the guideline also potentially applies to applicants for generic versions of existing products. On one level, an applicant for a generic medicine might assume that the active substance in their medicine is "out of scope," as clearly such a medicine has a significant preexisting period of use such that its safety is known. However, this assumption relies upon the generic active pharmaceutical ingredient and medicinal product having the same quality and impurity profile as the existing drug substance and drug product. This may or may not be the case, as even if similar chemistry is used, subtleties of manufacture or formulation can lead to potentially significant differences in impurity profile, especially when "significant" is no longer being considered as reflecting ICH unspecified impurity control limits (e.g. in the order of 0.1%—i.e. parts per thousand), but at the levels of TTC-based controls (which can be in the order of parts per million). And, of course. other interesting and important questions arise when considering the development of generic products. How can a generic applicant assure themselves they have introduced no new risk factors with respect to previously approved materials? Can they simply meet the preexisting European Pharmacopoeia (Ph.Eur.) monograph for the active substance (if one exists)? This may *not* be sufficient: these monographs rarely include controls on potential GIs at low levels. Even where they do, they relate to a specific process (usually the innovators). Maybe the generic applicant could simply test their drug substance against the previously approved drug substance? But what analytical methods should be used? Of course, this lack of transparency relates not only to the generic manufacturer; the regulator charged with assuring the suitability of the new product faces a similar challenge.

Of course, if the generic applicant decided to do a comprehensive and independent risk assessment of their drug substance or drug product, and their manufacturing processes and establish TTC-based controls for any potentially GIs (on the basis of structural alerts, etc.), then no doubt the regulatory agencies will be presented with a potentially approvable drug substance, associated specification and manufacturing process. Will the Agency then turn to the previously approved marketing application holders and demand that they too test their preexisting supplies for the potentially GIs that the subsequent applicant has determined to be potentially present, even though the existing marketing application holders (MAHs) and products have not changed the risk profile of their products? One can imagine how wonderfully complex such considerations of implementation quickly could become.

1.6.7 Control Expectations for Excipients

The guideline formally is not stated to apply to excipients used in pharmaceutical manufacture, this being addressed by a separate EMEA publication[7] (discussed further below—see Section 9.1). This might be considered ironic when one of the apparent triggers leading to the guideline was the potential presence of a genotoxic impurity in a novel cyclodextrin excipient. One could wonder why these materials are excluded, as some excipients are also manufactured by chemical synthesis, and may also be exposed to routes of manufacture that contain reactive and "at risk" reagents and intermediates. The Ph.Eur. contains many excipients, for example that are polymers of epoxides, or use epoxides to derivatize other materials (e.g. cyclodextrins), and of course epoxides are alkylating materials and hence are potentially genotoxic potential impurities in the excipients. Clearly, with excipients often being a more significant percentage in weight terms of a medicine than the active substance, the potential risk associated with excipient impurities might also be of concern. However, many of the excipients in the Ph.Eur. have a significant period of safe use, many indeed are listed within the FDA GRAS list,[9] and hence the guidance would, on balance, conclude that there are no fresh risks to bring their quality into the scope of the guideline.

But what of the potential risk associated with manufacturing process changes related to excipient manufacture? What of the (admittedly relatively infrequent) case of a novel excipient being developed? The guideline makes no comment as to how such examples should be handled. Should these "new risks" be in scope or out of scope?

1.6.8   Control Expectations for Natural/Herbal Products

Pharmaceuticals are in the majority of cases well-characterized small molecules manufactured by well-defined chemical synthesis. However, the situation can be quite different in relation to some medicines derived from natural products. Some of these natural product-derived medicines, including herbal medicines, can be less well-characterized materials that can subject to significant variability in terms of composition, depending on their source. Of course, the control of impurities in such medicines is also important, and, by extension, one perhaps should consider whether such medicines too might contain potentially GIs. It is, however, practically impossible to apply the same degree of risk management to the manufacture/isolation of a natural product, nor the same degree of process selection and design. How should one approach the management of potential genotoxic risk in such active substances? The guideline provides no specific guidance. This would be later addressed through a specific guideline covering herbal products, this is explored in Section 9.2.

1.6.9   Identification of Potential Impurities

As highlighted earlier, the guideline noted that risk assessment of manufacturing processes should be undertaken to identify potential GIs, and that impurity structures should be risk assessed (using e.g. predictive databases like DEREK or MCASE that link structural motifs to potential toxicological responses). This sounds very reasonable and practicable. However, one could find two "experts" in the field who might draw up two different lists of potential impurities associated with a particular manufacturing process. After all, what is considered reasonable when defining impurities?

It is also very unclear as to how many steps within a process should be taken into consideration when performing such an assessment. Thus, even apparently very reasonable risk management processes suggested in the guideline become difficult to implement in a consistent manner.

1.6.10 Concerns Related to the Principle of Avoidance

The guidance also contained very specific expectations that the pharmaceutical development efforts should first and foremost "avoid" genotoxic materials or impurities and take every effort to select a manufacturing process that avoids there being potential genotoxic risks associated with the product.

> *A justification needs to be provided that no viable alternative exists, including alternative routes of synthesis …*

> *If a genotoxic impurity is considered to be unavoidable in a drug substance, technical efforts (e.g. purification steps) should be undertaken to reduce the amount of the genotoxic residues in the final product in compliance with safety needs or to a level as low as reasonably practicable.*

These were elements of the guideline that had provoked considerable comment during the drafting process. Assembling drug substances by chemical synthesis is predicated on the combination of simple chemicals into more complex drug substance structures. This synthesis involves chemical reactions, often driven by reactive functional groups that, as a consequence of their reactivity (e.g. alkylating functionality), can be potentially toxic and indeed potentially genotoxic. Thus, to have "complete avoidance" as the fundamental principle of chemical process development would be extremely problematic. *In extremis*, the effect of such an approach could be that many important, necessary (and well understood) reactions would suddenly be declared unsuitable or at the very least subject to intense scrutiny. Not only would avoidance be problematic as a fundamental principle, but avoidance can also be appreciated to be inherently unnecessary, in risk management terms, when one considers that a manufacturing process can be designed in such a way as to ensure that the residues of these reactive materials are not significantly present in the drug substance.

An important consequence of the intrinsic reactivity of some of the materials "to be avoided" is that they can easily break down to innocuous materials during isolation of intermediates, for example, by hydrolysis. This would mean that one would be being told to avoid a useful synthetic material that would anyway be destroyed and removed during manufacture. This removal would make "avoidance" unnecessary. Furthermore, manufacturing processes can be designed with the removal of potential genotoxic reagents, intermediates, or impurities in mind, either by using such reagents early in a multi-step manufacturing process, or by designing isolation processes or purification processes specifically to remove materials of concern. Thus, having "avoidance" as a fundamental design criterion for drug substance manufacture could be considered to be an overreaction and extremely precautionary. When all aspects of risk management and scientific understanding are considered, avoidance can be seen to be nonscientific. The risks being avoided can be managed in other scientifically sound ways, and furthermore can also be controlled, if need be, by analytical testing. The primary consideration of the chemical manufacture of drug substances (and medicinal products) should be the safety (and efficacy) of the medicine, and since the adoption of the TTC-principle establishes a basis of adequate safety (or acceptable risk), then control strategies and control tests on specifications can be established to "control" the adequate safety of manufactured drug substances without imposing a "ban" on the use of many important reagent and reaction types.

Let us be sure we are absolutely precise and fair to the wording of the guideline. In the guideline, "avoidance" was stated to be a fundamental principle, but was not required if the applicant had shown that no other manufacturing process free of attendant genotoxic risk factors could be employed

> A justification needs to be provided that no viable alternative exists ...
> If a genotoxic impurity is considered to be unavoidable ...

While on the face of it a seemingly reasonable request, in practice, this particular aspect of guidance is in reality a case of "how long is a piece of string?" in terms of the expected extent of such investigations. It is virtually impossible to make this objective and hence to consistently implement. How many alternative routes of synthesis need to be evaluated and discarded before one can conclude "there is no viable alternative"? How many potential routes should one explore if a drug substance is made by a manufacturing process that uses "risky" reagents like alkylating reagents, but contains no trace of the impurity that would have potential genotoxicity? If a route of synthesis not employing "at risk" materials can be shown to be feasible but the drug substance cannot be made economically, or in an environmentally acceptable manner, by that route should that potential medicine be "avoided"? Having development chemists chasing alternative routes to one medicine is a surefire way to prevent development chemists developing other medicines. Thus, this guidance, by placing "avoidance" above "control" could very well prevent the innovation of new medicines or new manufacturing routes (with improved environmental benefits). Despite the later helpful clarification provided through the Q&A document[8] around many other issues, the specific issue of the necessity for avoidance remains unclear.

1.6.11 Concerns Related to the ALARP Principle

The guideline also suggested that if avoidance was not possible, then residues of any genotoxic materials to be used should be removed to a level that was "as low as reasonably practicable" (the so-called "ALARP" concept). This concept too sounds immediately reasonable, especially in the context of the original request to control to as low as technically feasible, but is flawed when one begins to consider aspects of its implementation. Consider a case when an applicant has developed a process to deliver an active ingredient that contains a measurable, but low level, of a potentially genotoxic impurity. The applicant has established a control strategy in accordance with a TTC-based limit. Should the assessor approve this application or require the applicant to further modify the process to lower the residual level yet further? How much more work would be required to be considered "reasonably practicable"? Can such a judgment be consistently applied, by all assessors, to all applicants? Will some applicants or assessors expect more to be done than others?

All such considerations could introduce inconsistencies in what needs to be a level regulatory landscape. Given the conservative nature of the guideline, there should simply be no *need* to further improve quality if a TTC-based control strategy has been established. After all, the TTC is considered a virtually safe dose. These concerns were later addressed through the EFPIA Q&A document, see Section 7.4.

1.6.12   Overall

Potentially, the most troublesome aspect of the guideline is the scope for inconsistent interpretation even in relation to the many apparently "well-developed" concepts. It is therefore perhaps not surprising that regulators and industry alike struggled and are still struggling to fully understand how to interpret and apply it in its entirety.

To begin to resolve the difficulties described, much further work and discussion has taken place after the final publication of the guidance in both regulatory circles (CHMP Safety Working Party [SWP] and European Directorate for the Quality of Medicines [EDQM]) and in industry and industry trade associations (European Federation of Pharmaceutical Industry Associations–EFPIA) as all parties involved looked to examine these important topics in depth. As a result, some significant steps forward have been taken since the first publication in January 2007, which we will look in at detail here.

Since the publication of the final guideline, significant clarifications of several key topics have been issued, via an SWP Question/Answers publication,[8] and, separately, by the EDQM regarding the implementation requirements of the guidance for Pharmacopoeial monographs.[10]

1.7   SWP Q&A DOCUMENT

1.7.1   The Application of the Guideline in the Investigational Phase and Acceptable Limits for GIs Where Applied to Studies of Limited Duration

It has been clarified and confirmed that it is important to ensure that investigational medicinal products are of appropriate quality with respect to potential GIs. Importantly, it has been clarified, via an SWP Q/A[8] (published originally June 26, 2008 as EMEA/CHMP/SWP/431994/2007), that durational adjustments to the TTC limit are acceptable for investigational studies. This approach of extrapolating the lifetime-based TTC limit to shorter duration exposures had been proposed by a PhRMA[5] cross-industry workgroup (led by Lutz Mueller—Roche), who, as described earlier, proposed a set of "staged" TTC limit dependent upon study duration. The SWP have accepted the principle of such duration-dependent modifications to the TTC, but have published a set of durational limits that are slightly different from the original PhRMA proposal. These are shown below (Table 1.2):

> *The acceptable limits for daily intake of genotoxic impurities are 5, 10, 20, and 60 µg/day for a duration of exposure of 6–12 months, 3–6 months, 1–3 months, and less than 1 month, respectively. For a single dose an intake up to 120 µg*

TABLE 1.2 Staged TTC Limits

	Duration of exposure				
	Single dose	≤1 month	≤3 months	≤6 months	≤12 months
Allowable daily intake	120 μg	60 μg	20 μg	10 μg	5 μg

is acceptable. Compared to the proposal of a staged TTC in the Mueller et al. (Reg Tox & Pharm, 2006, 44, 198–211) paper these values incorporate a dose rate correction factor of 2 to account for deviations from the linear extrapolation model.

The scientific basis/driver behind the need to apply a correction factor to the linear model is unclear given the conservative nature of the linear extrapolation model itself, as is the rationale that requires restricting the 120 μg/day to a single dose.

In the published Q/As, the SWP have stated that these modified limits can be applied in the investigational phase only, and cannot be automatically presumed to apply to commercial products that are used for short durations. The applicant for such an acute-use therapy can however propose amended control limits in their MAA, and the approval of product-specific limits for the commercial product will be established during the review process, considering the full product-specific risk benefit of the product.

1.7.2 Application of the Guideline to Existing Products

The guideline had originally, and very reasonably, limited the application to existing products to "known causes for concern" and to "change management." However, the lack of a definition of what constituted a "cause for concern" was a real shortfall in the guidance. This shortfall led to difficulty in interpretation and potentially to inconsistent application of the guidance both by regulatory agencies and industry. This has led to the SWP looking to provide a clarification, again via the official Q/A publication, that a "cause of concern" is a material with either a preexisting or new genetic toxicology findings (and in their answer, the SWP give one example class of impurity that would be considered as constituting a cause for concern—mesylates and alkyl mesylates).

If a manufacturing procedure for API remains essentially unchanged a re-evaluation with respect to the presence of potentially genotoxic impurities is generally not needed. However, new knowledge may indicate a previously unknown cause for concern. One example is the mesylate salt drug substances for which a few years ago, a concern regarding the potential for formation of genotoxic alkyl mesylates was raised. This concern resulted in the "Production Statement" requesting a specific evaluation of the potential for formation of these highly toxic products now included as part of the PhEur monographs for all the mesylates salts.

The EDQM have further extended the clarity on this point by noting, in a PharmEuropa publication,[10] that structurally alerting functionality alone does not constitute a cause for concern without actual toxicology data.

> *Structural alert does not automatically imply genotoxicity.*
>
> *Action is needed only where there is study data demonstrating genotoxicity of the impurity. The existence of structural alerts alone is considered insufficient to trigger follow-up measures.*

Furthermore at present, there has been limited clarification provided on the second key concern in terms of implementation of the guideline to existing products, that is what constitutes a significant change to a manufacturing process that should trigger risk assessment of the product? It had been assumed by industry that route and process changes that might significantly affect the potential presence or level of potentially GIs in the active pharmaceutical ingredient or medicinal product would be in scope and would merit risk assessment but that Variations that constitute less impactful changes (e.g. changing the site of manufacture with no other route or process changes) would not require genotoxic risk assessment. However podium presentations by individual assessors from competent authorities have emphasized that it is not clear what constitutes a significant change. Indeed, it appears that any variation, irrespective of its likely impact on quality, might draw a request from the assessor for the applicant to provide a risk assessment for potential GIs in the product. As in many cases the Variation does not result from a significant route or process change, this regulatory request for risk assessment seems to be inconsistent with the intent of the guideline as it effectively means that the guideline is being retrospectively applied to the existing product.

EDQM also addressed this issue through its PharmEuropa publication, discussing the applicability of the guideline to pharmaceutical monographs. The statement made provides a very useful, risk-based approach to managing the application of the guideline to monographed materials. The EDQM article stated that *"Substances included in medicinal products authorised in recent years have been thoroughly evaluated for safety and in view of the experience with their use the need for retrospective application of a policy on genotoxic impurities is not considered necessary unless there is specific cause for concern,"* again emphasizing the role of prior clinical exposure and pharmacovigilance in their management of the existing products. The detailed Appendix table from this EDQM publication provides a variety of tiers of potential change and the action considered necessary to support each "change." This very helpful table (Table 1.3) is reproduced below.

The most recent version of the Q&A document—revision 2 (December 2009), has now confirmed that the principles outlined in the EDQM document can also be applied to existing products that at present have no monograph, stating that in such instances:

> *For active substances included in medicinal products authorized by the competent authorities before implementation of the CHMP guideline, the specifications as described in the dossier for marketing authorization should be followed.*

TABLE 1.3   EDQM Decision Table for Use during Elaboration or Revision of Monographs

Status	Action
Substance included in a medicinal product authorized after Issuance of the CHMP guideline	Monograph should be based on marketing authorization(s)
Substance included in a medicinal product authorized before issuance of the CHMP guideline: No PGI expected from synthetic route	No action needed, monograph based on marketing authorization
Substance included in a medicinal product authorized before issuance of the CHMP guideline: PGI expected from synthetic route of first authorized product Subsequently authorized products (if any) have no expected PGI or same PGI as the first authorized product at same or lower level No data showing genotoxicity	No action needed during elaboration of monograph (based on marketing authorization), no revision of existing monographs
Substance included in a medicinal product authorized before issuance of the CHMP guideline: PGI expected from synthetic route of an authorized product Data showing genotoxicity of an expected PGI	Monograph should be elaborated or revised based on evaluation by the Competent Authority
Substance included in a medicinal product authorized before issuance of the CHMP guideline: PGI expected from synthetic route of first authorized product Subsequently authorized products have a new expected PGI or same PGI as innovator product at a higher level Data showing genotoxicity of an expected PGI	Monograph should be elaborated or revised based on evaluation of new PGI or higher level of previously known PGI by the Competent Authority
Substance included in a medicinal product authorized before issuance of the CHMP guideline: PGI not expected from synthetic route of first authorized product Subsequently authorized product(s) have a new expected PGI Data showing genotoxicity of an expected PGI	Monograph should be elaborated or revised based on evaluation of new PGI by the Competent Authority

Reproduced with the kind permission of PharmEuropa.

1.7.3   Control of Multiple GIs

There has also been further consideration of what should be done to manage instances where more than one potentially genotoxic impurity is associated with the route of synthesis. The SWP opinion outlined in the Q&A document states that:

> *When more than one genotoxic impurity is present in the drug substance, the TTC value of 1.5 μg/day can be applied to each individual impurity only if the impurities are structurally unrelated.*

This is based on the assumption that the impurities act by the same genotoxic mode of action and have the same molecular target, and thus might exert effects in an additive manner.

It is attractive to believe that this position can be stated in the simple way described. However, this is probably *too* simple to fully address the complexity of the topic in full. There are both toxicological and quality aspects that have to be considered when thinking about control strategies when more than one impurity is involved.

For example, from a "quality" perspective, two impurities containing similar structural motifs might not be equally likely to survive the manufacturing process and be present in API. There may be no need to control one of these, as it is effectively purged by the process, therefore the control method may not need to be capable of controlling both to low levels.

From a safety perspective, it could be that the built-in conservatism of the TTC approach can accommodate there being more than one risk factor present without impacting significantly upon the overall risk. Bercu et al.,[11] in a recent publication, has suggested that low numbers of impurities with genotoxic potential all controlled at individual TTC limits would not have a statistically appreciable impact on the risks associated with the medicine compared with if all impurities were controlled to one total limit.

Nevertheless, one might consider it reasonable that two impurities that are known or suspected to be genotoxic via a particular common mechanism of action *in vivo* and which both might survive to be present in an active substance might best be controlled in total as a pair to one cumulative limit. However, it is a simplification to immediately relate simple structural similarity (based on e.g. the impurities bearing the same DEREK alerting motif for genotoxicity) to toxicological similarity. The link between structural alerts and actual toxicology needs careful risk assessment and requires considerable expertise. Clearly, structure activity relationships provide the underlying basis of, for example DEREK risk evaluation, and very close structural relationships to materials of known toxicology are an important aspect to consider in risk evaluation. Within such assessment, though there are many subtleties that need to be considered when evaluating the structural basis of genotoxicity— small structural differences in secondary features can have a very significant impact on toxicology.

In DEREK risk assessment, the actual structural environment of an alert has to be considered, as this can have a profound affect on actual genotoxicity (e.g. the reactivity and toxicity of alkyl halides can be determined by structural, steric, and electronic factors), such that one alkyl halide will be genotoxic but another not.

Similarly, the genotoxicity of aromatic materials is significantly affected by substitution patterns (see toluene and benzene for a very simple example). These effects are real, but still leave two materials with the same apparent structural alert.

It is also important to note that DEREK and other similar SAR programs that focus on a specific structural alert overpredict for genotoxicity. They are designed to be overpredictive in order not to miss a potentially alerting structure.

(In reality, only around 50%–60% of molecules are actually found to test positive when Ames tested). Thus, it is very difficult to absolutely predict toxicology from structural alerts alone. So, suggesting structural similarity is an "assessable surrogate" of toxicological similarity can be an oversimplification, even before considering the relative likelihood of two structurally similar materials being actually present in a drug substance at similar levels. The risk of presence of both at similar levels of concern is very dependent on the point that the impurities in question are first introduced/formed within the process and the subsequent downstream processing conditions. In most cases, the associated risk potential will differ significantly.

For these reasons, it is unlikely that families of structurally similar potential impurities associated with a manufacturing process actually need cumulative control as families and subdivision of a limit between all members of the family, as their actual presence will likely be different, and their actual toxicity will likely be dissimilar.

These considerations challenge the "one-size-fits-all" generic guidance on this complex topic of how best to control the product if more than one GI is present. It may be that case-by-case evaluation would be a better approach where there is appreciable risk/probability of multiple potentially GIs present in an active substance or medicinal product.

1.7.4   Avoidance and ALARP

It has been confirmed by the SWP in a Q/A that if a product or substance has been shown to be controlled (e.g. to have any GIs associated with the product controlled to an appropriate safety based limit), then it is not necessary to conduct further work to further reduce the levels of GIs present. Thus, the driver to have ALARP principles drive further process development of an acceptably safe product has been agreed as unnecessary. However, currently, the stated need to "avoid" the use of genotoxic materials or to avoid genotoxic residues in substances and/or products has not been formally addressed and removed by an SWP Q/A. Thus, even though the Q/A provided on ALARP would seem to have established that control can acceptably guarantee the quality and safety of a product, and hence establishes that control and not avoidance should be the fundamental need for product and process development, this clarification has not been issued to remove the stated primary and fundamental need for "avoidance." This is somewhat disappointing as the need for "avoidance" is unnecessary as a requirement, provided effective process development and robust control strategies are implemented.

1.7.5   ICH Identification Threshold and Its Relation to GIs Assessment

One other topic that had been raised by some as a potential concern (and has now been addressed within the EMEA Q&A document) was the question as to how to relate the ICH identification threshold to unknown impurities and how this related to GI assessments. The answer provided by SWP was to confirm that the identification threshold outlined in ICH Q3a remained appropriate, presumably because the overall quality of drug substance is supported by a well-defined and reasoned risk assessment of the manufacturing process that serves to identify significant potential major concerns. This focused risk assessment is employed to assure the quality of the drug substance and should mean that any unknown impurity present below the identification threshold has a low probability of being potentially genotoxic.

Despite the progress described, there nevertheless remain a number of other topics/areas that still need clarification. One area of uncertainty that is not currently fully addressed relates to oncology candidates (which themselves can possess genotoxicity). Is the guideline applicable in such cases? It certainly would have been helpful if it were made clear that in some cases, the medicinal product can be seen as essentially "out of scope" of the guideline. It is very difficult to see the benefit, in risk terms, of applying the guideline in the context of advanced stages of disease where life expectancy is diminished, and the patient is exposed, often in combination with other treatments, to cytotoxic agents that themselves represent an appreciable risk. It seems very likely that this will be re-examined in the context of the ICH S9 guideline—Non-Clinical Evaluation for Anti-Cancer Pharmaceuticals,[12] which notes that the risk assessment requirements applied to GT impurities can differ for this class of medicines (discussed further below).

It is therefore imperative that the clarification mechanism, established through the Q&A Process by the SWP, remains in place for some time to come.

The EMEA guideline and subsequent Q&A document of course technically relate only to Europe. Up to the end of 2008, the FDA's position remained somewhat unclear, although it was clear from podium presentations that the FDA supported the underlying principles, for example the TTC, of the EMEA guideline. In December 2008, the FDA finally published their long-anticipated draft guideline addressing the topic of GIs.[13]

1.8   FDA DRAFT GUIDELINE

Unsurprisingly, there are significant similarities between this FDA draft guideline and the EMEA guideline, certainly in terms of the key principles such as the TTC, the acceptance of a staged approach where study duration is limited, and the use of SAR evaluation. There are, though, some significant differences, most notably the suggestion of the need to introduce lower limits for different patient populations; specifically pediatric populations. Additional safety factors of 3 and 10 are mentioned and suggested for consideration. The need for this additional level of control for pediatric medicines is unclear when considered in the context of the extremely conservative assumptions that form the basis of the calculated TTC control.

Another relates to the FDA's apparent stance toward the qualification process. The section of the guideline that addresses this is difficult to interpret and thus open to variable interpretation as a result. It appears to suggest that for any impurity above the ICH qualification threshold, irrespective of whether or not it has any structural alert, specific genotoxicity testing should be performed on the isolated impurity. This would appear to be inconsistent with ICH Q3A.

Also of concern is the utilization of the avoidance—ALARP—TTC hierarchy recently modified within the EMEA guideline. Unfortunately, the FDA draft guideline seems to refer directly to the original EU guideline rather than to the SWP Q&A clarifications.

Additionally, other subtler differences also exist, including differences in staged TTC values in relation to very short (less than 14 days) studies, the FDA favoring the extension of the $120\,\mu g/day$ for the whole of this period.

Taken together, the differences between the two guidelines would present anyone faced with having to comply with both with a challenge, even before any issues associated with practical application of the FDA guideline come to the fore. It is to be hoped that the public round of comments will result in some useful modifications to the FDA draft guideline, and that remaining anomalies between the two guidelines can be addressed through dialogue with both agencies simultaneously, resulting in a common standard. At the time of writing this chapter, the topic of management of GIs is being considered as an ICH topic for harmonized guidance development.

1.9   OTHER RELEVANT GUIDANCE

As well as the main guidelines and supporting documents described, there are a short series of other documents that relate to this area that warrant comment.

It has certainly been interesting to follow recent publications on two related topics—the control of potential GT impurities in herbal medicines, and, second, a paper considering the degree of risk associated with GIs in pharmaceutical excipients. Even more recently, the issue of the ICH S9 guideline has drawn considerable comment/interest. Each of these is briefly examined below.

1.9.1   Excipients

The EMEA's CHMP has responded to a request from the European Commission to provide an opinion on the potential risks associated with carcinogens, mutagens, and substances toxic to health when these substances are used as excipients of medicinal products for human use. This is clearly linked to the general wider considerations of such risks in pharmaceuticals (and their impurities) in general. The CHMP published this opinion (in a joint paper from the Quality and Safety Working Parties, published as EMEA/CHMP/SWP/146166/2007 on October 18, 2007).[7] The conclusion of this evaluation was that the accumulated safety and pharmacovigilance data regarding well-known, established, and standard excipients that meet EP requirements for quality served to provide a generally acceptable proof of acceptable quality. This is well aligned with the GTI guidelines position on the accepted safety of existing drug products/drug substances. The opinion also noted that novel excipients (but not necessarily changes in the process of manufacture of established excipients) would be subject to comprehensive evaluation, including both pharmaceutical quality and toxicological evaluation.

1.9.2 Herbals

It has been intriguing to see a draft guideline published by the EMEA's Committee of Herbal Medicine (EMEA/HMPC/107079/2007, dated October 31, 2007)[14] addressing how GTI management of herbal medicines should potentially be approached. This proposes a very simple approach—a herbal medicine and its source and manufacturing process should simply be evaluated in genotoxicity studies, and if the material is free of genotoxic response, then the impurity profile needs no further risk assessment. This seems a very reasonable position and one that could, in theory, have been adopted for synthetic pharmaceuticals if no known genotoxicants are present or are associated with manufacture. It would be very straightforward to adopt the same approach for such synthetic materials and simply test material and manufacturing process in genetic toxicology studies. Indeed, such testing, and often carcinogenicity studies on the active substance, are conducted as a matter of course. It is interesting that this reliance on a "clean" genotoxicity study is not accepted as sufficient for synthetic materials for a number of reasons, one of which may be perhaps that as more can be done for synthetic materials (e.g. requirements for "avoidance" can be imposed, low-level detection for potential genotoxic impurities can be imposed, etc.), so more should be done. Equally interesting, it has been stated[15] that for genotoxic tests like the Ames test to be effective in determining the true risk of an impurity being genotoxic, there needs to be a particular level of exposure to the impurity in the test ($250 \,\mu g$/plate as a stated recommended threshold). An impurity below this threshold in the test cannot be deemed to be nongenotoxic if the test comes back without adverse findings.

1.9.3 ICH S9

ICH S9—Nonclinical Evaluation for Anticancer Pharmaceuticals reached step 4 in late 2009.[12] This, as the title suggests, aims to provide guidance relating to the level of safety testing required to support the use of anticancer pharmaceuticals, particularly in the context of the stage of disease. It suggests a reduced package of testing where treatment is associated with advanced disease, recognizing the inconsequential impact any toxicity related issues would have in terms of patient risk/benefit. This, in many ways, reflects the comments made in the EMEA guideline, where it states that factors such as limited life expectancy and seriousness of disease can be used as the basis for establishing alternative limits to those defined simply by the TTC. ICH S9 goes further though through the specific statement

> *It is recognised that impurities are not expected to have any therapeutic benefit, that impurity standards have been based on a negligible risk (e.g. an increase in lifetime risk of cancer of one in 10^5 or 10^6 for genotoxic impurities) and that such standards might not be appropriate for anticancer pharmaceuticals intended to treat advanced stage patients.*

This seems to clearly suggest that treatments used in advanced stages of disease can be considered to be outside of the scope of genotoxic guidelines. Another interesting aspect of this is the question as to whether the Oncology therapy area is a "special case," or whether the same logic applies to other treatments of life-threatening conditions.

1.10 CONCLUSIONS

Since the original EU position paper, marked progress has been made in terms of appropriate guidance relating to GIs and yet, as described, there still remains uncertainty associated with this area. Undoubtedly, these remaining issues will only ultimately be resolved through continued dialogue between industry and regulators. It is also hoped that this dialogue will not only address current concerns, but will also provide a means by which, in the long term, both industry and regulators can develop a better understanding of the actual real risks associated with the presence of low-level GIs.

REFERENCES

1. European Directorate for the Quality of Medicines and Healthcare. 2000. Enquiry: Alkyl mesilate (methane sulfonate) impurities in mesilate salts. *PharmEuropa* 12:27.
2. Committee for Proprietary Medicinal Products. Position paper on the limits of genotoxic impurities. London, December 18, 2002. CPMP/SWP/5199/02/draft 2.
3. Committee for Medicinal Products for Human Use (CHMP). Guidelines on the limits of genotoxic impurities. London, June 23, 2004. CPMP/SWP/5199/02.
4. Bos PMJ, Baars B, Marcel TM, van Raaji TM. 2004. Risk assessment of peak exposure to genotoxic carcinogens. *Toxicology Letters* 151:43–50.
5. Muller L, Mauthe RJ, Riley CM, et al. 2006. A rationale for determining, testing and controlling specific impurities in pharmaceuticals that possess potential for genotoxicity. *Regulatory Toxicology and Pharmacology* 44:198–211.
6. Committee for Medicinal Products for Human Use (CHMP) Guidelines on the limits of genotoxic impurities. London, June 26, 2006. CPMP/SWP/5199/02.
7. CHMP Scientific article 5(3) Opinion on the potential risks of carcinogens, mutagens and substances toxic to reproduction when these substances are used as excipients of medicinal products for human use. London, October 18, 2007. EMEA/CHMP/SWP/146166/2007.
8. CHMP Safety Working Party (SWP). Question & answers on the CHMP guideline on the limits of genotoxic impurities. London, December 17, 2009. EMEA/CHMP/QWP/251344/2006Q&A.
9. *GRAS List*. Available at http://www.accessdata.fda.gov/scripts/fcn/fcnNavigation.cfm?rpt=grasListing (accessed September 2010).
10. European Directorate on Quality of Medicines (EDQM). 2008. Potentially genotoxic impurities and European pharmacopoeia monographs on substances for human use. *PharmEuropa* 20(3):426–427.
11. Bercu J. 2008. Quantitative assessment of cumulative risk for multiple genotoxic impurities in a new drug substance. *Regulatory Toxicology and Pharmacology* 51(3):270–277.
12. ICH Topic S9: Non-clinical evaluation for anticancer pharmaceuticals, Step 4 (2009). EMEA/CHMP/ICH/646107/2008.
13. Guidance for industry genotoxic and carcinogenic impurities in drug substances and products: Recommended approaches draft. Center for Drug Evaluation and Research (CDER) December 2008.

14. Concept paper on the development of a guideline on the assessment of genotoxic constituents in herbal substances/preparations. Committee for Medicinal Products (CHMP), European Medicines Agency, London, October 25, 2006. EMEA/HPPC/413271/2006.

15. Kenyon MO, Cheung JR, Dobo KL, Ku WW. 2007. An evaluation of the sensitivity of the Ames assay to discern low-level mutagenic impurities. *Regulatory Toxicology and Pharmacology* 75–86.

CHAPTER 2

DEVELOPMENT OF THE THRESHOLD OF TOXICOLOGICAL CONCERN CONCEPT AND ITS RELATIONSHIP TO DURATION OF EXPOSURE

Alessandro Brigo
Lutz Müller

2.1 HISTORY AND DEVELOPMENT OF THRESHOLD OF TOXICOLOGICAL CONCERN (TTC)

The TTC has its basis in the concept that it is possible to identify "safe levels of exposure" for chemicals with known toxicological profiles. The TTC is a pragmatic risk assessment approach that aims to establish a human exposure threshold value below which there is a very low probability of an appreciable risk to human health. The concept is based on extrapolation of toxicity data from one or more available databases to a chemical compound for which the chemical structure is known, but for which no or limited toxicity data is available. In addition, the human exposure to such compound has to be so low that carrying out toxicity studies is not justified.

The TTC concept began its evolution process in 1958 and 1960, when legislative amendments to the Food, Drug, and Cosmetic Act of 1938 were passed by the U.S. Congress requiring manufacturers to establish the safety of food additives (in foods) and color additives (in foods, drugs, and cosmetics). A controversial provision included in each of them was the "Delaney Clause," which specified that no additive could be deemed safe (or given FDA approval) if found to cause cancer in man, or, experimentally, in animals. This provision was initially opposed by FDA and by scientists who agreed that an additive present in food at very low levels should not necessarily be forbidden solely on the basis of its capability to cause cancer in animals dosed at very high levels. Nonetheless, political supporters justified the Delaney

Genotoxic Impurities: Strategies for Identification and Control, Edited by Andrew Teasdale
Copyright © 2010 by John Wiley & Sons, Inc.

Clause on the grounds that cancer experts were unable to determine an absolutely safe level for any known carcinogen. With passage of the amendments, FDA was required by law to apply a "zero-risk tolerance" standard for potential carcinogens in food. By the late 1980s, however, improvements in analytical methodologies had made obvious the fact that numerous substances possessing known or unknown potential to cause cancer in animals under experimental conditions (such as pesticides and chemical residues from food contact materials) could be quantitatively measured in foodstuffs. Leading scientific experts in the fields of carcinogenesis and cancer-risk analysis recognize that there is no "absolutely safe" level for carcinogens, because carcinogenesis is based on statistical events involving multiple stages.[1] Thus, even if extremely improbable, any single point mutation to a given cell's DNA at the wrong time and place is, in theory, capable of playing a significant role in the carcinogenesis cascade of events. Recently, the history of how this became the default approach for risk assessment for carcinogens has been reviewed and at the same time heavily criticized.[2]

A big impulse for change was given by a U.S. Federal Court case decision, in *Monsanto vs. Kennedy* (D.C. Cir. 1979). The Monsanto Company proved that no detectable leaching of an acrylonitrile copolymer resulted from use of their beverage container product, and as such, that the copolymer did not have to be regulated as a food additive. In its decision, the court pointed out that the FDA Commissioner had the discretion to determine if the contamination level of food with a particular substance is so negligible as to present no public health or safety concerns. During the 1980s and early 1990s, data analysis was also being conducted on a set of carcinogens known at the time, and an effort was being made to characterize a dose limit below which a daily exposure to any carcinogen (either known or unknown) could be justified as being "virtually safe," that is, a TTC. Following the work of Rulis[3] and Gold et al.[4], the TD$_{50}$ doses (*the daily dose required to halve the probability of an experimental animal of remaining without tumors at the end of its standard lifespan*) of 343 orally administered rodent carcinogens were used to calculate the distribution of exposures required to give a constant of 1 in 1,000,000 lifetime cancer risk. Subsequent work carried out by Munro in 1990[5] extended the analysis and came to the conclusion that a dietary level of 1 ppb of a substance of unknown toxicity presents low probability of a cancer risk higher than 1 in 1,000,000.[6–8]

Based on published reports of the TTC concept and its own analyses, the FDA established thereafter a "threshold of regulation (ToR)" for trace substances coming from food contact materials, a level below which the risk of all forms of toxicity (including lifetime risk of cancer if the substance was later found to be a carcinogen) was considered to be less than 1 in 1,000,000, thereby rendering the risk negligible. For substances with the potential to leach from food contact materials, a threshold of 0.5 ppb was chosen, which, based on an assumed 3000 g ingestion of food and beverages, is equal to a daily intake of 1.5 μg. Hence, by setting a threshold of regulation, FDA had justified the use of an abbreviated application process that allowed trace substances with unknown carcinogenic potential arising from food contact materials to be present in food below a specified limit, without having to go through an act of Congress to repeal and revise the 1958 amendment containing the Delaney Clause.

One of the latest, most comprehensive TTC analysis, based on the Rodent Carcinogenic Potency Database, was described by Kroes et al.[9] The work applied a

TABLE 2.1   Conservative Assumptions Applied in the Use of the Rodent Carcinogenic Potency Database to derive TTC Values[9]

- Establishment of the dose giving a 50% tumor incidence in (TD_{50}) using data for the most sensitive species and most sensitive site.[12]
- Based on a selected subset of the database containing 730 carcinogenic substances which had adequate estimates of the TD_{50} following oral dosage.
- Simple linear extrapolation from the TD_{50} to a 1 in 1,000,000 incidence.
- The approach assumes that all biological processes involved in the generation of tumors at high dosages are linear over a 500,000-fold range of extrapolation.
- The possible effects of cyto-protective, DNA repair, apoptotic and cell cycle control processes are not taken into account.
- All of the compounds were analyzed assuming there is no threshold in the dose response.

number of conservative assumptions (see Table 2.1) without emphasising though that humans are known to possess more efficient DNA repair mechanisms compared to rodents.[10,11]

The concentrations of the several hundreds of rodent carcinogens that have been analyzed for the derivation of the TTC limit of 1.5 µg (one in a million risk) form an approximate Gaussian distribution spanning about seven orders of magnitude. Based on the rodent data model, the statistical upper-bound lifetime risk of cancer at 1.5 µg daily exposure is actually much less than 1 in 1,000,000 for all but the most potent known carcinogens (e.g. N-nitroso, azoxy, benzidine- and aflatoxin-like chemicals).

Before the work of Kroes and colleagues in 2004,[9] Cheeseman and co-workers extended in 1999[12] the ToR concept of the U.S. FDA by incorporating acute and short-term toxicity data, the results of genotoxicity testing, and structural alerts to discriminate between potent and nonpotent carcinogens. The authors evaluated 709 rodent carcinogens, and linearly extrapolated the dose corresponding to an upper-bound limit of a lifetime cancer risk of 10^{-6}, which confirmed the validity of a ToR of 0.5 ppb in food for most rodent carcinogens. Based on the information collected from the Registry of Toxic Effects of Chemical Substances (RTECS) on oral reproductive toxicity and other repeat-dose toxicity studies data, Cheeseman and colleagues suggested a tiered approach (not yet adopted by FDA) in which structural alerts, genotoxicity test results, and short-term toxicity data could be used to modulate the existing FDA's ToR approach:

- 1.5 µg/person/day (0.5 ppb): General threshold for substances possessing positive Ames test results or certain structure alerts such as N-nitroso or benzidine-like chemicals.
- 15 µg/person/day (5 ppb): Threshold for chemicals without structural alerts for carcinogenicity or with negative mutagenicity test (Ames test).
- 45 µg/person/day (15 ppb): Threshold for chemicals without structural alerts for carcinogenicity or with negative mutagenicity test (Ames test) and with an appropriate acute toxicity test with $LD_{50} > 1000$ mg/kg bodyweight.

Although the ToR/TTC is currently used by FDA with focus on possible carcinogenic effects, Munro and co-workers in 1996[6] made an evaluation of the use of TTC for different endpoints using structural information based on an algorithm developed in 1978 by Cramer et al.[13] A decision tree approach was developed based on 33 specific questions. Each answer led to another question through to a final classification into one of the three structural classes (I, II, and III), corresponding to a supposed low, moderate, or significant toxicity. Human exposure thresholds of 1800, 540, and 90 μg/person/day were proposed for class I, II, and III, respectively (Fig. 2.1).

In summary, the TTC concept was originally employed to justify FDA's "threshold of regulation", a mechanism created to reconcile FDA's legal responsibility to uphold the Delaney Clause with the realities that:

1. trace substances of unknown genotoxicity potential from food contact materials may exist in food without danger; and

2. an "absolutely safe" level for a carcinogen does not exist.

In practical terms, the "zero risk" standard has been replaced with a 1.5 μg "virtually zero risk" standard, a threshold limit below which lifetime cancer risk across the entire U.S. population could be considered as negligible.

2.2 CURRENT APPLICATIONS OF THE TTC CONCEPT

2.2.1 Risk Assessment

Kroes et al. in 2004[9] affirmed that "the TTC approach should be used only in cases where the available chemical-specific data are inadequate for normal risk characterization. Any available information on the compound should be considered to ensure that any decision is compatible with the available data." This may include, for example read-across, *in silico* methods, such as QSAR models and knowledge base applications, preliminary testing results, and all other relevant safety information.

Since humans are exposed to chemicals via ingestion, inhalation, or dermal absorption, the dose at the target organ becomes critical for the TTC concept application. Due to the high variability in the population (consumers, workers, general population exposed in the environment, children) and in routes of exposure (i.e. ingestion, inhalation, dermal uptake), the typical assumption is that absorption is always 100% via the preferred route, unless specific data indicates otherwise. When being confronted with a risk assessment of a particular substance, it is essential to identify all potential exposure routes and sources, especially for those chemicals that may be present in food packaging, cosmetic products, and as contaminants in the air. As already mentioned, the TTC principle has been developed from toxicity databases, which mainly comprise data derived from studies with oral administration (gavage or in the feed or drinking water). At this point in time, no methodology is reliable enough to assess combined multiroute exposures; therefore, the estimation of exposure should be carried out in the most appropriate way in order to provide sensible and conservative exposure values. An additional

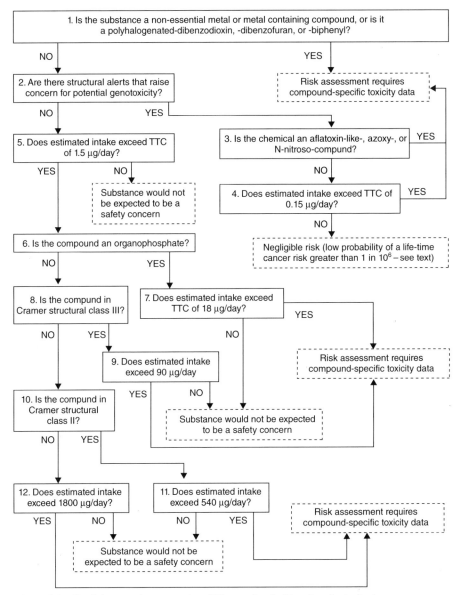

Figure 2.1   Decision tree incorporating different thresholds of toxicological concern as a function of the structural class.[9] Reprinted from Kroes et al., *Food and Chemical Toxicology* 42:65–83. Copyright 2004, with permission from ILSI Europe.

layer of complexity is added by those chemicals that are known or highly likely to accumulate in the body: for such molecules, the TTC approach should not be used, as it is not possible to give an estimation of their concentrations at the target organ.

2.2.2 Food

The regulation of chemicals that may be present in food as contaminants (e.g. migrating from packaging/contact material) or additives (e.g. flavoring substances) via a TTC-like approach was introduced by the U.S. FDA in 1995. Currently, should the dietary concentration of a substance present in food contact material be equal or below 0.5 ppb (25 ng/kg bw/day), a request for exemption from regulation can be submitted. However, such a request must be corroborated by a detailed discussion of how the estimation of the dietary concentration was assessed along with existing toxicological data on the substance. Such information will be used to assess whether there is any carcinogenicity or other toxicity risks associated with the substance(s) under evaluation.

Unlike in the United States, the TTC approach is not used in the European Union for approval of food contact materials. The former Scientific Committee on Food (SCF) advised the European Commission that, despite the fact that the ToR concept provides "reasonable assurance that no adverse effect would occur in man," there is insufficient data concerning endpoints such as neurotoxicity, immunotoxicity, developmental toxicity, and endocrine-active compounds. Even though the TTC concept per se is not used, a similar tiered approach is applied by the European Food Safety Authority's Panel.[14-16] For example, if a substance that migrates from the packaging material does not exceed 50 ppb in food, only three *in vitro* genotoxicity tests are required, and if all of them are negative, then no adverse effect is expected.

On the other hand, as far as flavoring substances are concerned, the Joint FAO/WHO Expert Committee on Food Additives (JECFA) in 1995 decided to apply the TTC principle. The procedure described by Dr. Munro[6,7] and finally endorsed with modifications in 1996 was based on cumulative distributions of no-effect levels (NOELs) of compounds in the database of reference divided into the three Cramer structural classes.[13] EFSA and JECFA have the goal to compile a list of chemically characterized flavoring substances in food.[17] The procedure adopted for the evaluation of flavoring substances is schematically depicted in Figure 2.2.

The current database contains 2800 flavoring substances added to food and beverages in Europe and the United States. Most of them, 400 of which are natural compounds, are structurally well characterized. In 1999, SCF[18] decided that flavoring compounds should be assessed for the presence of structural alerts for genotoxicity and for experimental data suggesting potential genotoxic activity. In cases where evidence of genotoxicity is found, the procedure described should not be used.

2.2.3 Pharmaceuticals

2.2.3.1 Genotoxic Impurities in Pharmaceuticals
The synthesis of active pharmaceutical ingredients (API) frequently involves the use of reactive reagents forming intermediates and by-products, which, at the end of the process, may still be present in the final drug substance as impurities. A subset of these impurities may present a potential for genotoxicity and carcinogenicity, posing an additional safety concern to patients and clinical subjects. Delaney in 2007[19] estimated that up to 25% of all intermediates used in the synthetic processes of APIs would test positive in

Procedure for Safety Evaluation of Chemically Defined Flavouring Substances

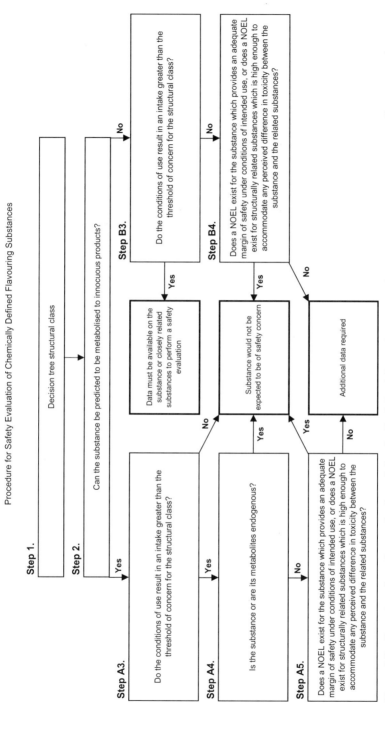

Figure 2.2 Procedure for safety evaluation of chemically defined flavouring substances (Scientific Committee on Food[18] and Larsen[1]).

33

the Ames assay, that is behave as bacterial mutagens due to their reactivity. Yet this characteristic is needed to make them useful for organic synthesis. In such a framework, pharmaceutical industry and its regulators are well aware of the potential hazard, and significant efforts are put in place to control and limit all impurities down to safe concentrations.

From a regulatory point of view, control of impurities in the drug substance and degradants in APIs are addressed in the International Conference of Harmonization Quality Guidelines Q3A(R)[20] and Q3B(R),[21] respectively, and the Q3C[22] guideline that deals with residual solvents. However, these documents do not provide any specific guidance for determining acceptable levels for genotoxic impurities. In these guidelines, one sentence elaborates on identification and control of unusually toxic impurities as follows: "For impurities known to be unusually potent or to produce toxic or unexpected pharmacological effects, the quantitation/detection limit of the analytical procedures should be commensurate with the level at which the impurities should be controlled." This sentence could be interpreted in a way that, for example immunogenic, carcinogenic, and genotoxic impurities would potentially need lower specification limits than those given by these guidelines for ordinary impurities. However, the guidelines do not give any specifics as to how to do that in practice. In this context, the process for highly toxic "group 1" residual solvents as described in the ICH guideline Q3C[22] is helpful. In this guideline, for instance, a general limit of 2 ppm is imposed on the genotoxic and carcinogenic solvent benzene. However, the guideline does not address the fact that the limit of 2 ppm for benzene translates into large differences in human exposure whether the daily dose of a drug were 1 mg or 2 g, not to speak of the impact of duration of use, which is also ignored. Hence, for limitations of risk based on total daily dose, a generic ppm limit does not make scientific sense. Yet they may be very useful for technical development due to their practicality and applicability across projects.

The European Medicines Agency Committee for Medicinal Products for Human Use (CHMP) released in 2006,[23] a "Guideline on the Limits of Genotoxic Impurities," which describes an approach for assessing genotoxic impurities of unknown carcinogenic potential based on the TTC concept. In 2007, a Question & Answer document was published on the EMEA website addressing several practical aspects relating to implementation of the recommendations contained in the guideline.

Genotoxicity is a broad term that typically describes a deleterious action on cellular genetic material. Chemicals may induce DNA damage by directly interacting with it (e.g. alkylating agents) or by acting on non-DNA targets (e.g. mitotic spindle poisons, inhibitors of topoisomerase, etc.). For DNA-reactive genotoxins, the mechanism by which they induce genetic damage is assumed to follow a linear no-threshold model; on the other hand, for molecules not interacting directly with DNA, the existence of a threshold concentration required to induce the damage is by and large accepted (see Section 2.2.3.1 for an extensive example). Impurities that belong to the second category of substances can be regulated according to the ICH Quality Guideline Q3C,[22] which includes Class 2 solvents. The thresholds or permissible daily exposures (PDE) are calculated from the no observed effect level (NOEL) obtained in the most relevant animal studies with the use of conservative conversion factors used to extrapolate the animal data to humans.

The CHMP guideline suggests that the TTC concept should be applied to those genotoxic impurities that do not have sufficient evidence of a threshold-related mechanism of action. The reference values are taken from Kroes et al.,[9] where a TTC of 0.15 µg/day is proposed for impurities presenting a structural alert for genotoxicity, corresponding to a 10^{-6} lifetime risk of cancer. In the case of pharmaceuticals, the guideline suggests a 1 in 100,000 risk be applied, resulting in a TTC of 1.5 µg/day.

2.2.3.2 Classification of Potential Genotoxic Impurities in APIs

For drug substances, the identification thresholds above which impurities are required to be identified are within the range of 0.05% and 0.1%. ICH Guidelines Q3A(R)[20] and Q3B(R)[21] state that even though the identification of impurities is not necessary at levels lower than or equal to the identification threshold, "analytical procedures should be developed for those potential impurities that are expected to be unusually potent, producing toxic or pharmacological effects at a level not higher than the identification threshold." In order to provide more accurate information on potential genotoxicity of impurities, the guideline recommends carrying out a thorough evaluation of the synthetic route, along with chemical reactions and conditions, with the aim of identifying reagents, intermediates, starting materials, and readily predicted side products that may be of potential concern. Once all potential impurities are theoretically identified and listed, an initial assessment for genotoxicity is carried out by a scientific expert using computer tools such as QSAR and knowledge base expert systems. A thorough literature and internal archive (when applicable) search also needs to be completed, as a number of intermediates and reagents have often been tested in genotoxicity or carcinogenicity assays. It goes without saying that reliable experimental data overrule the predictions given by *in silico* systems. The potential genotoxic impurities that may be present in an API are then classified into one of five classes;[24] the purpose is to clearly identify those impurities that pose a high risk and need to be limited to very low concentrations:

- *Class 1: Impurities known to be both genotoxic (mutagenic) and carcinogenic.* This group includes known animal carcinogens with adequate data for genotoxic mechanism and human carcinogens. In such cases, the best option is to try to avoid the presence of these impurities by modifying the synthetic process either changing starting materials or introducing additional purging steps. Often, though, a radical change in a nearly optimized synthetic process is not feasible, and specifications should be determined. Compound-specific risk calculations can be conducted when sufficient 2-year rodent bioassay data is available. The TD_{50} or the maximum tolerated dose (MTD) can be used to calculate the maximum daily intake.[25]

- *Class 2: Impurities known to be genotoxic (mutagenic), but with unknown carcinogenic potential.* This group includes impurities tested positive in reliable genotoxicity tests, but with unknown potential for carcinogenicity. Mutagenic impurities should be evaluated as to whether they present any evidence for a threshold-mediated mechanism. If they do, exposure levels can be determined as a function of the NOEL or lowest observed effect levels

TABLE 2.2   Acceptable Qualification Thresholds for Genotoxic and Carcinogenic Impurities

	Duration of clinical trial exposure					
	<14 days	14 days to 1 months	1–3 months	3–6 months	6–12 months	>12 months
Genotoxic and carcinogenic impurity threshold (µg/day)	120	60	20	10	5	1.5

(LOEL). In the case of impurities that show direct interaction with DNA (e.g. DNA adduct formation or DNA binding), their limits will have to be controlled using the staged TTC approach (see Section 2.2.3.3 and Table 2.2).

- *Class 3: Alerting structure, unrelated to the structure of the API and of unknown genotoxic (mutagenic) potential.* This group includes impurities containing functional moieties that trigger structural alerts for genotoxicity in knowledge-base or in quantitative structure-activity expert systems but for which there is no experimental data. A Class 3 impurity may trigger one of the following actions: (1) test the isolated impurity in an Ames assay, or, alternatively, spike the API with the impurity and test the mixture in an Ames assay; (2) quantify the amount of the impurity effectively present within the API down to ppm level; and (3) if suitable, provide a sound chemical reasoning that could prove that the impurity cannot possibly be present within the API (e.g. because it is unstable in the subsequent reaction conditions).

- *Class 4: Alerting structure, related to the API.* This group includes impurities containing functional moieties that are shared with the API structure. Albeit the genotoxicity of the isolated impurity is not known, the genotoxicity of the API has been characterized through the standard genotoxicity battery of tests; therefore, no further action should be required.

- *Class 5: No alerting structure or sufficient evidence for absence of genotoxicity.* Treat as a normal impurity.

2.2.3.3   Staged TTC Approach   In agreement with the CHMP Guideline on Genotoxic Impurities, the TTC concept[7,8,26,27] is used to establish a limit of 1.5 µg/day as a virtually safe dose for most genotoxic compounds, while some highly potent genotoxic compounds (specifically N-nitroso compounds, azoxy-compounds and aflatoxin-like compounds) may require even lower levels.[9] However, during investigational stages, due to the high variability in the duration of exposure, that is from single day to years, this threshold may be modified to take into consideration duration of exposure.

Bos et al.[28] reviewed the derived cancer risk from short-term, high-dose exposure to a genotoxic carcinogen relative to the same cumulative dose distributed over a lifetime (virtually safe dose). The authors suggest that the most pragmatic approach to calculate acceptable short-term exposures to known genotoxic carcinogens is to linearly extrapolate the short-term exposure from the acceptable lifetime exposure or virtually safe dose.

This concept was developed further by Müller et al. through the publication of the stage TTC concept.[24]

The values described within the Müller paper were ultimately effectively halved by Regulatory Agencies (EMEA and FDA), even though no clear rationale has been provided for this decision. Table 2.2 shows the acceptable daily intakes of genotoxic impurities during clinical development[29] as a function of the duration of exposure.

2.3 GROUP CHEMICALS AND LINEAR EXTRAPOLATION AT LOW DOSE

Over 30 year ago, U.S. EPA decided that chemical carcinogens should be assumed to act following a linear model at low doses. This decision continues to have a big impact on how risk assessment is being carried out, and the background supporting such approach has been extensively reviewed and challenged in a recent publication.[2] The main argument presented in the review is that the scientific evidence supporting such approach is far from being conclusive: some of the guiding principles to low-dose linearity were based on claims such as: (1) only one or two changes in a cell are needed to irreversibly transform the cell and lead to cancer; (2) exposure would be directly additive to the background if acting via the same mechanism; (3) if the mechanism involves mutation, there will be no threshold.[2] Recently, very significant scientific evidence has been published, suggesting that the straightforward application to potential carcinogens of the linear extrapolation to low dose might be too conservative, with the consequence of overestimating the carcinogenicity risk. Extensive preclinical studies carried out on the well-known genotoxic carcinogen ethyl methanesulfonate (EMS) (see Section 2.3.1) demonstrated that its mechanism of action follows a threshold mechanism (*Toxicology Letters* 190[3]:239–340, 12 November 2009[30,31]). Additional data suggesting non-linear behavior at low doses of the potent environmental carcinogen dibenzo[*a,l*]pyrene (DBP) have been published by Bailey and co-workers using the Shasta strain rainbow trout as *in vivo* model.[32] DBP induces tumors in multiple target organs in a number of species, including rat, mouse, trout and medaka.[33–35] The study protocol described by Bailey and colleagues included 40,800 trout, which was fed 0–225 ppm of DBP for 4 weeks. The observed liver and stomach tumor incidences were plotted in a log–log scale and modeled to visualize ultralow dose exposures. Figure 2.3 shows the extrapolations of the dose-response portion from models well-fitting the tumor incidence data.[32]

None of the models that accurately fit the liver data is compatible with the linear default EPA extrapolation methods. Furthermore, the virtually safe dose is estimated to be between 500 and 1500-fold higher than that predicted by the linear default extrapolation (i.e. DBP is less hazardous). In the case of stomach data, the virtually safe doses estimated by the three nonlinear models are between 360 and 5500 times greater than the dose calculated by the conservative EPA linear method.[32]

A. liver

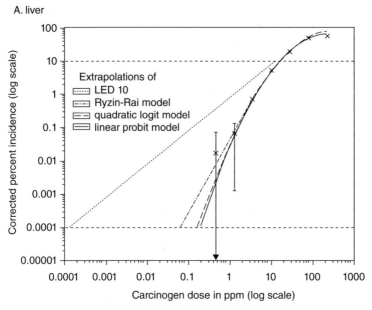

B. Stomach

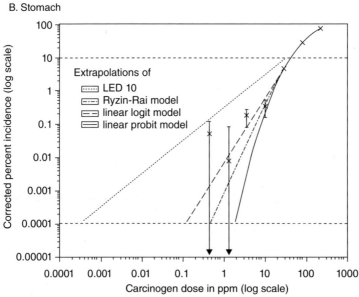

Figure 2.3 Extrapolations of the dose-response portion from well-fitting models for trout tumor incidence in liver (A) and stomach (B) data and from the linear model from the effective dose of carcinogen achieving 10% incidence (LED$_{10}$). The dotted lines represent default linear extrapolations from LED$_{10}$ points of departure, which were established using a standard linear logit model fit to the incidences from the highest three doses.[32] Figure reprinted from Bailey et al., *Chemical Research in Toxicology* 22:1264–1276. Copyright 2009, with permission from American Chemical Society via Rightslink.

These data show that when sampling tumor incidences at very low doses, which is not the typical case in the rodent bioassay, the linear back extrapolation from high dose to levels expected to cause one additional cancer in a million individuals is likely to significantly overestimate the hazard posed by the studied carcinogen. The data presented by Bailey and colleagues represent an additional challenge to the conservatism of the default application of linear extrapolation to low dose and advocates the consideration of new approaches in cancer risk assessment.

In the following paragraphs, the pros and cons for a linear extrapolation of tumor data for genotoxic compounds in order to define a (very) low level to control human exposure shall be put forward. The following section looks to examine this through the investigation of selected chemical groups that possess well-known genotoxic properties.

2.3.1 EMS

In the context of the debate on whether linear default extrapolations for cancer risk into the low dose/exposure range are appropriate for genotoxic carcinogens, a recent case of contamination of a drug product with the alkylating carcinogen EMS plays a major role. The protease inhibitor nelfinavir mesylate (Viracept®, F. Hoffmann-La Roche Ltd., Basel, Switzerland), produced between March 2007 and June 2007, was found to contain elevated levels of EMS, a known mutagen (alkylator)—leading to a global recall of the drug. EMS levels in a daily dose (2500 mg Viracept/day) were predicted not to exceed a dose of ~2.75 mg/day (~0.055 mg/kg/day based on a 50 kg patient). As existing toxicology data on EMS did not permit an adequate patient risk assessment, a comprehensive animal toxicology evaluation of EMS was conducted. General toxicity of EMS was investigated in rats over 28 days. Two studies for DNA damage were performed in mice; chromosomal damage was assessed using a micronucleus assay, and gene mutations were detected using the MutaMouse transgenic model. In addition, experiments designed to extrapolate animal exposure to humans were undertaken. A general toxicity study showed that the toxicity of EMS occurred only at doses ≥60 mg/kg/day, which is far above that received by patients. Studies for chromosomal damage and mutations in mice demonstrated a clear threshold effect with EMS at 25 mg/kg/day, under chronic dosing conditions. Exposure analysis (C_{max}) demonstrated that ~370-fold higher levels of EMS than that ingested by patients are needed to saturate known, highly conserved, error-free, mammalian DNA repair mechanisms for alkylation. Details of these investigations, the associated risk assessment, and the risk management process with regulatory authorities, prescribing doctors, and patients, can be found in a special issue of *Toxicology Letters*: "Assessment of human toxicological risk of Viracept patients accidentally exposed to ethyl methanesulfonate (EMS) based on preclinical investigations with EMS and ethylnitrosourea" (190[3]:239–340, 12 November 2009[30,31,36–38]). In summary, the animal studies suggested that patients who took Nelfinavir mesylate with elevated levels of EMS are at no increased risk for carcinogenicity or teratogenicity over their background risk, since mutations are prerequisites for such downstream events. These findings are potentially relevant to >40 marketed drugs that are mesylate salts. As biomarkers of exposure to EMS such as adducts on globin or DNA do generally follow linear dose-response relationships, these data clearly show that such biomarkers cannot be used for risk assessment or risk management processes. While hints for nonlinear behavior of mutations *in vivo* over a critical dose range already existed, these data give the first reliable experimental basis for a proper risk management in a low-dose exposure scenario. Two key essential elements of risk assessment based on the data for EMS shall be mentioned here:

1. A reasoned assumption that DNA adducts produced by EMS can be repaired error free.
2. The use of exposure assessment to free EMS in several species as a basis for human exposure modeling.

To this end, traditional cross-species exposure scaling methods together with safety margin calculations to balance uncertainties about the exact threshold dose can be used for risk management for a genotoxic carcinogen. The direct nature of the genetic damage by EMS, which does not involve any major metabolic step, makes cross-species scaling and risk assessment less complicated than in many other cases, in which metabolic activation or detoxification processes have to be taken into account. In summary, this case study demonstrates that the default assumption of linearity as basis of the TTC concept for genotoxic carcinogens may be overly conservative.

2.3.2   Mesylates

Following the example of EMS elaborated on in the previous section, one could ague that similar principles of nonlinearity must exist for compounds producing similar DNA damage. Hence, a permitted daily exposure argument as proposed for EMS,[30] may be applicable to other sulfonate esters, for example mesylates, besylates, and tosylates. When querying the Carcinogenic Potency Database (CPDB, http://www.epa.gov/ncct/dsstox/sdf_cpdbas.html) for mesylates, tosylates, and besylates, a total of nine substances are found. Within the mesylates subgroup, methyl methanesulfonate (MMS, CAS No. 66-27-7), Myleran (CAS No. 55-98-1) and improsulfan hydrochloride (3,3'-Iminobis-1-propanoldimethanesulfonate(ester) hydrochloride, CAS No. 3458-22-8) are included (see Fig. 2.4).

Using EMS as a reference, the closest analogue is methyl methanesulfonate (MMS), with a reported TD_{50} value in mouse of 31.8 mg/kg/day. As a genotoxic carcinogen, linear back extrapolation to a cancer incidence of 1 out of 100,000 leads to daily dose of 0.64 μg/kg or 31.8 μg for a 50 kg person, which is already over 20 times above the generic TTC value of 1.5 μg/day.[30] An analysis carried out by Swenberg and coworkers[39] on data obtained with MMS suggested that the mutagenic response was not following a linear model at low doses. Doak and coworkers[40] compared MMS low dose effects in the *Hprt* and *Tk* genes. In addition, Swenberg et al.[39] compared the molecular dose of the major DNA adduct, N7-methylguanine. Figure 2.5 shows that the shape of the mutation curves and the shape of the molecular dose of N7-methylguanine are different. DNA adducts are linear over the entire dose response, whereas *Hprt* and *Tk* mutations, as well as micronuclei inductions, are highly sublinear.[40]

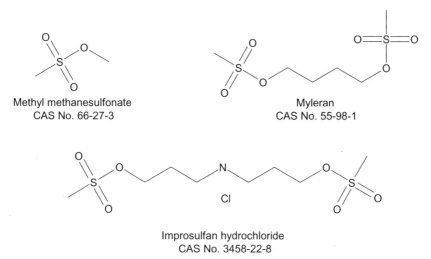

Methyl methanesulfonate
CAS No. 66-27-3

Myleran
CAS No. 55-98-1

Improsulfan hydrochloride
CAS No. 3458-22-8

Figure 2.4   Mesylates subgroup represented in the Gold Carcinogenicity Database.

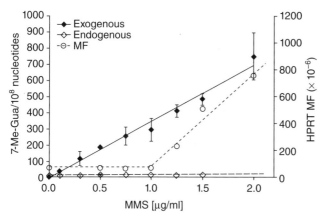

Figure 2.5   Comparison of N7-methyl guanine DNA adducts and *Hprt* mutations in HH-1 cells exposed to MMS for 24 h. The endogenous adducts are N-7Me-G (◊), while the exogenous adducts are [13C2H3]-7Me-G (♦). The *Hprt* mutant frequency is shown as (O).[39] Figure reprinted from Swenberg et al., *Chemical Research in Toxicology* 21:253–265. Copyright 2008, with permission from American Chemical Society via Rightslink.

Myleran is active in the Ames assay, but showed no carcinogenic activity in male rats, the only species and sex that the molecule was tested in. Improsulfan hydrochloride, an alkylating agent tested in the past as anticancer agent in patients with measurable, surgically incurable colorectal carcinoma,[41] showed also no carcinogenic activity in rats or mice. Even though these substances represent a very limited number of examples within the chemical class of mesylates, their related genotoxicity and carcinogenicity data suggests that the straight application of the principle of linear extrapolation to compounds belonging to this chemical class, without a case by case evaluation, is most likely to overestimate the risk that they may actually represent.

2.3.3 Phosphonates

Alkyl esters of phosphorus acids are typically classified as mutagenic by *in silico* expert systems. They are electrophilic compounds that can alkylate and phosphorylate cellular nucleophilic groups. A number of them are active in the Ames assay and their activity is thought to be induced by DNA alkylation.[42] Other reports suggested that an oxidative stress mechanism may play an important role[43,44] in their genotoxicity. This class of compounds is represented by three substances in the Carcinogenicity Potency Database (CPDB): diethyl-β,γ-epoxypropylphosphonate (CAS 7316-37-2), dimethyl methylphosphonate (CAS No. 756-79-6) and trichlorophone (CAS No. 52-68-6). Diethyl-β,γ-epoxypropylphosphonate was tested only in female mice, in which it did not show any carcinogenic activity at a dosage up to 28.6 mg/kg/day. Dimethyl methylphosphonate induced kidney tumors in male rats, whereas it showed no activity in female rats or female mice. The TD_{50} calculated for the findings in male rats is 700 mg/kg/day, which, via linear back extrapolation to a cancer incidence of 1 out of 100,000, leads to a virtually safe daily dose of 14.0 μg/kg or 700 μg for a 50 kg person, which is over 460 times above the TTC level of 1.5 μg. Given the fact that dimethyl methylphosphonate is also Ames negative, a nonlinear mechanism of carcinogenicity can be assumed. Trichlorphone is positive in the Ames assay and showed no carcinogenic activity in male and female mice (experimental results reported for both sexes together).

Diethyl benzylphosphonate (CAS No. 1080-32-6) has been tested in the Ames assay at F. Hoffmann-La Roche (Fig. 2.6) and found to be devoid of any mutagenic activity; the same results had been found with the mono- and diethyl-derivatives of diethyl benzylphosphonate (CAS Nos. 33973-50-1 and 33973-25-0 in Fig. 2.6). Furthermore, (2-cyclopropyl-2-oxo-ethyl)-phosphonic acid dimethyl ester (CAS No. 866406-01-1) was also tested in house in the Ames assay and showed no mutagenic activity. The data from these molecules suggests that a permitted daily exposure approach may be considered for this class of compounds, since they seem to show little evidence of mutagenic activity and a rather unclear carcinogenicity risk.

2.3.4 Alkyl Chlorides

Alkyl chlorides represent a very important class of compounds in chemical synthesis. They can be used as solvents (e.g. chloroform, dichloromethane, trichloroethane), in polymer synthesis (e.g. vinyl chloride for PVC synthesis), and in the synthesis of pharmaceutical ingredients. The chemical reactivity that makes them useful in chemical synthesis brings about the risk that a number of such molecules may react with DNA, leading to carcinogenesis. The Carcinogenicity Potency Database (CPDB) contains 31 derivatives with a molecular weight lower than 250 Da: our arbitrary choice of a molecular weight cutoff is made mainly to try to limit the molecular complexity of the compounds belonging to this class, in order to avoid any confounding factors (e.g. multiple potentially mutagenic/carcinogenic

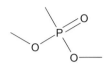

Diethyl-beta,gamma-epoxypropylphosphonat
CAS No. 7316-37-2

Dimethyl methylphosphonate
CAS No. 756-79-6

Trichlorophone
CAS No. 52-68-6

Diethyl benzylphosphonate
CAS No. 1080-32-6

Monoethylated diethyl benzylphosphonate
CAS No. 33973-50-1

Diethylated diethyl benzylphosphonate
CAS No. 33973-25-0

(2-Cyclopropyl-2-oxo-ethyl)-phosphonic
acid dimethyl ester
CAS No. 866406-01-1

Figure 2.6 Phosphonates represented in the Gold Carcinogenicity Database (first three compounds) and tested in the Ames assay at F. Hoffmann—La Roche (benzylphosphonates).

functional groups, larger compounds designed as anticancer drugs, mixed mechanisms of action, etc.). Table 2.3 gives an overview of the carcinogenicity and mutagenicity data that are available for such substances. Among the 20 low molecular weight compounds that tested positive in the Ames assay, only five have a TD_{50} value that will lead, by linear back extrapolation to a cancer incidence of 1 out of 100,000, to a virtually safe daily dose in the same order of magnitude or lower as the generic TTC value (see Table 2.3, compounds 5, 11, 14, 15, and 20, in boldface).

TABLE 2.3   Overview of Alkyl Chlorides Represented in the Carcinogenicity Potency Database with a MW Lower than 250 Da

No.	Structure	Name/CAS No.	Ames assay	TD_{50} rat mg/kg/day	TD_{50} mouse mg/kg/day	Daily dose in μg[a]
1		Chloroethane, 75-00-3	+	No positive	1810 (female)	1810
2		Allyl chloride, 107-05-1	+	Inadequate	No positive	–
3		Chloroacetaldehyde, 107-20-0	+	n.d.	36.1	36.1
4		563-47-3	+	113	77.7	77.7
5		**Epichlorohydrin, 106-89-8**	+	**2.96**	**No positive (only female)**	**2.96**
6		127-00-4	+	No positive	No positive	–
7		1,2-Dichloroethane, 107-06-2	+	14.6	138	14.6
8		Glycerol alpha-monochlorohydrin, 96-24-2	+	No positive	n.d.	
9		Telone II, 542-75-6	+	100 (only positive in male)	118 (only positive in male)	100
10		1,2-Dichloropropane 78-87-5	+	No positive	276	276
11		**Trans-1,4-Dicholorobutene-2, 110-57-6**	+	**0.297**	**1.52**	**0.297**
12		Benzyl chloride, 100-44-7	+	No positive	61.5	61.5
13		Bis-2-chloroethylether, 111-44-4	+	n.d.	11.7	11.7

TABLE 2.3 (*continued*)

No.	Structure	Name/CAS No.	Ames assay	TD_{50} rat mg/kg/day	TD_{50} mouse mg/kg/day	Daily dose in μg^a
14		**1,2,3-Trichloropropane, 96-18-4**	+	**1.35**	**0.875**	**0.875**
15		**Nitrogen mustard, 51-75-2**	+	**0.0114**	**n.d.**	**0.0114**
16		6959-47-3	+	No positive	No positive	–
17		6959-48-4	+	433	229	229
18		108-60-1	+	No positive	191	191
19		4'-(Chloroacetyl)-acetanilide, 140-49-8	+	No positive	No positive	–
20		**1,2-Dibromo-3-chloropropane, 96-12-8**	+	**0.259**	**2.72**	**0.259**
21		n-Butyl chloride, 109-69-3	–	No positive	No positive	–
22		Monochloroacetic acid, 79-11-8	–	No positive	No positive	–
23		2-Chloro-1,1,1-trifluoroethane, 75-88-7	–	87.3	n.d.	87.3
24		1,1,2-Trichloroethane, 79-00-5	–	No positive	55	55

(*continued*)

TABLE 2.3   (*continued*)

No.	Structure	Name/CAS No.	Ames assay	TD_{50} rat mg/kg/day	TD_{50} mouse mg/kg/day	Daily dose in μg^a
25		2-Chloroacetophenone 532-27-4	–	No positive	No positive	–
26		999-81-5	–	No positive	No positive	–
27		1,1,1,2-Tetrachloroethane, 630-20-6	–	No positive	182	182

^{a} Virtually safe daily dose for a 50 kg person, calculated from the lowest TD_{50} value observed in the most sensitive species as linear back extrapolation to a cancer incidence of 1 out of 100,000.

An observation that can be made on these five molecules is that they all bear more than one potential DNA alkylating function, and one of them, nitrogen mustard (compound 15, CAS No. 51-75-2), is an anticancer agent that was purposefully designed to strongly alkylate DNA.

Compounds with higher MW belonging to this chemical class and represented in the Gold Carcinogenicity database include nitrosoamines (e.g. CAS Nos. 96806-34-7, 96806-35-8, 110559-85-8, Chlorozotocin) and potent antineoplastic drugs, such as Cyclophosphamide and Isophosphamide, Chlorambucil, Mannitol nitrogen mustard, Melphalan, and Prednimustine. With the exception of Mannitol nitrogen mustard, all of the listed antineoplastic drugs showed, as expected, TD_{50} values leading to a virtually safe daily dose in the same order of magnitude as the TTC or lower. These data appear to verify the comment made by Delaney in 2007,[19] that the systematic application of the TTC concept to alerting monofunctional alkyl chlorides typically used in the synthesis of active pharmaceutical ingredients may be too restrictive, as the high-level analysis presented herein suggests. As a matter of fact, all the monofunctional alkyl chlorides depicted in Table 2.3 have TD_{50} values leading to safe daily doses at least one order of magnitude greater than the default TTC value of 1.5 μg/day. In the pharmaceutical industry, as described in Section 2.2.3.2, a molecule bearing an alkyl chloride moiety is normally flagged by the most commonly used *in silico* systems, and, consequently, an Ames assay is carried out. If the compound shows mutagenic activity, potential genotoxic carcinogenicity is assumed, and, in clinical development, the staged TTC concept is applied. The carcinogenicity data shown in this paragraph for this particular class of molecules is far from being exhaustive; however, it should make the readers reflect on the fact that monofunctional alkyl chlorides tend to be toward the weaker side of carcinogenicity potency in rodents, and that alternative ways of de-risking such chemicals as impurities may be more appropriate. From our experience at Roche with alkyl chlorides and alkyl bromides tested in the Ames assay (data not shown), we could observe, in some cases rather surprisingly, that many of the compounds that were expected to be positive turned out to be negative, and that small structural variations in simple molecules (i.e. low molecular weight) have a major impact in their mutagenic activity. It is of course common knowledge that changes in the overall molecular properties, even leaving the "alerting" alkylating moiety untouched, can completely change the biological activity of the compound, including its capability to induce DNA damage. A way to approach such topics may be to work on QSAR *in silico* models, which focus on specific chemical classes whose members have a limited chemical diversity. With such an approach, combined with the widely used method of structural alerts, better results can be achieved as a wider range of molecular properties are considered, patterns of activity may be found more easily, and predictions based on such patterns made more reliable. It goes without saying, though, that more experimental data will be necessary in order to generate robust models that can be comfortably used in risk assessment.

In the context of impurities present in APIs, it is highly unlikely that significant amount of rodent carcinogenicity data will be generated; on the other hand, a vast amount of mutagenicity data are generated every year in the pharmaceutical industry, encompassing a large portion of the most synthetically useful intermediates and reactants. Efforts aiming at bringing the main pharmaceutical industries together and share their mutagenicity data on nonproprietary intermediates and reactants have already been started by the firm Lhasa Limited, and the results included, to the benefit of the participating members, into VITIC, a database for the management of toxicological information (http://www.lhasalimited.org); however, more has to be done in this direction, as every single company will ultimately benefit from shared knowledge, in particular, by saving significant resources in testing potential impurities, which may have already been tested by competitors and hence reducing the time required for risk assessment.

2.3.5 Aromatic Amines

Aromatic amines represent one of the most important classes of industrial and environmental chemicals. Many of them exhibit mutagenicity in the Ames assay,[45–50] and have been reported to be strong carcinogens.[51–53] The exposure to such molecules can occur from several sources, including tobacco smoking, industrial and agricultural activities; therefore, many studies have been carried out on a number of derivatives for safety assessment purposes and for the identification of those structural features that are most critical for their potential mutagenic and carcinogenic activity.[54] The biochemical mechanism by which aromatic amines may induce cancer has been extensively studied:[55–57] the mechanism of action thought to be responsible for the carcinogenicity of aryl amines involves an activation reaction that leads to the formation of the corresponding N-hydroxylamine. Under certain conditions, such as acidic pH or through enzymatic oxidation, aryl hydroxylamines form the reactive nitrenium ions, which can react with cellular macromolecules, in particular with DNA, thus leading to toxicity and carcinogenicity.[58]

In many pharmaceutical syntheses, simple and complex aromatic amines are rather common, and, according to the CHMP guideline, they need to be classified following the criteria described in paragraph 2.3.2. In most cases, aromatic amines are alerting in the routinely used *in silico* tools (e.g. Derek for Windows—http://www.lhasalimited.net and MC4PC—http://www.multicase.com), and when tested in the Ames assay, it is not unusual that they give a positive response. Similarly to alkyl chlorides and mesylates, all the N-unsubstituted aryl amines (with the exclusion of hetero-aromatic derivatives) have been extracted from the Carcinogenicity Potency Database, along with their available Ames and TD_{50} data. The search returned a total of 108 compounds; after disregarding proflavine hydrochloride hemi-hydrate (CAS No. 952-23-8) for an inadequate NTP carcinogenicity assay, and four coloring substances (C.I. direct black 38, CAS No. 1937-37-7; C.I. direct blue 6, CAS No. 2602-46-2; C.I. direct blue 15, CAS No. 2429-74-5; C.I. direct blue 218, CAS No. 28407-37-6) due to their complex structures (i.e. MW between 781 and 1087 Da), 103 compounds were retained for the subsequent analysis (see Table 2.4). The selected molecules were submitted to Derek for Windows version 11.0.0, taking only the mutagenicity and chromosome damage alerts into consideration. Table 2.4 depicts the results: out of 103 compounds, 71 were alerting for mutagenicity, and two (see Table 2.4) were alerting only for chromosome damage. Of the 71 alerting molecules for mutagenicity, 50 had been tested in the Ames assay, and all of them gave a positive response (Table 2.4). All the lowest available TD_{50} values for the most sensitive species were used to extrapolate the allowed daily dose for a 50 kg person. Among the 103 chemicals, only 19 (18%) showed an allowed daily dose for a 50 kg person in the same order of magnitude of the generic TTC value of 1.5 μg/day (Table 2.4 in boldface).

Of these 19 chemicals, 10 are multifunctional (i.e. 2-hydrazino-4-(p-aminophenyl) thiazole, CAS No. 26049-71-8; o-aminoazotoluene, CAS No. 97-56-3; benzidine, CAS No. 92-87-5; 4,4'-oxydianiline CAS No. 101-80-4; 4,4'-thiodianiline, CAS No. 139-65-1; 2,4-diaminotoluene, CAS No. 95-80-7; 2,4-diaminotoluene.2HCl, CAS No. 636–23-7; 4,4'-methylene-bis(2-methylaniline), CAS No.838-88-0; 3,3'-dimethylbenzidine.2HCl, CAS No. 612-82-8; 3,3'-dimethoxybenzidine.2HCl, CAS No. 20325-40-0). Hence, only about 10% of the 103 analyzed molecules can be classified as mono-functional potent carcinogens. This analysis pointed out also the fact that the carcinogenicity potency of this class of molecules is very difficult to predict with the most frequently used *in silico* tools. As a matter of fact, among the 30 nonalerting compounds in Derek nine were positive in the Ames assay, and two (i.e. p-Chloroaniline.HCl, CAS No. 20265-96-7 and 2,4,6-Trimethylaniline. HCl, CAS No. 6334-11-8) had a one-digit TD_{50} value (Table 2.4). Among the alerting structures, it can be observed that most of them are positive in the Ames assay and show carcinogenic activity in rodents. However, when looking at the carcinogenic potency of this class of compounds, their TD_{50} values span four orders of magnitude, indicating that more efforts should be made in order to identify

TABLE 2.4 Aromatic Amines with the Exclusion of N-Alkyl-Arylamines Represented in the Carcinogenicity Potency Database

Name/CAS No.	TD_{50} rat mg/kg/day	TD_{50} mouse mg/kg/day	Ames	Derek alerts mutagenicity	Derek alerts chromosome damage	Daily dose in μg[a]
N-Phenyl-p-phenylenediamine.HCl 2198-59-6	No positive	No positive	n.d.	No alert	para-Phenylenediamine	–
2,2'-[(4-Aminophenyl)imino] bisethanol sulfate 54381-16-7	No positive (male)	n.d.	n.d.	No alert	para-Phenylenediamine	–
2-Hydrazino-4-(p-aminophenyl)thiazole 26049-71-8	**1.03**	**11.3**	**n.d.**	**Arylhydrazine and Aromatic amine or amide**	**Arylhydrazine**	**1.03**
p-Nitroaniline 100-01-6	No positive	No Positive	n.d.	Aromatic nitro compound	Aromatic nitro compound	–
5-Nitro-o-anisidine 99-59-2	53.9	3720	+	Aromatic amine or amide and Aromatic nitro compound	Aromatic nitro compound	53.9
4-Nitroanthranilic acid 619-17-0	No positive	No positive	n.d.	Aromatic amine or amide and Aromatic nitro compound	Aromatic nitro compound	–
HC red no. 3 2871-01-4	No positive	No positive	n.d.	Aromatic amine or amide and Aromatic nitro compound	Aromatic nitro compound	–
2,6-Dichloro-4-nitroaniline 99-30-9	n.d.	No positive	n.d.	Aromatic nitro compound	Aromatic nitro compound	–
4,4'-Diaminoazobenzene 538-41-0	n.d.	No positive	n.d.	Aromatic azo compound and Aromatic amine or amide	No alert	–
o-Aminoazotoluene 97-56-3	**4.04**	**No positive (male)**	**+**	**Aromatic azo compound and Aromatic amine or amide**	**No alert**	**4.04**
2-Methoxy-4-aminoazobenzene 80830-39-3	n.d.	No positive	n.d.	Aromatic azo compound and Aromatic amine or amide	No alert	–

(continued)

TABLE 2.4 (continued)

Name/CAS No.	TD$_{50}$ rat mg/kg/day	TD$_{50}$ mouse mg/kg/day	Ames	Derek alerts mutagenicity	Derek alerts chromosome damage	Daily dose in µg[a]
3-Methoxy-4-aminoazobenzene 3544-23-8	n.d.	60.2	+	Aromatic azo compound and Aromatic amine or amide	No alert	60.2
m-Phenylenediamine 108-45-2	n.d.	No positive	n.d.	Aromatic amine or amide	No alert	–
p-Phenylenediamine 106-50-3	No positive	n.d.	n.d.	Aromatic amine or amide	para-Phenylenediamine	–
4-Aminodiphenyl 92-67-1	**n.d.**	**2.1**	**+**	**Aromatic amine or amide**	**No alert**	**2.1**
m-Phenylenediamine.2HCl 541-69-5	No positive	No positive	n.d.	Aromatic amine or amide	No alert	–
o-Phenylenediamine.2HCl 615-28-1	248	735	+	Aromatic amine or amide	No alert	248
p-Phenylenediamine.2HCl 624-18-0	No positive	No positive	n.d.	Aromatic amine or amide	para-Phenylenediamine	–
Benzidine 92-87-5	**1.73**	**19.9**	**+**	**Aromatic amine or amide**	**No alert**	**1.73**
4'-Fluoro-4-aminodiphenyl 324-93-6	**n.d.**	**1.14**	**n.d.**	**Aromatic amine or amide**	**No alert**	**1.14**
4,4'-Oxydianiline 101-80-4	**9.51**	**33.6**	**+**	**Aromatic amine or amide**	**No alert**	**9.51**
4-Aminodiphenyl.HCl 2113-61-3	**0.98**	**n.d.**	**+**	**Aromatic amine or amide**	**No alert**	**0.98**
3,4,4'-Triaminodiphenyl ether 6264-66-0	n.d.	13.3	n.d.	Aromatic amine or amide	No alert	13.3
4,4'-Thiodianiline 139-65-1	**3.71**	**33.2**	**+**	**Aromatic amine or amide**	**No alert**	**3.7**

Compound (CAS No.)						
4-Chloro-4'-aminodiphenylether 101-79-1	37.6	346	n.d.	Aromatic amine or amide	No alert	37.6
2,5-Dimethoxy-4'-aminostilbene 5803-51-0	**0.721**	**95.9**	**n.d.**	**Aromatic amine or amide**	**No alert**	**0.72**
Benzidine.2HCl 531-85-1	n.d.	19.7	+	Aromatic amine or amide	No alert	19.7
4,4'-Methylenedianiline.2HCl 13552-44-8	20	32.4	+	Aromatic amine or amide	No alert	20
2,4-Diaminotoluene 95-80-7	**2.47**	**26.7**	**+**	**Aromatic amine or amide**	**No alert**	**2.47**
2,4,5-Trimethylaniline 137-17-7	**33.6**	**6.13**	**+**	**Aromatic amine or amide**	**No alert**	**6.13**
p-Cresidine 120-71-8	98	54.3	+	Aromatic amine or amide	No alert	54.3
4-Chloro-m-phenylenediamine 5131-60-2	315	1230	+	Aromatic amine or amide	No alert	315
4-Chloro-o-phenylenediamine 95-83-0	214	1340	+	Aromatic amine or amide	No alert	214
5-Nitro-o-toluidine 99-55-8	No positive	277	+	Aromatic amine or amide and Aromatic nitro compound	Aromatic nitro compound	277
2-Nitro-p-phenylenediamine 5307-14-2	No positive	614	+	Aromatic amine or amide and Aromatic nitro compound	Aromatic nitro compound	614
4-Nitro-o-phenylenediamine 99-56-9	No positive	No positive	n.d.	Aromatic amine or amide and Aromatic nitro compound	Aromatic nitro compound	–
2-Amino-4-nitrophenol 99-57-0	839	No positive	+	Aromatic amine or amide and Aromatic nitro compound	Aromatic nitro compound	839
2-Amino-5-nitrophenol 121-88-0	111	No positive	+	Aromatic amine or amide and Aromatic nitro compound	Aromatic nitro compound	111

(continued)

TABLE 2.4 (continued)

Name/CAS No.	TD$_{50}$ rat mg/kg/day	TD$_{50}$ mouse mg/kg/day	Ames	Derek alerts mutagenicity	Derek alerts chromosome damage	Daily dose in µg[a]
4-Amino-2-nitrophenol 119-34-6	309	No positive	+	Aromatic amine or amide and Aromatic nitro compound	Aromatic nitro compound	309
2,4-Xylidine.HCl 21436-96-4	No positive (male)	12.4	+	Aromatic amine or amide	No alert	12.4
2,5-Xylidine.HCl 51786-53-9	152	626	+	Aromatic amine or amide	No alert	152
2,4,5-Trimethylaniline.HCl 21436-97-5	98.5	45.5	+	Aromatic amine or amide	No alert	45.5
2,6-Dichloro-p-phenylenediamine 609-20-1	No positive	803	+	Aromatic amine or amide	No alert	803
2,4-Dimethoxyaniline.HCl 54150-69-5	No positive	No Positive	n.d.	Aromatic amine or amide	No alert	–
3-Amino-4-ethoxyacetanilide 17026-81-2	No positive	2070	+	Aromatic amine or amide	No alert	2070
2,4-Diaminotoluene.2HCl 636-23-7	**4.42**	**203**	**+**	**Aromatic amine or amide**	**No alert**	**4.42**
2,6-Diaminotoluene.2HCl 15481-70-6	No positive	No positive	n.d.	Aromatic amine or amide	No alert	–
2,4-Diaminophenol.2HCl 137-09-7	No positive	143	+	Aromatic amine or amide	No alert	143
Chloramben 133-90-4	No positive	5230	+	Aromatic amine or amide	No alert	5230
2,5-Diaminotoluene sulfate 6369-59-1	No positive	No positive	n.d.	Aromatic amine or amide	para-Phenylenediamine	–
2-Aminoanthraquinone 117-79-3	101	1190	+	Aromatic amine or amide	No alert	101

Compound						
4,4'-Methylene-bis(2-methylaniline) 838-88-0	**7.38**	**n.d.**	+	**Aromatic amine or amide**	**No alert**	**7.38**
2,4-Diaminoanisole sulfate 39156-41-7	183	906	+	Aromatic amine or amide	No alert	183
2-Chloro-p-phenylenediamine sulfate 61702-44-1	No positive	No Positive	n.d.	Aromatic amine or amide	No alert	–
Tetrafluoro-m-phenylenediamine.2HCl 63886-77-1	No positive (male)	86.3	n.d.	Aromatic amine or amide	No alert	86.3
3,3'-Dichlorobenzidine 91-94-1	28.1	n.d.	+	Aromatic amine or amide	No alert	28.1
4,4'-Methylene-bis(2-chloroaniline) 101-14-4	19.3	n.d.	+	Aromatic amine or amide	No alert	19.3
3,3'-Dimethylbenzidine.2HCl 612-82-8	**0.629**	**28.6**	+	**Aromatic amine or amide**	**No alert**	**0.629**
3,3'-Dimethoxybenzidine.2HCl 20325-40-0	**1.04**	**73.8**	+	**Aromatic amine or amide**	**No alert**	**1.04**
2,2',5,5'-Tetrachlorobenzidine 15721-02-5	No positive	No positive	n.d.	Aromatic amine or amide	No alert	–
3,3'-Dichlorobenzidine.2HCl 612-83-9	n.d.	12.3	n.d.	Aromatic amine or amide	No alert	12.3
Rosaniline.HCl 632-99-5	No positive	n.d.	n.d.	Aromatic amine or amide	No alert	–
4,4'-Methylene-bis(2-chloroaniline).2HCl 64049-29-2	No positive (male)	66.6	+	Aromatic amine or amide	No alert	66.6

(continued)

TABLE 2.4 (continued)

Name/CAS No.	TD$_{50}$ rat mg/kg/day	TD$_{50}$ mouse mg/kg/day	Ames	Derek alerts mutagenicity	Derek alerts chromosome damage	Daily dose in μg[a]
C.I. disperse blue 1 2475-45-8	156	No positive	+	Aromatic amine or amide	No alert	156
3,3',4,4'-Tetraaminobiphenyl.4HCl 7411-49-6	395	288	n.d.	Aromatic amine or amide	No alert	288
1-Naphthylamine 134-32-7	No positive	67.3	n.d.	Aromatic amine or amide	No alert	67.3
2-Naphthylamine 91-59-8	61.6	39.4	+	Aromatic amine or amide	No alert	39.4
1,5-Naphthalenediamine 2243-62-1	69.6	162	+	Aromatic amine or amide	No alert	69.6
2-Aminodiphenylene oxide 3693-22-9	**No positive**	**4.24**	**n.d.**	**Aromatic amine or amide**	**No alert**	**4.24**
3-Dibenzofuranamine 4106-66-5	**2.48**	**No positive**	**n.d.**	**Aromatic amine or amide**	**No alert**	**2.48**
3-Amino-9-ethylcarbazole mixture	26.4	38	n.d.	Aromatic amine or amide	No alert	26.4
2-Methoxy-3-aminodibenzofuran 5834-17-3	29	No positive	n.d.	Aromatic amine or amide	No alert	29
3-Amino-9-ethylcarbazole.HCl 6109-97-3	57.2	38.6	+	Aromatic amine or amide	No alert	38.6
Aniline 62-53-3	No positive (male)	n.d.	n.d.	No alert	No alert	–
2,6-Dimethylaniline 87-62-7	No positive (male)	n.d.	n.d.	No alert	No alert	–
p-Chloroaniline 106-47-8	No positive	No positive	n.d.	No alert	No alert	–

Compound						
Aniline.HCl 142-04-1	269	No positive	–	No alert	No alert	269
Anthranilic acid 118-92-3	No positive	No positive	n.d.	No alert	No alert	–
m-Cresidine 102-50-1	470	No positive (female)	+	No alert	No alert	470
3-Chloro-p-toluidine 95-74-9	No positive	No positive	n.d.	No alert	No alert	–
5-Chloro-o-toluidine 95-79-4	No positive	195	–	No alert	No alert	195
m-Toluidine.HCl 638-03-9	No positive (male)	1440	–	No alert	No alert	1440
o-Toluidine.HCl 636-21-5	43.6	840	+	No alert	No alert	43.6
p-Toluidine.HCl 540-23-8	No positive (male)	83.5	+	No alert	No alert	83.5
o-Anisidine.HCl 134-29-2	29.7	966	+	No alert	No alert	29.7
p-Anisidine.HCl 20265-97-8	No positive	No Positive	n.d.	No alert	No alert	–
p-Chloroaniline.HCl 20265-96-7	**7.62**	**89.5**	**+**	**No alert**	**No alert**	**7.62**
2,4,6-Trimethylaniline.HCl 6334-11-8	**5.17**	**24.8**	**n.d.**	**No alert**	**No alert**	**5.17**
4-Chloro-o-toluidine.HCl 3165-93-3	No positive	25.8	–	No alert	No alert	25.8
3-Hydroxy-4-aminobiphenyl 4363-03-5	No positive (female)	n.d.	n.d.	No alert	No alert	–

(continued)

55

TABLE 2.4 (continued)

Name/CAS No.	TD$_{50}$ rat mg/kg/day	TD$_{50}$ mouse mg/kg/day	Ames	Derek alerts mutagenicity	Derek alerts chromosome damage	Daily dose in µg[a]
2,4,6-Trichloroaniline 634-93-5	No positive (male)	259	–	No alert	No alert	259
2-Biphenylamine.HCl 2185-92-4	No positive	1120	+	No alert	No alert	1120
2-Naphthylamino,1-sulfonic acid 81-16-3	n.d.	No Positive	n.d.	No alert	No alert	–
4,4'-Diaminobenzanilide 785-30-8	n.d.	No Positive	n.d.	No alert	No alert	–
1-Amino-2-methylanthraquinone 82-28-0	59.2	174	+	No alert	No alert	59.2
Dapsone 80-08-0	22.4	No Positive	–	No alert	No alert	22.4
Cinnamyl anthranilate 87-29-6	12,100	2580	–	No alert	No alert	2580
Sulfisoxazole 127-69-5	No positive	No positive	n.d.	No alert	No alert	–
Sulfamethazine 57-68-1	n.d.	1510	–	No alert	No alert	1510
3,3'-Dihydroxybenzidine.2HCl 1592-36-5	No positive	353	n.d.	No alert	No alert	353
p-Rosaniline.HCl 569-61-9	39.4	51.5	+	No alert	No alert	39.4
1-Amino-2,4-dibromoanthraquinone 81-49-2	46	477	+	No alert	No alert	46
4,4'-Diamino-2,2'-stilbenedisulfonic acid, disodium salt 7336-20-1	No positive	No positive	n.d.	No alert	No alert	–

[a] Virtually safe daily dose for a 50 kg person, calculated from the lowest TD$_{50}$ value observed in the most sensitive species as linear back extrapolation to a cancer incidence of 1 out of 100,000.

subgroups of arylamines with specific substitution patterns or molecular properties that consistently correlate with high or low potency levels. This would allow the application of "corrected" TTC values as a function of the carcinogenicity potency subclass, which the compound to be assessed belongs to.

2.4   CUMULATION VERSUS ADDITION

The synthesis of drug substances usually involves steps of alkylation, conjugation, oxidation, and reduction until the final drug substance is obtained. It is understandable that these steps may imply a carry over of not only one but several intermediates or by-products with a genotoxic potential into the final product. Hence, any risk assessment for genotoxic impurities in drug substances and drug products may have to address the issue of whether several genotoxic impurities can act synergistically or not.

Neither the TTC nor the staged TTC concepts have specifically addressed this problem. Yet one could argue that the origin of the TTC concept is in the area of food and food additives,[5,59] and that any risk assessment for an individual food ingredient or contaminant usually has to work under the assumption that the total human burden from food and other sources will include additional exposures to genotoxic carcinogens. ICH guidelines that describe the appropriate studies to cover impurities in drug substances and drug products implicitly take care of this issue because their general principle is that any final product will be tested in appropriate toxicity tests, including all of its impurities. Hence, any testing of such material will directly assess the genotoxicity of a combination of impurities in the drug substance of drug product material. However, the regulatory guidelines for genotoxic impurities in drugs work under the assumption that genotoxicity tests on drug material, including its impurities may not be sensitive enough to detect the genotoxic potential of impurities, and require other means to identify and control their risk. The FDA draft guideline for genotoxic impurities in drugs recommends conducting genotoxicity assays with the impurity in isolation.

Regarding an appropriate approach for a drug that may contain several genotoxic impurities, the FDA draft guideline reads as follows:

> "The threshold approach for genotoxic or carcinogenic impurities limits the likelihood that any individual impurity in a given drug product will present more than a 10^{-5} excess cancer risk, but the approach is not intended to ensure an aggregate excess cancer risk of less than 10^{-5}. This means the threshold approach to individual impurities is not intended to limit the overall excess cancer risk to 10^{-5} from all impurities in a single drug product or from multiple drug products concomitantly administered." In conclusion, this means that the sum of several genotoxic impurities could be higher than what is defined as "Threshold of Toxicological Concern." Yet, the FDA draft guideline also states: "However, in cases where a class or family of structurally similar impurities is identified and is expected to have similar mechanisms resulting in their genotoxic or carcinogenic potential, the total daily exposure to the related compounds should be evaluated relative to the recommended threshold exposure." Similarly, the CHMP Q&A document states the following: "When

more than one genotoxic impurity is present in the drug substance, the TTC
value of 1.5 μg/day can be applied to each individual impurity only if the
impurities are structurally unrelated. In case of structural similarity, it can be
assumed that the impurities act by the same genotoxic mode of action and have
the same molecular target and thus might exert effects in an additive manner. In
such a situation, a limitation of the sum of the genotoxic impurities at 1.5 μg/day
is recommended."

While this may be a logical assumption, there is little experimental data to prove
that a combination of structurally related mutagens is additive (or cumulative) in
their genotoxic and carcinogenic potential relative to the same dose of a single
mutagen/carcinogen. First of all, the TTC concept was based on a linear extrapolation of rodent cancer data to low doses. The authors of this chapter are not aware
of any single rodent carcinogenicity study with a combination of structurally similar
mutagens to prove this hypothesis experimentally. If combination studies have been
conducted, they involved tests of structurally dissimilar compounds, aimed at
proving anticarcinogenic potential, activation pathways of chemical carcinogens via,
for example UVB light, or, for example the anticancer activity of a combination of
chemotherapeutic agents.[60] There are also data published that show an enhanced
mutagenicity if zidovudine–didanosine co-exposure potentiates DNA incorporation
of zidovudine and mutagenesis in human cells.[61] Most published data, however, refer
to testing of complex, often unidentified, mixtures.[62] When one looks into the details
of the feasibility of a proper assessment of how several genotoxic agents do react
in combination and how to use this information in risk assessment, many issues
become apparent:

1. Structural similarity is a loosely defined term. In terms of mutagenicity, it may
   mean that two compounds are structurally similar only if they produce similar
   lesions in the DNA, and these lesions are processed by similar repair mechanisms. Such knowledge is usually not available, and if it is available, like for
   EMS and MMS, it shows distinct differences between the two in terms of
   DNA adducts and their removal.[39,63] Hence, even for the structurally very
   similar mutagens EMS and MMS, additivity in their mutagenic and carcinogenic action cannot be easily claimed.

2. Structurally very dissimilar agents such as γ-radiation and EMS can have
   additive or even supra-additive effects in genotoxicity tests, partly because
   they may use similar pathways to process the DNA damage or to repair it.[64]

3. Structural similarity in terms of drug substances is very often defined based
   on their pharmacology, which cannot be a criterion for control of genotoxic
   impurities.

4. Structural similarity for more complex structures of usually higher molecular
   weight may be used in terms of shared biotransformation pathways. In this
   context, quite dissimilar compounds, as defined in terms of chemical structure,
   may behave similarly. This can be very important for mutagenicity, that is
   structurally very dissimilar compounds may share only one small substructural
   element, which is important for their mutagenicity/carcinogenicity, for example
   an aromatic amine moiety. These may behave similar in an Ames test under

forced solubility enhancing conditions (via e.g. using DMSO as solubilizing agent), but can differ quite fundamentally *in vivo* with regard to absorption, tissue distribution and elimination.

5. In looking at the mutagenic and carcinogenic potency of structurally very similar compounds, very different dose-response curves become apparent. A detailed analysis of the effect of combining multiple impurities that are in similar or different chemical classes[65] indicated that the risk estimates were not substantially affected.

6. In reality, many mutagens may display sublinear and nonlinear dose-response curves at low doses. Under such circumstances, a combination effect could appear supra-additive because the increment in the effect caused by the second agent produces a different (e.g. steeper) slope of the dose response of the first.[66]

Linear-low dose extrapolation, which calculates a 10^{-5} excess cancer risk, is based on the conservative one-hit hypothesis. It is unlikely at low doses that exposure to one compound would influence the probability of developing cancer for another compound regardless of mechanism. This is in contrast to high doses, where the toxicity of one compound can influence effects of another. It is possible that the carcinogenic risks of two structurally similar compounds are correlated. However, simulations for the additive risk of multiple genotoxic impurities show that an increase in total carcinogenic risk over background for compounds with correlated carcinogenic potencies were no greater than uncorrelated compounds.[65]

In essence, the authors of this chapter feel that more experimental work needs to be carried out to provide an experimental basis for judgment of mutagenicity of combinations of structurally similar compounds and how to use these data in risk assessment and control. We also note that the extremely conservative assumptions made in deriving the TTC, and the errors involved in the extrapolations, mean there is no practical difference between 1.5 and 4.5 µg/day, for example for 1 versus 3 impurities. Also, as outlined above, in practice, it is difficult to predict that chemicals with structural similarities will have similar potencies.

2.5 CONCLUSIONS AND PERSPECTIVES

Within this chapter, the authors have gone through the history of the TTC concept and its development during the last years. A high level analysis of some chemical classes with considerable industrial and environmental importance have been carried out, with a particular focus on the available carcinogenicity data and on how the TTC concept is typically applied to such substances. In addition, some criticism—corroborated by most recent publications—to the linear back extrapolation of virtual safe dose from animal carcinogenicity data obtained at high dose levels has been outlined. The special issue of *Toxicology Letters*, published on November 12, 2009 describing all the preclinical studies that led to the conclusion that the well-known genotoxin EMS exerts its toxic activity via a threshold mechanism, opened new perspectives in understanding the low-dose effects of DNA-reactive chemicals and the approaches used for risk estimation. It has been generally assumed that one single molecule of a genotoxin directly acting on DNA (e.g. EMS or ethyl nitrosourea) could induce a mutation ultimately responsible for tumor development.[67] According to this theory, any exposure, regardless of the dose, represents a cancer risk.[68,69] However, as Calabrese[2] rightly shows, this assumption may be flawed in many aspects and is not compatible with experimental reality, if one looks with detailed sophisticated multi-dose experiments into the response *in vivo* in suitable test organisms.[31,39] However, additional work is required to show wider applicability of risk assessment based on nonlinear extrapolation models. Alternatively, the TTC concept can still be applied to limited datasets, but the intervention level needs to be adjusted. Currently, the regulatory guidelines for pharmaceuticals have put this generic intervention level at 1 additional cancer case in 100,000 exposed persons with a lifetime exposure dimension. In practice, appropriate control of risk may be already achieved with an intervention level that is at least 10-fold higher. A generic TTC of at least 15 µg/day for genotoxic impurities in drug substances may hence be arguably a sufficient level of control as the data of the chemical classes examined in this chapter showed.

The intention of the present contribution is to encourage the readers to reflect on how the decision to unequivocally apply certain approaches in risk assessment have been made, and to envision which efforts should be made in order to consider alternative methods, keeping always in mind the safety of exposed people. In our view, more activities should be focused on analyzing group chemicals in order to obtain subclasses with specified concentration limits as a function of their experimental values (e.g. subclasses of arylamines or phosphonates). It goes without saying that often, the available data is not sufficient to lead to unequivocal conclusions regarding the potential risk of specific chemical classes, therefore we would strongly encourage chemical and pharmaceutical companies to share the genotoxicity data on nonsensitive /proprietary structures (such as potential genotoxic impurities). Such an initiative would bring enormous benefits to regulatory institutions, allowing them to generate risk assessments faster and with a higher level of confidence. Moreover, on the industry side, significantly higher amounts of data will allow to save lab resources, avoiding the testing of already tested compounds and to improve modeling techniques, which in the long term will provide invaluable help in the risk assessment procedures.

REFERENCES

1. McMichael AJ, Woodward A. 1999. Quantitative estimation and prediction of human cancer risk: Its history and role in cancer prevention. In: *IARC Scientific Publication no.131*, edited by S Moolgavkar, D Krewski, L Zeise, E Cardis, H Møller. International Agency for Research on Cancer, Lyon, pp. 1–10.
2. Calabrese EJ. 2009. The road to linearity: Why linearity at low doses became the basis for carcinogen risk assessment. *Archives of Toxicology* 83(3):203–225.
3. Felix CW. (ed.) 1986. De minimis and the threshold of regulation. In: *Food Protection Technology*, Lewis, Chelsea, MI, pp. 29–37, Rulis, AM.
4. Gold LS, Sawyer CB, Magaw R, et al. A carcinogenic potency database of the standardized results of animal bioassays. *Environmental Health Perspectives* 58:9–319.

5. Munro IC. 1990. Safety assessment procedures for indirect food additives: An overview. Report of a workshop. *Regulatory Toxicology and Pharmacology* 12:2–12.

6. Munro IC, Ford RA, Kennepohl E, Sprenger JG. 1996. Correlation of structural class with no-observed-effect levels: A proposal for establishing a threshold of concern. *Food and Chemical Toxicology* 34:829–867.

7. Munro IC, Kennepohl E, Kroes R. 1999. A procedure for the safety evaluation of flavoring substances. *Food and Chemical Toxicology* 37(2–3):207–232.

8. Kroes R, Kozianowski G. 2002. Threshold of toxicological concern (TTC) in food safety assessment. *Toxicology Letters* 127:43–46.

9. Kroes R, Renwick AG, Cheesemann M, et al. 2004. Structure-based thresholds of toxicological concern (TTC): Guidance for application to substances present at low levels in the diet. *Food and Chemical Toxicology* 42:65–83.

10. Allen BC, Crump KS, Shipp AM. 1998. Correlation between carcinogenic potency of chemicals in animals and humans. *Risk Analysis* 8:531–544.

11. Goodman G, Wilson R. 1991. Predicting the carcinogenicity of chemicals in humans from rodent bioassay data. *Environmental Health Perspectives* 94:195–218.

12. Cheeseman MA, Machuga EJ, Bailey AB. 1999. A tiered approach to threshold of regulation. *Food and Chemical Toxicology* 37:387–412.

13. Cramer GM, Ford RA, Hall RL. 1978. Estimation of toxic hazard—A decision tree approach. *Food and Cosmetics Toxicology* 16:255–276.

14. Barlow SM. 1994. The role of the Scientific Committee for Food in evaluating plastics for packaging. *Food Additives and Contaminants* 11:249–259.

15. SCF. 1992. *Guidelines for Presentation of Data for Toxicological Evaluation of A Substance to Be Used in Materials and Articles Intended to Come into Contact with Foodstuffs.* European Commission Directorate General—Internal Market and Industrial Affairs, Luxembourg. Available at http://ec.europa.eu/food/fs/sc/scf/reports/scf_reports_26.pdf (accessed on September 20, 2010).

16. SCF. 2001. *Guidelines of the Scientific Committee on Food for the Presentation of an Application for a Safety Assessment of a Substance to be Used in Food Contact Materials Prior to Its Authorization.* Available at http://ec.europa.eu/food/fs/sc/scf/out82_en.pdf (accessed December 13, 2001).

17. Larsen JC. 2006. Risk assessment of chemicals in European traditional foods. *Trends in Food Science and Technology* 17:471–481.

18. SCF. 1999. *Opinion on a Programme for the Evaluation of Flavouring Substances.* Available at http://ec.europa.eu/food/fs/sc/scf/out45_en.pdf (accessed September 20, 2010).

19. Delaney EJ. 2007. An impact analysis of the application of the threshold of toxicological concern concept to pharmaceuticals. *Regulatory Toxicology and Pharmacology* 49:107–124.

20. ICH. 2002. Impurities testing guideline: Impurities in new drug products (revision). *International Conference on Harmonisation of Technical Requirements for Registration of Pharmaceuticals for Human Use (ICH). Topic Q3A(R2).* CPMP/ICH/2737/99 Rev. 2. Available at http://www.ema.europa.eu/docs/en_GB/document_library/Scientific_guideline/2009/09/WC500002675.pdf (accessed September 20, 2010).

21. ICH. 2003. Q3B(R2): Impurities in New Drug Products. *International Conference on Harmonisation of Technical Requirements for Registration of Pharmaceuticals for Human Use (ICH). Topic Q3B(R).* CPMP/ICH/2738/99. Available at http://www.ema.europa.eu/docs/en_GB/document_library/Scientific_guideline/2009/09/WC500002676.pdf (accessed September 20, 2010).

22. ICH. 1998. Impurities: Residual solvents. *International Conference on Harmonisation of Technical Requirements for Registration of Pharmaceuticals for Human Use (ICH). Topic Q3C.* CPMP. Available at http://www.ema.europa.eu/docs/en_GB/document_library/Scientific_guideline/2009/09/WC500002674.pdf (accessed September 20, 2010).

23. EMEA Guideline. *Guideline on the Limits of Genotoxic Impurities.* CPMP/SWP/5199/02. Available at http://www.ema.europa.eu/docs/en_GB/document_library/Scientific_guideline/2009/09/WC500002903.pdf (accessed September 20, 2010).

24. Müller L, Mauthe RJ, Riley CM, et al. 2006. A rationale for determining, testing, and controlling specific impurities in pharmaceuticals that possess potential for genotoxicity. *Regulatory Toxicology and Pharmacology* 44:198–211.

25. Gaylor DW, Gold LS. 1995. Quick estimate of the regulatory virtually safe dose based on the maximum tolerated dose for rodent bioassays. *Regulatory Toxicology and Pharmacology* 22:57–63.

26. Kroes R, Galli C, Munro I, et al. 2000. Threshold of toxicological concern for chemical substances present in the diet: A practical tool for assessing the need for toxicity testing. *Food and Chemical Toxicology* 38:255–312.

27. Barlow SM, Kozianowski G, Wurtzen G, Schlatter J. 2001. Threshold of toxicological concern for chemical substances in the diet. *Food and Chemical Toxicology* 39:893–905.

28. Bos PMJ, Baars B, Marcel TM, van Raaji TM. 2004. Risk assessment of peak exposure to genotoxic carcinogens. *Toxicology Letters* 151:43–50.

29. FDA. 2008. *Draft Guidance on Genotoxic and Carcinogenic Impurities in Drug Substances and Products: Recommended Approaches.* CDER, http://www.fda.gov/downloads/Drugs/Guidance ComplianceRegulatoryInformation/Guidances/ucm079235.pdf (accessed on September 20, 2010).

30. Müller L, Gocke E. 2009. Considerations regarding a permitted daily exposure calculations for ethyl methanesulfonate. *Toxicology Letters* 190(3):330–332.

31. Müller L, Gocke E, Lavé T, Pfister T. 2009. Ethyl methanesulfonate toxicity in Viracept—A comprehensive human risk assessment based on threshold data for genotoxicity. *Toxicology Letters* 190(3):317–329.

32. Bailey GS, Reddy AP, Pereira CB, et al. 2009. Nonlinear cancer response at ultralow dose: A 40800-animal ED(001) tumor and biomarker study. *Chemical Research in Toxicology* 22(7):1264–1276.

33. Cavalieri EL, Higginbotham S, RamaKrishna NV. 1991. Comparative dose-response tumorigenicity studies of dibenzo[alpha,l]pyrene versus 7,12-dimethylbenz[alpha]anthracene, benzo[alpha]pyrene and two dibenzo[alpha,l]pyrene dihydrodiols in mouse skin and rat mammary gland. *Carcinogenesis* 12:1939–1944.

34. Reddy AP, Harttig U, Barth MC, et al. 1999. Inhibition of dibenzo[a,l]pyrene-induced multi-organ carcinogenesis by dietary chlorophyllin in rainbow trout. *Carcinogenesis* 20:1919–1926.

35. Higginbotham S, RamaKrishna NV, Johansson SL, et al. 1993. Tumor-initiating activity and carcinogenicity of dibenzo[a,l]pyrene versus 7,12-dimethylbenz[a]anthracene and benzo[a]pyrene at low doses in mouse skin. *Carcinogenesis* 14:875–878.

36. Gocke E, Müller L, Pfister T. 2009. EMS in Viracept—Initial ("traditional") assessment of risk to patients based on linear dose response relations. *Toxicology Letters* 190(3):266–270.

37. Gocke E, Müller L. 2009. In vivo studies in the mouse to define a threshold for the genotoxicity of EMS and ENU. *Mutation Research/Genetic Toxicology and Environmental Mutagenesis* 678(2):101–107.

38. Gocke E, Ballantyne M, Whitwell J, Müller L. 2009. MNT and Muta™Mouse studies to define the in vivo dose response relations of the genotoxicity of EMS and ENU. *Toxicology Letters* 190(3):286–297.

39. Swenberg JA, Fryar-Tita T, Jenong Y-C, et al. 2008. Biomarkers in toxicology and risk assessment: Informing critical dose-response relationships. *Chemical Research in Toxicology* 21:253–265.

40. Doak SH, Jenkins GJ, Johnson GE, et al. 2007. Mechanistic influences for mutation induction curves after exposure to DNA-reactive carcinogens. *Cancer Research* 67:3904–3911.

41. Douglass HOJ, MacIntyre JM, Kaufman J, et al. 1985. Eastern Cooperative Oncology Group phase II studies in advanced measurable colorectal cancer. I. Razoxane, Yoshi-864, piperazinedione, and lomustine. *Cancer Treatment Reports* 69(5):543–545.

42. Woo YT, Lai DY, Argus MF, Arcos JC. 1996. Carcinogenicity of organo-phosphorus pesticides/compounds: An analysis of their structure-activity relationships. *Journal of Environmental Science and Health Part C: Environmental Carcinogenesis and Ecotoxicology Reviews* 14:1–42.

43. Cicchetti R, Argentin G. 2003. The role of oxidative stress in the in vitro induction of micronuclei by pesticides in mouse lung fibroblasts. *Mutagenesis* 18:127–132.

44. Wellmann SE, Kramer RE. 2004. Absence of DNA binding activity of methyl parathion and chlorpyrifos. *Toxicology Mechanisms and Methods* 14:247–251.

45. Zeiger E, Anderson B, Haworth S, et al. 1987. Salmonella mutagenicity tests: III. Results from the testing of 255 chemicals. *Environmental Mutagenesis* 9(Suppl. 9):1–109.

46. Zeiger E, Anderson B, Haworth S, et al. 1988. Salmonella mutagenicity tests: IV. Results from the testing of 300 chemicals. *Environmental and Molecular Mutagenesis* 11(Suppl. 12):1–158.

47. Zeiger E, Anderson B, Haworth S, et al. 1992. Salmonella mutagenicity tests: V. Results from the testing of 311 chemicals. *Environmental and Molecular Mutagenesis* 19(Suppl. 21):2–141.

48. Ashby J, Tennant RW. 1988. Chemical structure, Salmonella mutagenicity and extent of carcinogenicity as indicators of genotoxic carcinogenesis among 222 chemicals tested in rodents by the U.S. NCI/NTP. *Mutation Research* 204:17–115.

49. Haworth S, Lawlor T, Mortelmans K, et al. 1983. Salmonella mutagenicity test results for 250 chemicals. *Environmental Mutagenesis* 5(Suppl. 1):3–142.

50. Trieff NM, Biagi GL, Ramanujam VMS, et al. 1989. Aromatic amines and acetamides in *Salmonella typhimurium* TA98 and TA100: A quantitative structure-activity relation study. *Molecular Toxicology* 2:53–65.

51. Weisburger EK, Russfield AB, Homburger E, et al. 1978. Testing of twenty one environmental aromatic amines or derivatives for long-term toxicity or carcinogenicity. *Journal of Environmental Pathology and Toxicology* 2:325–356.

52. Kadlubar FF, Beland FA. 1985. *Chemical Properties of Ultimate Carcinogenic Metabolites of Arylamines and Arylamides*. American Chemical Society, Washington DC.

53. IARC. 1987. Overall evaluations of carcinogenicity: An updating of IARC Monographs volumes 1 to 42. *IARC Monographs on the Evaluation of Carcinogenic Risks to Humans* Suppl. 7:56–74.

54. Benigni R, Passerini L. 2002. Carcinogenicity of the aromatic amines: From structure-activity relationships to mechanisms of action and risk assessment. *Mutation Research* 511:191–206.

55. Beland FA, Kadlubar FF. 1990. Metabolic activation and DNA adducts of aromatic amines and nitro-aromatic hydrocarbons. In: *Handbook of Experimental Pharmacology. Chemical Carcinogenesis and Mutagenesis*, Vol. 94, edited by CS Cooper, PL Grover. Springer-Verlag, Heidelberg, pp. 267–325.

56. Kadlubar FF. 1990. IARC Scientific Publications No. 125, DNA adducts of carcinogenic aromatic amines. In: *DNA Adducts: Identification and Biological Significance*, edited by K Hemminki, A Dipple, DEG Shuker, et al. International Agency for Research on Cancer, Lyon, pp. 199–216.

57. Delclos KB, Kadlubar FF. 1990. Carcinogenic aromatic amines and amides. In: *Comprehensive Toxicology*, Vol. 12, *Chemical Carcinogens and Anticarcinogens*, edited by GT Bowden, SM Fischer. Elsevier Science, New York, pp. 141–170.

58. Doull J. 2001. *Casarett and Doull's Toxicology: The Basic Science of Poisons*. Pergamon, New York.

59. Renwick AG, Barlow SM, Hertz-Picciotto I, et al. 2003. Risk characterisation of chemicals in food and diet. *Food and Chemical Toxicology* 41(9):1211–1271.

60. Dobrzyńska MM. 2000. Micronucleus formation induced by the combination of low doses of X-rays and anti-neoplastic drugs in bone marrow of male mice. *Teratogenesis, Carcinogenesis, and Mutagenesis* 20:321–327.

61. Meng Q, Walker DM, Olivero OA, et al. 1990. Zidovudine–didanosine co-exposure potentiates DNA incorporation of zidovudine and mutagenesis in human cells. *Proceedings of the National Academy of Sciences* 97:12667–12671.

62. Claxton LD, Creason J, Leroux B, et al. 1992. Results of the IPCS collaborative study on complex mixtures. *Mutation Research* 276(1–2):23–32.

63. Beranek DT. 1990. Distribution of methyl and ethyl adducts following alkylation with monofunctional alkylating agents. *Mutation Research* 231(1):11–30.

64. Stopper H, Müller SO, Lutz WK. 2000. Supra-additive genotoxicity of a combination of γ-irradiation and ethyl methanesulfonate in mouse lymphoma L5178Y cells. *Mutagenesis* 15(3):235–238.

65. Bercu JP, Hoffman WP, Lee C, Ness DK. 2008. Quantitative assessment of cumulative carcinogenic risk for multiple genotoxic impurities in a new drug substance. *Regulatory Toxicology and Pharmacology* 51(3):270–277.

66. Burkart W, Jung T. 1998. Health risks from combined exposures: Mechanistic considerations on deviations from additivity. *Mutation Research/Reviews in Mutation Research* 411(2):119–128.

67. Walker VE, Casciano DA, Tweats DJ. 2009. The Viracept-EMS case: Impact and outlook. *Toxicology Letters* 190(3):333–339.

68. Butterworth BE, Bogdanffy MS. 1999. A comprehensive approach for integration of toxicity and cancer risk assessments. *Regulatory Toxicology and Pharmacology* 29:23–36.

69. Haber LT, Mmaier A, Zhao Q, et al. 2001. Applications of mechanistic data in risk assessment: The past, the present and future. *Toxicological Sciences* 61:32–39.

PART 2

EVALUATION OF GENOTOXIC RISK FROM A PRECLINICAL PERSPECTIVE

CHAPTER 3

GENETIC TOXICITY TESTING TO QUALIFY ALERTING IMPURITIES

Mike O'Donovan

3.1 INTRODUCTION

The purpose of this chapter is to describe the test methods that may be used to qualify potential genotoxic impurities. Regulatory guidelines covering genotoxic impurities do not definitively specify the tests to be used; the Committee for Medicinal Products for Human Use (CHMP) Guideline[1] simply states that when a potential impurity contains structural alerts, additional testing, typically in a bacterial reverse mutation assay, should be considered. However, the draft FDA Guidance[2] gives slightly more detail, as follows

> *If an impurity that is present at levels below the ICH quantification thresholds is identified, the impurity should be evaluated for genotoxicity and carcinogenicity based on structural activity relationship (SAR) assessments (i.e. whether there is a structural alert). This evaluation can be conducted via a review of the available literature or through a computational toxicology assessment: commonly used software includes MDL-QSAR, MC4PC and Derek for Windows. The conduct of an in vitro mutation assay (i.e. bacterial reverse mutation assay) generally would be an acceptable initial screen for impurities with an identified alert, since positive signals in computational toxicology programs are often derived from the results of bacterial mutation assays and mutagenic carcinogens are considered to operate through nonthreshold-related mechanisms. An assessment in a mammalian cell assay may be needed for impurities with specific structural groups, such as carbamates, that are not well characterised in bacterial assays, or for compounds that are toxic to E. coli and Salmonella, such as antibiotics.*

> *If the initial evaluation of the genotoxic potential of an impurity is negative, no further genotoxicity studies are recommended and the impurity should be considered adequately qualified regarding its genotoxic potential."*

The CHMP Q&A document[3] on the CHMP Guideline also agrees that an adequate bacterial mutation test, if negative, is sufficient to qualify a structurally alerting impurity.

Genotoxic Impurities: Strategies for Identification and Control, Edited by Andrew Teasdale
Copyright © 2010 by John Wiley & Sons, Inc.

TABLE 3.1 REACH[a] Requirements for Transport of Bulk Chemicals within the European Union

Annual amount	Tests required
1–10 tons	Skin irritation *in vitro* Eye irritation *in vitro* Skin sensitization **Mutagenicity *in vitro*, bacteria** **(Further mutagenicity shall be considered in case of a positive result)** Acute oral toxicity
10–100 tons	Skin irritation *in vivo* Eye irritation *in vivo* **Mutagenicity *in vitro*, mammalian cells or micronucleus** **(Appropriate *in vivo*) mutagenicity studies shall be considered in case of a positive result)** Acute toxicity, inhalation or dermal 28 day toxicity Reproductive toxicity
100–1000 tons	28 days toxicity, if not provided earlier 90 days toxicity Reproductive toxicity
>1000 tons	Further studies depending on chemical safety assessment

[a] Regulation (EC) No. 1907/2006 of the European Parliament and of the Council of December 18, 2006 concerning the Registration, Evaluation, Authorization, and Restriction of Chemicals (REACH).

Boldface indicates genetic toxicity tests, as opposed to general toxicity tests.

Because of its importance as the primary screen, the bacterial reverse mutation assay and modifications of it, are considered in greatest detail in this review. The *in vitro* mammalian cell assays are described because they can also be required to qualify impurities, and the standard rodent *in vivo* tests are prescribed by legislation for the transport of bulk chemicals such as process intermediates within the European Union (see Table 3.1); data generated for an intermediate can be significant if it is subsequently found to be an impurity. The *in vivo* tests may also be used to assess the risk of compounds, giving positive results in an *in vitro* assay, but it should be noted that in most cases, those giving positive results in the bacterial mutation assay will be assumed to be DNA reactive, and, hence, require control to prescribed threshold limits.

Finally, neither the United States nor the European guidelines specify practical details of the genotoxicity tests required to qualify impurities, so it is assumed that the criteria identified in the ICH S2A and S2B[4,5] guidelines for pharmaceuticals apply.

3.2 *IN VITRO* GENOTOXICITY TESTS

3.2.1 Background

The ability of chemicals to cause mutations was first realized during the Second World War, when Auerbach and Robson showed mustard gas to be mutagenic in

Drosophila.[6,7] Mutagenicity has also been studied in bacteria for over 50 years, with the initial work aiming to understand the function of DNA after it had been found to be the hereditary material in all organisms. However, it was not until the early 1970s that the possible use of bacterial tests to predict carcinogenicity was seriously considered, and, in 1973, this led Bruce Ames to publish his paper, titled "Carcinogens are mutagens."[8] A few years afterwards, Lijinsky described this as "An overenthusiastic interpretation of the available evidence,"[9] but the field of what became to be known as genetic toxicology had become established.

The use of bacteria for screening chemicals for potential mutagenicity, and, hence, carcinogenicity, is based on the observation that the primary structure of DNA is the same throughout the living world. There is a considerable amount of evidence that DNA damage in germ cells can cause heritable genetic defects, and in somatic cells can be critical in both the initiation of cancer and subsequent steps in the progression of the disease. A large range of different sorts of genetic damage may have adverse effects on living organisms, but induction of mutation in bacteria is taken as a sensitive indicator that an agent may be capable of causing damage to DNA. The nature of the damage may not be the same as those causing cancer or birth defects in man, but mutagenicity in bacteria does indicate that a chemical has the intrinsic ability to interact with DNA and modify its function, not simply to destroy it.

Early in the development of genetic toxicology, it was appreciated that many carcinogens require metabolism to produce the DNA-reactive, electrophilic species, and it was shown that binding of polycyclic aromatic hydrocarbons to DNA was dependent on metabolism by microsomes.[10,11] It was quickly appreciated that the bacteria used for mutation tests had limited capacity for metabolism, and liver homogenates were used to overcome this. To increase the metabolic capability, liver homogenates (S9) were prepared from rats that had been treated with enzyme inducers, initially phenobarbital, and the activity of several carcinogens, including aflatoxin B_1, benzo(a)pyrene, and benzidine, were shown to require S9 activation.[8] Subsequently, inducers with a broader spectrum of induction have been used, including polychlorinated biphenyls, such as Aroclor 1254,[12] or a combination of phenobarbital and β-naphthoflavone. The S9 mix is supplemented with cofactors for NADPH generation, so it is very efficient at cytochrome p450-mediated phase 1 metabolism; however, phase 2 metabolism is generally very poor, unless cofactors for conjugation are also added.

Similar S9 systems are used in all *in vitro* genotoxicity test systems.

3.2.2 Bacterial Reverse Mutation or "Ames" Test

The bacterial mutation assay examines mutation in specific strains of *Salmonella typhimurium* and *Escherichia coli* constructed to detect a range of mutagens, and is commonly referred to as the "Ames" test, after Professor Bruce Ames (University of California, Berkeley), who developed the *Salmonella* strains.[12] Technically, however, this term is incorrect if any of the *E. coli* strains are included, since these were developed independently by Green and Muriel.[13]

A standard test uses five different strains, and the ICH S2A Guideline[4] gives the following options.

- S. *typhimurium* TA1535;
- S. *typhimurium* TA98;
- S. *typhimurium* TA1100;
- S. *typhimurium* TA1537 *or* TA97 *or* TA97a; and
- S. *typhimurium* TA102 *or* E. *coli* WP2 uvrA *or* WP2 uvrA (pKM101).

The S. *typhimurium* and E. *coli* strains have mutations in the histidine and tryptophan operons, respectively, and reversion of these mutations is measured by the ability of colonies to grow in medium lacking these amino acids. The target sequences in the mutations mean the strains detect agents acting through different mechanisms, namely, those illustrated in Table 3.2.

In addition, the strains have other characteristics influencing their response to mutagens: all the S. *typhimurium* strains except TA102 are DNA repair deficient with the *uvrB* gene deleted, and the E. *coli* strain has a similar deletion, *uvrA*; TA98, TA100, and the E. *coli* strain all contain the pKM101 plasmid, conferring error-prone repair; all the strains also have deficient lipopolysaccharide walls, allowing greater permeability to test agents.

Compounds are tested in both the presence and absence of metabolic activation comprising the S9 fraction of livers from rats pretreated with enzyme inducers, supplemented with cofactors for NADPH generation. The enzyme inducers are used to increase the activity of a wide range of cytochrome p450s. Originally polychlorinated biphenyls (PCB) such as Aroclor 1254 were used, but, subsequently, a combination of phenobarbital and β-naphthoflavone was found to be an effective alternative to PCBs;[14,15] either inducing regime is now accepted. In the standard plate-incorporation test, bacteria and test compound, with or without S9, are mixed with agar before plating onto agar plates, incubated for three days, then numbers of revertant colonies are scored. In the preincubation method, bacteria and test compound ±S9 are incubated together for 60 min before mixing with agar and plating as before. The preincubation method is preferred for volatile test compounds. Experimental procedures for the assay are described in greater detail by Maron and Ames,[16] and Mortelmans and Zeiger[17] for the *Salmonella* strains, and Mortelmans and Riccio[18] for E. *coli*.

TABLE 3.2   Target DNA Sequences in the Common Bacterial Tester Strains

Strain	Mutation reverted by	Target DNA sequence
TA1535 & TA100	Base-pair substitution	–G–G–G–
TA1537	Frame shift	Near–C–C–C–run
TA98	Frame shift	—G–C–G–C—G–C–G
TA102	Transition/transversion	–T–A–A–
WP2 uvrA WP2 uvrA (pKM101)	Base-pair substitution	–T–A–A–

S. *typhimurium* sequences taken from Mortelmans and Zeiger (2000)[17].

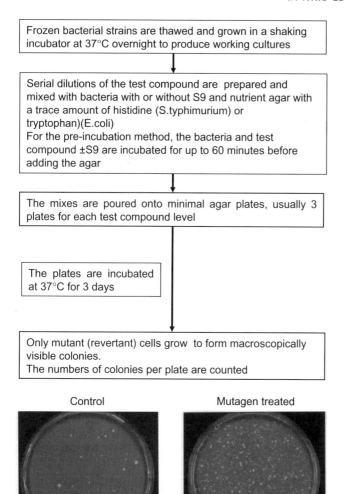

Figure 3.1   Flow chart illustrating the standard Ames test.

A test for regulatory submission should comply with OECD Guideline 471,[19] and the highest level used is 5000 µg/plate, unless limited by toxicity to the indicator strains, or by solubility in either the initial solvent, routinely dimethyl sulphoxide (DMSO), or the aqueous agar medium. Although DMSO is the default organic solvent used in most laboratories, several others have been shown to be compatible, including dimethyl formamide, acetonitrile, acetone and 95% ethanol.[20] A flow chart illustrating the Ames test is shown in Figure 3.1.

3.2.3 Modifications to the Standard Ames Test

It is presumed that for impurities, a five-strain Ames test performed according to ICH Guidelines will be accepted by regulatory authorities worldwide. In terms of the design of the test itself, it is believed that some regulatory authorities are satisfied with a two-strain test, TA98 and TA100, but others require all five strains to be used. The effects of limiting the numbers of tester strains are considered below.

For screening early pharmaceutical research compounds where compound supply can be critical, several modifications in the scale of the Ames test have been explored, and various high throughput screens have been developed. These are considered below, but experience at AstraZeneca (AZ) has shown that the number of impurities is not large enough to require a screen with genuinely high-throughput capability, and supply of test material is not usually limiting.

Because of the practical manipulations involved in mixing bacteria with drug, S9 mix, and agar before spreading onto agar plates, there is no way of completely automating the standard Ames test, although, for the strains with high control revertant numbers, plates are usually read with a video colony counter.

Since compound availability can be critical in early discovery, methods to reduce the amount of material for screening Ames tests have been investigated in the 30 years since the original methods were published. Approximately 300 mg is required for a single five-strain test performed to regulatory submission standards (without allowing material for formulation analysis), and this amount can only be reduced in the following ways: restricting the number of strains, limiting the highest test level, reducing the number of plates per dose, reducing the size of the plates, and performing the test only in the presence of S9. Considering these possibilities in order:

3.2.3.1 Restricting the Number of Strains Of all the available strains, TA98 and TA100 are considered to respond to the majority of bacterial mutagens. Individually, they have been shown to detect 69% and 67%, respectively, of 103 direct acting mutagens, and, used in combination, detected 83% of these.[21] A survey of European laboratories showed that, of 414 positive results from 1275 tests, 17 (4.1%) were positive for only TA1535, and 11 (2.7%) were positive only for TA1537,[22] and of the direct-acting mutagens above, 1% and 3%, respectively, were uniquely positive in these strains.[21] Out of 659 chemicals judged to be mutagenic in the NTP screening protocol, 36 (5%) were positive for TA1535 but not TA100, and 31 of these were detected by no other strain.[23] Data for 28 novel pharmaceuticals showed that two gave positive results with TA1537, but no other strain.[24] It should be noted that these analyses compared only responses between the *Salmonella* strains and do not include *E. coli*. There are limited published comparisons of the sensitivities of the *E. coli* and *Salmonella* strains,[25] but analysis of data held by the Japanese Ministry of Labour on 5526 compounds has shown that approximately 7.5% of the mutagens are identified by *E. coli* WP2 uvrA, but not by the four standard salmonella strains.[4] This is supported by smaller databases held by various pharmaceutical companies that contributed to the ICH process, and AZ has an example of a unique positive in this strain, 2-chloro-N,N-diethylacetamide. The percentage of compounds that would be missed by using only TA98 and TA100 is difficult to estimate, but it is now generally considered that both used together should detect around 90% of all compounds that would be positive using five strains.

It may be possible to limit the strains used to follow up specific alerts. For example, all known mutagenic aromatic amines and nitroaromatics are detected by TA98 and/or TA100, and alkyl halides typically revert TA1535 and/or TA100.

3.2.3.2   Limiting the Highest Test Level   OECD and ICH Guidelines require compounds to be tested to a maximum of 5000 μg/plate if allowed by solubility and toxicity to the indicator strains. A typical concentration range is 5000, 1600, 500, 160, 50, and 16 μg/plate, requiring 300 mg of test compound, so the amount could obviously be reduced by factors of 3 or 10 by limiting the maximum to 1600 or 500 μg/plate, respectively. However, this would miss some compounds, and analysis of 97 positive compounds arbitrarily chosen from 18 diverse research projects within AZ showed that 35 (36%) of these were positive only at ≥1600 μg/plate, and 14 (14%) only at 5000 μg/plate.

3.2.3.3   Reducing the Number of Test Plates per Dose Level   A standard good laboratory practice (GLP) Ames test uses three plates at each level of test compound and three control. The current AZ 2-strain screen (TA98 and TA100) test uses two plates per treatment, with four solvent controls common with other compounds tested concurrently; this requires 80 mg compound. Further reduction to one plate could be done, but test sensitivity and reproducibility would be compromised.

3.2.3.4   Reducing the Size of Individual Test Plates   The standard test uses 9 cm Petri dishes; smaller plates would reduce the amount of compound in proportion to their surface area; a "Miniscreen" utilizing this approach was published some time ago.[26] However, the number of revertant colonies per plate is also proportional to surface area, and this significantly affects the statistical power of the test. For example, TA98 has a control revertant frequency of 30–40 colonies per 9 cm (64 cm^2) plate that would be reduced to two to three colonies on the 4 cm^2 dishes used in the mini screen. Nevertheless, it is possible to make some reduction in plate size although sensitivity is, inevitably, reduced to some extent.

3.2.3.5   Performing Tests Only in the Presence of S9   The large majority of mutagens require metabolic activation and omitting the test without S9 would obviously halve the amount of compound required. Although S9 often reduces the mutagenicity of compounds that do not require activation, of >400 compounds found to be positive at AZ, only one was active only in the absence of S9.

3.2.4   High Throughput Bacterial Screens

Various screens have been used in the pharmaceutical industry to predict the outcome of the definitive Ames test. The aim of these is to provide information at a very early stage in order to direct chemical synthesis programs and the main criteria in the development of them all are to have very high throughput (thousands of compounds per year) and very small compound requirements, typically <5 mg. Several of these assays are summarized below, but all have the limitation that the results they generate differ, to a greater or lesser extent, from the Ames test. Although they can have value in drug discovery, the benefit of high throughput is not usually a major consideration for testing process intermediates and impurities. Similarly, supplies of process intermediates are not usually limited, although it can be difficult to isolate sufficient quantities of some impurities. Although performance of some of the tests is actually quite good, none predicts the activity in the Ames test with greater than about 80% accuracy.

3.2.5   Microscale Fluctuation Test

It is possible to perform a bacterial mutation test using *S. typhimurium* and *E. coli* strains using a modification of the classic fluctuation test devised by Luria and Delbruck.[27] A method using liquid exposure in microtitre plates was first published over 25 years ago at Glaxo[28,29] and has the potential be automated. It was progressively refined at GlaxoWellcome then GSK, but has the limitation that, using only TA98 and TA100, it is not able to detect the ~10% compounds positive only in the other strains. Nevertheless, the method has been shown to be reproducible in other laboratories, and may be a useful alternative if testing is necessary with only very limited amounts of compound; ~10 mg gives a concentration equivalent to 5000 µg/plate.

3.2.5.1   SOS/umu Test

The SOS/*umu* test is considered in detail here because it was used for screening purposes at AZ for a period of about 8 years. It uses a genetically modified version of one of the standard Ames strains, TA1535, containing plasmid pSK1002. This plasmid carries a fused *umu*C'-'*lacZ*, which allows *lacZ* to function as a reporter for *umu*C. Recognition of DNA damage by the bacterial SOS repair system results in expression of the *umu* operon, together with *lacZ*, which is then assayed spectrophotometrically by measuring β-galactosidase activity. It must be noted that the system measures only a bacterial DNA-repair response, not subsequent processing of DNA damage that may result in mutation, as in the Ames test. Approximately 5 mg compound is required to test at levels corresponding to 5000 µg/plate in the Ames test.

The decision to introduce the SOS/*umu* test was influenced by the extensive validation database[30] in which, for 274 compounds, an overall concordance of 90% with Ames test results was achieved. Also, unusual for this sort of validation exercise, a reasonable number of compounds, 88 (32%), were inactive, that is gave negative results in the Ames test. An in-house trial of 20 compounds gave exact correspondence with published results, and a subsequent comparison for 83 chemicals in the NTP carcinogenicity database again gave 83% concordance with the Ames test.[31]

Although the published validation data for the SOS*umu* test are considerably more extensive than for most other high-throughput bacterial screens and show very good agreement with Ames test results, the correlation between the two test systems for AZ research compounds was disappointing. A total of 1474 compounds were

TABLE 3.3   Results for 103 Novel Compounds in the Ames and SOS/*umu* Tests

		Ames	
		Positive	Negative
SOS/*umu*	Positive	2	9
	Negative	9	83

tested in the SOS/*umu* test, of which 112 (7.6%) were positive, directly comparable with the incidence of positive in the Ames test in this laboratory. However, the concordance for positive results was poor (see Table 3.3).

The reasons for the difference between the two tests are not known, but it is possible that duration of exposure to the test compound may be a factor in some cases. In the Ames test, the test compound, bacteria, and activation system are in contact from the start of treatment until the plates are scored 3 days later; in practice, possible DNA damage occurring in the first ~24 h may result in a scoreable mutant colony. In contrast, the SOS/*umu* test is completed in a total of 2–3 h, allowing a much shorter period of time for compound and/or S9-generated metabolites to interact with DNA. Results with 3-amino-9-ethylcarbazole (AEC), a genotoxic rodent carcinogen, support this possibility. AEC is clearly mutagenic in the Ames test, but gives negative results in SOS/*umu*; however, the activity in the former can be dramatically reduced if the bacteria are incubated with AEC and S9 for only 60 min then washed before plating. The Ames bacterial strains are known to have acetylation capacity, and it is possible that the longer period of exposure also allows better opportunity for critical bacterial metabolism. In agreement with this hypothesis, at least three proprietary aromatic amines have been shown to be positive in the Ames test but negative in SOS/*umu*. It is also possible that DNA damage is recognized by the repair system reported in the SOS/*umu* test, but does not result in mutation. Findings with compounds from an infection project, where the pharmacological target is a bacterial topoisomerase, support this hypothesis; six compounds were active in SOS/*umu*, but six closely related structures were all inactive in the Ames test.

Because of its apparent poor predictivity for the Ames test with AZ compounds, use of the SOS/*umu* assay was discontinued.

3.2.5.2   SOS/lux Tests   A variant of the SOS/*umu* test in which the *lacZ* reporter is replaced by luciferase has also been developed.[32] This has considerably increased sensitivity in terms of lowest detectable concentrations in comparison with SOS/*umu*, and this is a potential advantage for waste-water monitoring, its intended use. Although this system was briefly investigated at GSK, it does not appear to be used for screening purposes by any pharmaceutical company.

A similar SOS/*lux* assay in E.coli K12 was also developed for environmental monitoring,[33] but, again, it does not appear to be used by any pharmaceutical company.

3.2.5.3 SOS Chromotest

The SOS/chromotest is a bacterial DNA repair assay very similar to the SOS/*umu* test, but using *E. coli* rather than *S. typhimurium*. The mechanism is very similar with one of the SOS repair genes, in this case *sfiA*, also fused to a *lacZ* gene, which is again assayed spectrophotometrically by measuring β-galactosidase activity. Also, like the SOS/umu test, there is an extensive published database[34] with results for over 700 compounds. Ames test data are available for 452 of these, showing overall concordance with the Ames test is 82%, with sensitivity and specificity of the SOS chromotest of 80% (236/296) and 88% (137/156), respectively. It has also been used in the pharmaceutical industry for screening early stage compounds.

3.2.5.4 Xenometrix AmesII™

Despite its name, AmesII™ (Xenometrix, Allschwil, Switzerland) is not the Ames test but a proprietary version of a small-scale liquid incubation test in which numbers of revertant colonies are estimated by growth in microwell plates rather than on agar. In practice, this is effectively the same as reducing the size of the plates in a standard assay, and has the same limitation of reduced numbers of control revertants. Although it does have the advantage that the endpoint is mutation and it uses one of the standard Ames strains, TA98, the other indicator, TAMix is a mixture of six strains, TA7001-7006, none of which is from the standard set. Although the strains in TAMix all contain base-pair substitutions and are intended as an alternative to TA100, when results were compared with TA100 for 25 chemicals, concordance was seen for only 18.[35] Published data for AmesII are limited to a collaborative trial involving nine laboratories,[36] in which a total of 19 compounds were tested. Of the eight mutagens examined in all laboratories, only six gave uniformly positive results, and 2 out of 5 laboratories failed to detect cyclophosphamide as mutagenic. Although information from the Xenometrix website indicates that TA100 can now be included, this proprietary system appears to have no clear advantage over other reduced scale Ames tests that have been proposed. Although the compound requirement for AmesII is advertised to be 5 mg, in fact, 27.5 mg is needed to achieve 5 mg/mL, comparable with the limit level in the Ames test.

3.2.5.5 Midwest BioResearch MicroAmes Screen

Although it is difficult to determine the exact procedure from the limited amount of experimental detail made public, the MicroAmes screen appears to be a very small-scale version of the pre-incubation Ames test, with very small wells containing agar used to grow revertant colonies. Compound requirement is 5–10 mg, and it is claimed that the highest level tested, 250 µg/well, is equivalent to 5000 µg/plate in the standard Ames test; however, assuming a microwell contains 200 µL, this would be equivalent to only 1000 µg/plate, that is 25–50 mg would be needed to achieve 5000 µg/plate. More importantly, the reduced size of the agar growth area inevitably limits the number of control revertant colonies (as described above), and, for TA98, values of 1–2 mean that it is impossible to detect anything other than large increases. The validation dataset shown in the promotional literature comprises only 20 compounds, and none of the 13 mutagens requires S9 activation.

3.2.5.6 Pfizer In-House High-Throughput Ames Screen A method using genetically modified bioluminescent derivatives of TA98 and TA100 has recently been reported,[37] which is, in fact, a standard mutation assay, but bioluminescence is used to facilitate automated photographic scoring. After the trace amount of histidine has been depleted, histidine-dependent cells become metabolically starved and are not capable of maintaining high-level bioluminescent output. In contrast, revertant auxotrophs continue to produce measurable luminescence in the absence of histidine. However, the method uses 24-well plates, and, therefore, may have no advantage over the "mini screen" modification described previously,[26] and has the disadvantage that it uses bacterial strains that Pfizer appear to have patented. Although the validation study showed concordance of about 90% with Ames test results for 105 compounds in the NTP database, results of its performance with research compounds or process intermediates are not publicly available.

3.2.3 Mouse Lymphoma TK Cell Mutation Assay

The objective of the MLA is to determine the ability of a test compound to induce forward mutation at the thymidine kinase locus in L5178Y mouse lymphoma cells. Thymidine kinase (TK) allows cells to salvage thymidine for use in DNA synthesis; deficiency in this enzyme is not lethal because cells are able to survive using the *de novo* DNA synthetic pathway. Mouse lymphoma L5178Y 3.7.2C cells are heterozygous at the *tk* locus ($tk^{+/-}$), and may undergo forward mutation to the $tk^{-/-}$ genotype with little or no TK activity. Both $tk^{+/-}$ and $tk^{-/-}$ cells are viable in nonselective medium, but addition of a toxic thymidine analogue that can be phosphorylated, for example trifluorothymidine (TFT) to the culture medium results in killing of the $tk^{+/-}$ heterozygotes with preferential survival of the $tk^{-/-}$ mutants. The mutant frequency can thus be estimated by comparing the cloning efficiency of cells in medium with and without the selective agent, TFT, and mutagenic activity is determined by treating cultures with different concentrations of the test compound and examining the effect on mutant frequency.

The assay is designed to detect both multigenic deletions, encompassing the *tk* locus and mutations restricted to the thymidine kinase gene.[38] Thus, the mouse lymphoma assay will detect test compounds that give chromosome damage, in addition to those compounds that produce gene mutations.[39] Molecular analysis of the mutants has identified a wide spectrum of genetic alterations, including point mutations, deletions, translocations, recombination or gene conversion, and, possibly, nondisjunction (aneuploidy).[40]

The L5178Y TK$^{+/-}$ assay originally developed by Clive et al.[41] involved cloning in soft agar. It was subsequently modified to use cloning by limited dilution in microtitre plates to assess viability and mutant frequency.[42] The microtitre method is now more widely used in industrial laboratories than cloning in soft agar, but data generated using either method are acceptable to regulatory authorities.

Compounds are tested in both the presence and absence of an exogenous metabolic activation system comprising the S9 fraction of livers from rats pretreated with Aroclor 1254, or a combination of phenobarbital and β-naphthoflavone,

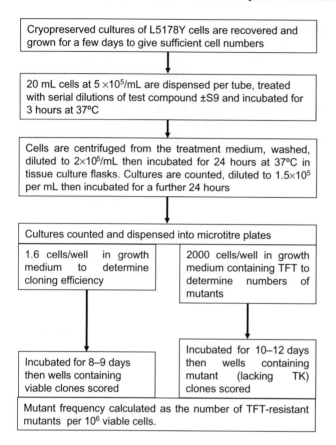

Cryopreserved cultures of L5178Y cells are recovered and grown for a few days to give sufficient cell numbers

20 mL cells at 5 ×10⁵/mL are dispensed per tube, treated with serial dilutions of test compound ±S9 and incubated for 3 hours at 37°C

Cells are centrifuged from the treatment medium, washed, diluted to 2×10⁵/mL then incubated for 24 hours at 37°C in tissue culture flasks. Cultures are counted, diluted to 1.5×10⁵ per mL then incubated for a further 24 hours

Cultures counted and dispensed into microtitre plates

1.6 cells/well in growth medium to determine cloning efficiency

2000 cells/well in growth medium containing TFT to determine numbers of mutants

Incubated for 8–9 days then wells containing viable clones scored

Incubated for 10–12 days then wells containing mutant (lacking TK) clones scored

Mutant frequency calculated as the number of TFT-resistant mutants per 10⁶ viable cells.

TK deficient cells are not killed by the toxic purine analogue TFT

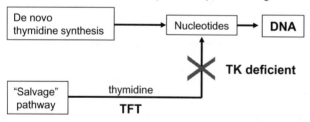

Figure 3.2   Flow chart illustrating the mouse lymphoma TK assay.

supplemented with cofactors for NADPH generation. The assay is described in greater detail by Clements.[43]

A GLP compliant study typically includes duplicate cultures tested using 3- and 24-h test compound exposure periods in the absence of S9 and 3 h exposure in the presence of S9. A test for regulatory submission must comply with OECD Guideline 476,[44] and the highest level used is 10 mmol/L unless limited by cytotoxicity, or solubility in the initial solvent (routinely DMSO) or the aqueous tissue culture medium. A flow chart illustrating the mouse lymphoma assay is shown in Figure 3.2.

3.2.4 *In Vitro* Cytogenetics Assays

The purpose of the *in vitro* chromosome aberration test (IVC) is to identify agents that cause structural chromosome aberrations in cultured mammalian cells.[45,46] Structural aberrations may be of two types, chromosome or chromatid; the majority of chemical mutagens induce aberrations predominantly of the chromatid type, but chromosome-type aberrations also occur. Further, an increase in polyploidy may indicate that a chemical has the potential to induce changes in chromosome number (aneuploidy).

Either primary cell cultures or established cell lines may be used for an IVC, and, for the past 20 or more years, the most widely used systems have been primary human peripheral lymphocytes, and Chinese hamster fibroblast lines originally derived from either ovary (CHO cells) or lung (CHL cells). The relative merits of lymphocytes, CHO and CHL cells have been discussed,[47,48] but a comprehensive review of all compounds tested did not show any clear difference between them.[49] However, recently, some evidence has been published to suggest that misleading results induced by non-DNA damaging agents are less likely to be generated in human lymphocytes than CHO cells.[50] It is possible that the more stringent checkpoint controls in primary lymphocytes than in the immortal CHO and CHL cells may prevent damaged cells reaching mitosis.

Human peripheral lymphocytes are obtained from prescreened donors, and cultured either in whole blood or as the mononuclear cell fraction separated by Ficoll density centrifugation or from the "buffy coat." In either case, the T-cells are stimulated to divide using phytohemagglutinin, and incubated for 2 days to allow significant numbers of cells to start cycling before the start of treatment. CHO and CHL cells are cultured according to standard procedures to give exponentially dividing cultures. Whichever system is used, in the first experiment the cells should be exposed to the test substance both with and without S9 (see the mouse lymphoma assay, above) for a period of 3–6 h, then sampled at about 1.5× the normal cell cycle time after the beginning of treatment (usually ~24 h for lymphocytes and ~20 h for (CHO/CHL cells). If negative results are obtained in the first experiment, a second experiment should be done without S9 with continuous treatment for about 1.5× the normal cell cycle time. Alternatively, all three treatments can be performed in a single experiment. In all cases, colcemide or colchicine is added 1 to 3 h before harvesting to block cell division at metaphase before chromosome preparations are made for microscopic analysis. Slides are scored to determine the number of metaphases showing chromosome damage, the number of mitoses, and the proportion of polyploid cells. Cytotoxicity can be estimated by reduction in cell confluency, cell count, or mitotic index, although it has recently been suggested that reduction in population doublings is the best measure.[51]

A test for regulatory submission must comply with OECD Guideline 473,[52] and, like the mouse lymphoma TK assay, the highest level used is 10 mmol/L unless limited by cytotoxicity, or solubility in the initial solvent (routinely DMSO) or the aqueous tissue culture medium. A flow chart illustrating the in vitro cytogenetics assay using human lymphocytes is shown in Figure 3.3.

10–20 mL blood sample is taken from a non-smoking volunteer and diluted with growth medium containing phytohaemagglutinin to stimulate lymphocytes to divide. Cultures are incubated at 37°C for 48 hours.

↓

Cultures are treated with serial dilutions of test compound for 3 hours ±S9 or 20 hours −S9. Colcemid is added 18 hours after the start of treatment to block cell division at metaphase. After a further 2 hours, microscope slides are prepared, fixed and stained.

↓

Slides are examined microscopically and metaphases scored for: a) mitotic index; b) chromosome aberrations; c) polyploid cells.

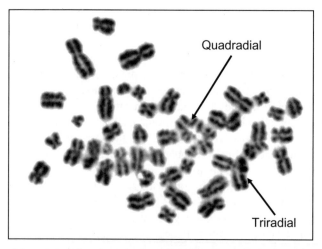

A human lymphocyte metaphase showing chromosome damage

Figure 3.3   Flow chart illustrating the *in vitro* cytogenetics assay using human lymphocytes.

3.3   *IN VIVO* GENOTOXICITY TESTS

3.3.1   Rodent Bone Marrow Micronucleus Test

Micronucleus tests can be applied to any population of dividing cells either *in vivo* or *in vitro*. Micronuclei are formed from chromosome fragments, or whole chromosomes, left behind during the anaphase stage of mitosis, and, therefore, may result from both clastogenic (chromosome breakage) and aneugenic (loss of whole chromosomes) events. They are visualized microscopically in cells that have gone through division as discrete small bodies of chromatin in the cytoplasm, and specialized staining techniques can distinguish whether they contain chromosome fragments or whole chromosomes.

The rodent bone-marrow micronucleus test provides an *in vivo* method for detecting agents that interfere with mitotic cell division,[53] and examines rapidly dividing erythropoietic cells that are exposed to plasma levels of drug and metabolites. Erythroblasts expel their nuclei a few hours after the last mitotic division, but micronuclei remain in the cytoplasm (see Fig. 3.4).

The bone-marrow must be sampled about 24 h after the animals have been treated in order to score immature erythrocytes (IE) that went through their final mitosis while exposed to the test compound. Samples are also taken 48 h after dosing to take into account any possible delay in the normal cell cycle time induced by the test compound. This can be achieved using either two sample times after a single dose, or one sample time after two doses.

After sampling the bone-marrow, slides must then be stained to allow mature and immature erythrocyes to be differentiated in order to score micronuclei in the latter. All the stains used rely on detecting the residual RNA in the immature erythrocytes (IE). For the mouse, the species originally used for the micronucleus test, the most common stain was May-Grunwald/Giemsa,[53] which identifies IE by their polychromatic appearance, hence the alternative term for IE, "polychromatic erythrocytes" (PCE). However, rat bone-marrow preparations contain mast cell granules that stain similarly to micronuclei with May-Grunwald/Giemsa, thus precluding its use. Consequently, modified staining procedures with hematoxylin and eosin,[54] or fluorescent dyes were introduced to allow the rat to be used routinely. Acridine orange[55] is now the most commonly used stain for rats, and is equally applicable to mice; the RNA in IE fluoresces orange in contrast to the green of DNA in the micronuclei. Whatever stain is used, the frequency of micronuclei in IE (PCE) is scored, and the ratio of IE to mature erythrocytes is used as an indicator of bone marrow toxicity.

Either the rat or the mouse can be used, and, for drug substances, the default species is often the rat in order to relate to other toxicology and toxicokinetic data. However, for impurities, this is unlikely to be a factor, and either species is equally acceptable.

The rodent bone-marrow micronucleus test can be performed by giving either a single dose and sampling groups after both 24 and 48 h, or by giving two doses 24 h apart and sampling 24 h after the second dose. In order to minimize animal numbers, the two-dose regimen is preferred for routine use, although a single dose may be more practicable if intravenous administration is required. A test for regulatory submission must comply with OECD Guideline 474,[56] and the highest dose must be the maximum tolerated up to a limit of 2000 mg/kg. A flow chart illustrating the rodent bone-marrow micronucleus test is shown in Figure 3.4.

3.3.2 Rodent Peripheral Blood Micronucleus Test

Although the rodent micronucleus assay was originally, and is still most commonly, performed by examining the bone marrow, it is possible to sample peripheral blood. The ICH S2A guideline[4] states that "*the measurement of micronucleated immature*

Rats or mice are given 2 doses of the test compound, 24 hours apart

Micronuclei are formed by chromosome breakage or loss of a whole chromosome at the final cell division of erythropoiesis. Nuclei are then expelled from the erythrocytes during maturation leaving any micronuclei in the immature erythrocytes (IE)

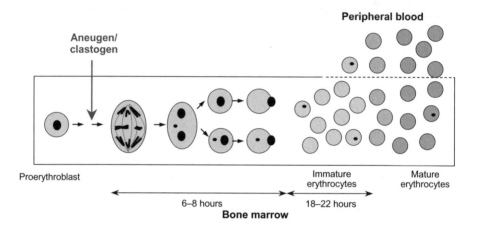

Peripheral blood

Aneugen/ clastogen

Proerythroblast

Immature erythrocytes

Mature erythrocytes

6–8 hours | 18–22 hours

Bone marrow

24 hours after the second dose the animals are killed and the femurs are removed. The bone marrow is aspirated and the cells are spread onto slides. After fixing and staining with acridine orange, the slides are examined microscopically. 2000 IE per animal are analysed and the numbers of IE containing micronuclei are recorded.

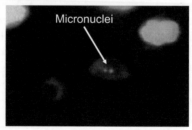

Micronuclei

An IE containing 2 micronuclei (acridine orange stain)

Figure 3.4   The rodent bone-marrow micronucleus test. (See color insert.)

Rats or mice are given 2 doses of the test compound, 24 hours apart

Micronuclei are formed by chromosome breakage or loss of a whole chromosome at the final cell division of erythropoiesis. Nuclei are then expelled from the erythrocytes during maturation leaving any micronuclei in the immature erythrocytes (IE)

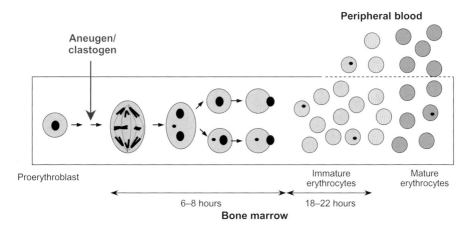

24 hours after the second dose the animals are killed and the femurs are removed. The bone marrow is aspirated and the cells are spread onto slides. After fixing and staining with acridine orange, the slides are examined microscopically. 2000 IE per animal are analysed and the numbers of IE containing micronuclei are recorded.

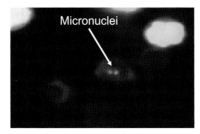

An IE containing 2 micronuclei (acridine orange stain)

Figure 3.4 The rodent bone -marrow micronucleus test.

(e.g. polychromatic) erythrocytes in peripheral blood is an acceptable alternative in the mouse, or in any other species in which the inability of the spleen to remove micronucleated erythrocytes has been demonstrated, or which has shown adequate sensitivity to detect clastogens/aneuploidy inducers in blood." At the time ICH S2A was written, it was not clear if peripheral blood could be sampled from rats, but with subsequent developments, the position is now summarized well in the Revised ICH S2 Guidelines (although only at Step 2 at the time of writing)[57] as follows. Although rats rapidly remove micronucleated erythrocytes from peripheral blood, it has been established that micronucleus induction by a range of clastogens and aneugens can be detected in blood reticulocytes.[58,59] Rat blood may be used for micronucleus analysis if methods are used to ensure that newly formed reticulocytes are analyzed,[60,61] and the sample size is sufficiently large to provide appropriate statistical power, given the lower micronucleus levels in rat blood than bone marrow.[62] Further, systems for automated analysis (image analysis or flow cytometry) can be used if appropriately validated.[56,60,63]

The major attraction of using peripheral blood from rats when testing pharmaceuticals is the potential to sample animals from pivotal 14/28 day toxicity studies, thus eliminating the need for a dedicated acute micronucleus test. Integration into repeat-dose studies is not likely to be a consideration when testing impurities or intermediates, but it is quite probable that automated analysis of peripheral blood samples from acute studies will become increasingly common.

3.3.3 Rat "Comet" Assay

The single-cell gel electrophoresis or "comet" assay is a method used to evaluate the ability of a test compound to cause DNA strand breaks and alkali labile sites, and can be applied *in vitro* or *in* vivo to virtually any eukaryotic cell population that can be obtained as a single cell suspension.[64–66] The rat comet assay has been gaining acceptance by regulatory authorities as the second *in vivo* study[67] in place of the rat liver unscheduled DNA synthesis (UDS) assay, which is now generally considered to lack sensitivity. As the second *in vivo* test, only the liver would be examined routinely, but methods are also available to analyze other tissues, including peripheral lymphocytes, stomach, and bone marrow.

After single cell suspensions have been prepared from the relevant tissue, they are embedded in agarose gel on glass microscope slides and lysed to rupture the cell membranes, extract the nuclear proteins, and leave supercoiled DNA. The DNA is unwound in strong alkaline buffer and then electrophoresed.[64] DNA damage is detected as an increase in the migration of DNA resulting from changes in the conformation and molecular weight of DNA and is measured as the amount of DNA present in the comet tail (Fig. 3.5). The method has been used for the detection of DNA damage in cells exposed to chemical and physical agents under *in vitro* and *in vivo* conditions.[64,68–70]

The rat comet assay requires samples to be analyzed at both 3–6h (or at C_{max}, if known) and approximately 24h after dosing. To minimize the number of animals used, doses are given on two consecutive days, and the tissues processed on the second day. If it is necessary to perform both the comet and bone marrow micronucleus tests,

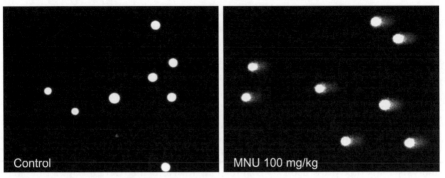

Figure 3.5   The comet assay. Hepatocyte nuclei from rats given an oral dose
of methylnitrosourea (MNU) showing DNA damage.

then it is possible to combine them. Methods are being developed in which the same
animals are given doses on three consecutive days, with both endpoints measured on
the third. An OECD Guideline has not yet been written, but, as for the micronucleus
assay, the highest dose must be the maximum tolerated up to a limit of 2000 mg/kg.

3.3.4   Rat Liver Unscheduled DNA Synthesis (UDS) Assay

Test for UDS measure excision repair of DNA following covalent adduct formation
by reactive chemicals, or, of less interest in this context, ionizing radiation. UDS
can be measured *in vitro* or *in vivo* using any population of cells that is not dividing;
the requirement for the cells to be nondividing is simply because the amount of DNA
synthesis resulting from excision repair is vastly exceeded by the amount synthesized during cell division. UDS is assessed by measuring uptake of radiolabeled
nucleotides, usually [³H]-thymidine. The amount of radiolabeled DNA can then be
quantified either by extraction and measuring the specific radioactivity by spectro-
photometry and scintillation counting, or by microautoradiography of cell or tissue
preparations.

The rat hepatocyte UDS test was originally developed as an *in vitro* screen in
which freshly isolated rat hepatocytes were treated with the test agent of interest.[71]
However, the established in vitro procedures were then modified to become an
ex vivo method in which the rats were dosed with the test agent and UDS measured
in vitro in hepatocytes obtained when the animals were killed shortly after
treatment.[72,73]

As in the rodent bone marrow micronucleus test, animals are treated with the
test compound up to the MTD or limit dose. At least two dose levels are normally
used because there are a few literature examples where the maximum UDS response
is seen below the MTD. The animals are killed 6 to 12 h after dosing, since most
genotoxic agents produce peak UDS activity at that time. The hepatocytes are isolated
by enzymic digestion, then allowed to attach to coverslips and cultured in medium
containing [³H]-thymidine for 3–4 h to label replicating DNA. They are then cultured
for a further period of about 20 h in medium containing unlabelled thymidine then

fixed and processed for autoradiography. After developing, radioactive labeling of the hepatocyte nuclei is measured microscopically by the deposition of silver grains in the overlying photographic emulsion. A test for regulatory submission must comply with OECD Guideline 486,[74] and as with the other *in vivo* tests, the highest dose must be the maximum tolerated up to a limit of 2000 mg/kg.

3.4 DNA BINDING ASSAYS

When developing pharmaceuticals, if positive results are found in any test, it can be important to determine whether or not the response is due to the formation of covalent adducts to DNA. Although it is usually assumed that positive results in the Ames test are due to DNA reactivity, the *in vitro* mammalian cell assays do have a relatively high incidence of positive results, some of which may be due to other factors. To evaluate further positive findings in any particular test, it may be useful to test for the ability of an agent to form DNA adducts. If adducts cannot be demonstrated, this can be used in a weight-of-evidence approach to support a nongenotoxic mode of action for which, consequently, thresholds and safety margins can be argued. Although a negative Ames test is usually sufficient to define an impurity as nongenotoxic (see test strategy, below), occasionally, additional tests, including in vitro mammalian cell tests, are performed to satisfy chemical registration and transportation requirements in various territories, and positive results in these may require further investigation.

There are numerous methods for the identification and quantification of DNA adducts, and these have recently been reviewed by Himmelstein et al.[75] The two most likely to be used in order to determine whether or not a positive genotoxic response is due to DNA adduct formation are ^{32}P postlabeling and radiolabel binding, and the following brief summaries are taken from Himmelstein et al.[75]

3.4.1 [32]P Postlabeling

[32]P postlabeling is a very sensitive technique that is applicable to an extensive range of DNA adducts and requires only microgram quantities of DNA; consequently, it is very widely used for DNA adduct analysis in vitro and in vivo.[76,77] DNA is isolated from the cells or tissue of interest and enzymatically digested to 3'-mononucleotides (occasionally dinucleotides), with, typically, micrococcal nuclease or spleen phosphodiesterase. Adducts are enriched from the normal nucleotides by n-butanol extraction, nuclease P1 treatment (which dephosphorylates normal 3'-mononucleotides leaving some adducted nucleotides intact), or immunoaffinity chromatography, and then phosphorylated with high specific activity ^{32}P-ATP and T4 polynucleotide kinase. The resultant, 3',5'-bisphosphates are then chromatographed by two-dimensional thin-layer chromatography or HPLC. No structural information on the nature of the adduct(s) is produced, but co-chromatography with suspected adducts if they can be synthesized can give a good indication of the probable structure. Attempts were made during the 1990s to standardize protocols for the assay through a series of workshops and collaborative trials, and these culminated in a recommended

set of procedures for the detection of adducts formed by polycyclic aromatic hydrocarbons, aromatic amines, and methylating agents.[78,79] A protocol including experience cumulated over a number of years has also been published recently.[80]

3.4.2 Radiolabel Binding

Radiolabel binding assays are used relatively commonly in the pharmaceutical industry to follow up positive results in mutagenicity assays, but have the obvious disadvantage that radiolabeled test material is required. While this is often available for drugs in development, it is frequently impracticable to provide radiolabeled impurities.

Like ^{32}P postlabeling, radiolabel binding assays can be performed *in vitro* and *in vivo* and compounds labeled with ^{3}H or ^{14}C are most commonly used. Labeling with ^{3}H has the advantage of allowing much higher specific activities, and, hence, higher sensitivities than ^{14}C, but the relatively rapid and easy exchange of radioactive ^{3}H with nonradioactive ^{1}H poses the risks of artifacts and may hamper accurate quantification.[81] After treatment, DNA is isolated from cells or tissues, purified to remove proteins and labeled adducts detected by scintillation counting to quantify the total amount of bound radioactivity. There is the potential to give false positive results due to artifactual presence of isotope in the DNA isolate, so the purity of the extracted DNA must be carefully considered (reviewed by Phillips et al.[82]).

3.5 TEST PERFORMANCE

The performance of a genetic toxicity test in predicting carcinogenicity is conventionally expressed in terms of "sensitivity," that is the proportion of carcinogens giving positive results, and "specificity," that is the proportion of carcinogens giving negative results.

The first extensive validation of the bacterial mutation assay reported from Ames' laboratory showed sensitivity of 90% (157/175) and specificity of 87% (94/108) for a total of nearly 300 compounds.[83] A few years later, data from a Japanese laboratory showed poorer performance with sensitivity and specificity of 85% and 74% for about 240 compounds,[84] and a subsequent European trial showed the values falling to only 76% and 57%, respectively.[85] However, the last trial included only seven noncarcinogens, so the specificity was, in fact, 4 out of 7 giving negative results. The figures above are presented in some detail to illustrate two important points about "validation" of test systems. First, initial comparisons tend to use compounds with well-defined activities, both positive and negative, which are likely to give very good correlations. Second, it is important to include similar numbers of compounds giving positive and negative results to avoid biasing estimates of sensitivity and specificity.

More recently, the performance of the most commonly used in vitro genotoxicity assays, including the Ames test, has been evaluated for the ability to discriminate between rodent carcinogens and noncarcinogens using data for over 700 chemicals compiled from the most reliable sources.[86] This dataset showed the Ames test to

TABLE 3.4   Ability of *In Vitro* Genotoxicity Test to Discriminate Rodent Carcinogens and Non-Carcinogens (from Kirkland et al. 2005)[86]

Assay	Sensitivity	Specificity
Bacterial mutation	59% (318/541)	74% (130/176)
Mouse lymphoma TK	73% (179/245)	39% (41/105)
In vitro cytogenetics	66% (231/352)	45% (61/136)

have sensitivity of about 59% for 541 carcinogens, and specificity of 74% for 176 noncarcinogens (Table 3.4). Although the sensitivity may appear relatively poor, the data include a large number of compounds known to be carcinogenic through mechanisms other than covalent binding to DNA. A positive result in the Ames test is now considered to be a very good indication that a compound is capable of forming covalent adducts to DNA in the conditions of the assay, although it is, of course, possible that those conditions are not replicated *in vivo*. Nevertheless, there are a number of factors that are known to be able to give artifactual positive results in bacterial mutation assays.[87] Since the *Salmonella* strains require mutation to allow them to grow in the absence of histidine, substances such as food samples or biological materials that supply a source of histidine can increase the numbers of countable colonies. Similarly, the *E. coli* WP2 strains, which are mutant at the TrpE locus, can grow if any intermediates that are formed after the point at which the synthetic sequence is blocked are added to the culture medium.

The review by Kirkland et al.[86] gave some concern that the specificity of the tests was relatively poor, and, therefore, a lot of noncarcinogenic agents would be wrongly classified. The specificity of the Ames test, 74%, in this analysis, was reasonable, but for the *in vitro* mammalian cell tests, this falls to around 40%, that is about 60% of compounds would be wrongly classified. However, this dataset included only compounds for which carcinogenicity data were publicly available, and, for obvious reasons, contained a disproportionate number of carcinogenic compounds. It is presumed, or hoped, that the majority of chemicals are not actually carcinogenic, and better indications of the specificities of individual assays can be obtained from the data for candidate or marketed drugs (see Table 3.5). Results have been compiled for all drugs submitted to the German regulatory authority during the 1990s,[88] and it is likely that this included some genotoxic, potentially carcinogenic oncology therapies. Similar data have also been compiled for marketed pharmaceuticals listed in the 2008 U.S. Physicians' Desk Reference, with cytotoxic anticancer and antiviral drugs, nucleosides (with known mechanistic genotoxicity), steroids with class-specific genotoxicity, and biologicals or peptide-based drugs all removed from the analysis.[89] It must be presumed that the majority of these drugs are not carcinogenic, and the incidence of positive results with them is much lower than reported by Kirkland et al.;[86] the Ames test has an incidence of 7%–8%, and the *in vitro* cells test around 20%–25%. Similar figures have been seen with AZ research compounds not intended to be carcinogenic, with ~8% of about 2000 Ames tests and 19% of >500 mouse lymphoma test giving positive results. Similar figures

TABLE 3.5   **Incidence of Positive Genotoxicity Results in Candidate and Marketed Pharmaceuticals**

	Number of positive tests			
Assay	German submissions[a] 1990–1997		PDR review[b] 2008	
Bacterial mutation	23/298	8%	38/525	7%
Mouse lymphoma TK	28/104	27%	32/163	19%
In vitro cytogenetics	77/266	29%	88/380	26%
In vivo cytogenetics	19/283	7%	49/438	11%

[a] Pharmaceuticals submitted to BfArM.[88]

[b] Marketed pharmaceuticals listed in the US Physicians' Desk Reference.[89]

were also obtained at Merck, with about 20% of all CHO cytogenetics tests giving positive results (Sheila Galloway, personal communication).

Data for the performance of the *in vivo* tests are more limited, but the incidence of positive results for *in vivo* cytogenetic tests, the large majority of which are the bone-marrow micronucleus assays, with pharmaceuticals is 7%–10% (Table 3.4). Similarly, data for the performance of the rat liver UDS or Comet assays are not yet available.

3.5   TEST STRATEGY

Only the actual tests for genotoxicity are considered in this section. Related topics such as the computational toxicology systems available, the staged threshold of toxicological concern (TTC) approach developed by Muller et al.,[90] and the ICH Q3C[91] approach for calculating permitted daily exposures (PDE) are discussed in detail elsewhere in this book.

The objective of a strategy to test potentially genotoxic impurities (PGI) is to define the levels to which they must be controlled in the API. If clearly nongenotoxic and not constrained by other limits such as those for residual solvents or heavy metals, the limits identified in ICH Q3A can be applied. If clearly genotoxic, the TTC will be applied in most cases. However, it may be able to provide data to mitigate against some positive genotoxicity findings and to justify levels higher than the TTC.

The first stage of the assessment of a PGI is to determine whether it contains a structural alert for genotoxicity as indicated in both the CPMP and draft FDA guidelines. This can be done by literature review, but, more typically, a computational toxicology assessment is made. The draft FDA Guideline identifies MDL-QSAR (MDL Information Systems, now part of Accelrys, Inc., San Diego, CA), MC4PC (MultiCase Inc., Beachwood, OH) and Derek for Windows (LHASA, Leeds, UK) as commonly used programs, and the FDA are known to use, or to have used, both Derek and MultiCase programs.

If it is decided that a structural alert for genotoxicity requires testing, a bacterial mutation assay is the usual first screen and is suggested in both the CHMP and draft FDA Guidelines. It is likely that negative results will be sufficient to dismiss the alert, and this is justified because (1) positive results in the various programs are often based primarily on results from bacterial mutation assays, and (2) as stated in the CHMP Guideline, mutagenic carcinogens are considered to have no established threshold. This view in endorsed in the recently published Questions and Answers document on the CHMP Guidelines,[3] which states that an adequately conducted negative Ames test will overrule a structural alert. There are no specified requirements for the design of the assay, except the comment in the CHMP Questions and Answers document that it must be "conducted to regulatory acceptable standards," but it is AZ practice to perform a standard five-strain Ames test in a GLP-compliant laboratory, but not necessarily to claim GLP compliance. For some classes of compound, it may be valid to limit the strains to those known to reliably detect them, for example TA 98 and TA100 for aromatic amines, and TA1535, TA100, and/or an *E. coli* strain for alkyl halides.

It is possible to perform the Ames test using samples containing an impurity at known levels or "spiked" with it to levels intended to exceed the highest levels likely to occur in production batches. However, it is recognized that the level must be such that most genotoxic agents would actually give positive results if present as an impurity. Based on literature results for approximately 450 mutagens, it appears that about 85% are detected at concentrations of 250 μg/plate or less.[92] Therefore, it was proposed that an impurity may be evaluated as part of the API as long as it is present to give a minimum concentration of 250 μg/plate,[90] that is 5% if the API can be tested to the limit level of 5000 μg/plate. This proposal has also been recently accepted by the CHMP.[3] However, it should be noted that some classes of bacterial mutagens e.g. many sulfonic acid esters may require higher concentrations to be detected, so consideration of the nature of an impurity is important if using this approach is to be used. Also, in principle, the same argument could be used to justify a maximum level of 250 μg/plate when an impurity is tested alone, but it is not certain whether this would be accepted by regulatory authorities.

If a PGI gives a positive result in the Ames test, it is very likely that there will be no alternative other than to control it to the TTC limits. There are a very few examples, such as sodium azide, that are clear bacterial mutagens but are not genotoxic in mammalian cells *in vitro* or *in vivo* because of differences in metabolism,[93] but it is unlikely that a similar explanation could be found for a novel impurity. Recently, a threshold and safety margins were established even for the DNA-reactive mutagenic carcinogen, ethyl methanesulphonate (EMS), after it was found to be an impurity in Viracept® (Pfizer, Inc., New York), and these allowed a human risk assessment to be made.[94] However, this required a significant number of *in vitro* and *in vivo* studies, with a compound for which there was already a large amount of data. This work was essential to perform the risk assessment after patients had been exposed, and it would generally be impracticable to generate similar data prospectively for an impurity in a drug in clinical development.

Although a negative Ames test will frequently be the only test used to qualify an impurity, there are occasions where a mammalian cell assay may be performed on a potential impurity, for example chemical registration—transportation requirements for a process intermediate, specific structural groups, such as carbamates, or compounds which are excessively toxic to the bacterial indicator strains. As was noted previously, the in vitro mammalian cell assays have a higher incidence of positive results than the Ames test, and at least some of these are known to result from mechanisms other than DNA reactivity and for which, therefore, threshold mechanisms can be argued. Examples of such thresholded mechanisms included in the CHMP Guideline on PGIs include interaction with the spindle apparatus of cell division leading to aneuploidy, topoisomerase inhibition, inhibition of DNA synthesis, overloading of defense mechanisms, and metabolic overload. If any of these mechanisms can be demonstrated to be responsible for an *in vitro* mammalian cell assay positive result, it is likely to be easier to justify levels of an impurity higher than the TTCs for genotoxins. If the mechanism is known to be able to cause chromosome breakage, assuming results in the Ames test are negative, the rodent bone marrow micronucleus test should provide sufficient data to justify a PDE using the ICH Q3C approach.

If a thresholded mechanism cannot be established, it is technically possible to perform DNA binding studies to show that an *in vitro* mammalian cell positive result is not a consequence of DNA reactivity. The ^{32}P postlabeling is likely to be more practical than radiolabel binding methods simply because radiolabeled material is not required, but either may be practical option to show an impurity is not DNA reactive. In practice, it is likely that performing two *in vivo* tests, that is the bone-marrow micronucleus test, and either the rat liver UDS test or Comet assay in rat liver would be the most practical solution, and then to use the weight of evidence approach to challenge the *in vivo* significance of the result of the cell assay.

For compounds with clear evidence of thresholded genotoxicity, the CHMP guideline accepts that exposure levels which are without appreciable risk of genotoxicity can be established according to the procedure for Class 2 solvents in the ICH Q3C Note for Guidance on Impurities: Residual Solvents. It would also seem reasonable to apply the same principle to compounds that give positive results only in an *in vitro* cell assay and for which the weight of evidence indicates no evidence of DNA reactivity. The ICH Q3C approach calculates a Permitted Daily Exposure (PDE) that is derived for the no observable effect level (NOEL), or, if it has not been established, the lowest observable effect level (LOEL) in the most relevant animal study (see Chapter 5 for more information on calculation of a PDE). In principle, the same calculation could be used to set PDEs for an Ames positive that gives negative results in two appropriate *in vivo* tests, but it is not certain that this would be accepted by regulatory authorities worldwide.

In conclusion, negative results in an adequately conducted Ames test should be sufficient to qualify a structurally alerting impurity for most regulatory authorities worldwide. Similarly, a clearly genotoxic impurity will almost certainly need to be controlled to the relevant TTCs at each stage of development, except for those potent agents for which specific lower limits may be required, that is N-nitrosamines. However, whether or not limits between these two extremes can be justified for chemicals that show some activity in *in vitro* tests but for which *in vivo* data are available, is not clear. It is essential that feedback is obtained from regulatory authorities for such examples in order for a generally accepted strategy to be developed.

GLOSSARY

Operon: A unit of genetic transcription comprising adjacent structural genes and a promoter region at one end, where the transcription of the structural genes into messenger RNA begins.

Gene mutation: A detectable permanent change within a single gene or its regulating sequences. The changes may be point mutations, frameshft mutations, insertions, or deletions.

Point mutation: Change in the genetic code, usually confined to a single DNA base pair.

Frameshift mutations: A mutation (change in the genetic code) in which one base or two adjacent bases are added to (inserted in) or deleted from the nucleotide sequence of a gene. This may lead to an altered or truncated protein.

Insertions: Insertions add one or more nucleotides into the DNA and may alter the gene product by affecting mRNA splicing or causing frame-shifts.

Deletions: Remove one or nucleotides from the DNA and may cause frame-shifts; large deletions can cause loss of most or all of a gene.

Translocation: A chromosome translocation is an abnormality caused by a rearrangement of parts between nonhomologous chromosomes; it can result in loss of gene function or altered gene expression.

Recombination: Breakage and balanced or unbalanced rejoining of DNA.

Clastogen: An agent that produces structural breakage of chromosomes, usually detectable by light microscopy.

Gene conversion: Gene conversion results from recombination; DNA sequence information is transferred from one DNA helix, which is not altered, to another helix the sequence of which is altered.

Nondisjunction: An error at mitosis that results in the two daughter cells not receiving the correct number of chromosomes so that both become aneuploid.

Aneuploidy: Small increases or decreases in the modal number of chromosomes in a cell or organism. It may arise spontaneously or be induced by an aneugen.

Polyploidy: A multiple of the total chromosome complement.

Chromosome: The individual thread-like structures in the cell nucleus comprising double helices of DNA complexed with proteins and RNA. They carry the genetic information in a linear array of functional units (genes).

Chromatid: The two halves into which a chromosome is longitudinally divided at mitosis. These are held together at the centromere and part from each to become daughter chromosomes at mitosis.

Mitosis: The process by which a cell nucleus divides into two daughter nuclei with chromosome numbers and genetic make-up identical to the parent cell.

Buffy coat: Is the fraction of an anticoagulated blood sample after density gradient centrifugation that contains most of the white blood cells and platelets.

Chromatin: The component of the nucleus which contains the genetic material; it describes the chromosomes visible at mitosis and the more diffuse arrangement of the genetic material in the interphase cell.

DNA strand breaks: Single or double strand scissions in DNA.

Excision repair: DNA excision repair is used when only one of the strands of the DNA helix has a defect and the other strand is used as a template to repair the damage. There are a number of excision repair mechanisms, that is base excision repair, nucleotide excision repair, and mismatch repair each responding to different types of DNA damage.

REFERENCES

1. Committee for Medicinal Products for Human Use (CHMP). 2006. *Guideline on the Limits of Genotoxic Impurities*. EMEA/CHMP/QWP/251344/2006, London, 28 June.
2. US Food and Drug Administration. Center for Drug Evaluation and Research. Guidance for Industry. 2008. *Genotoxic and Carcinogenic Impurities in Drug Substances and Products: Recommended Approaches*. Draft, December 2008.
3. CHMP Safety Working Party. 2009. *Questions and Answers on the CHMP Guideline on the limits of Genotoxic Impurities*. EMA/CHMP/SWP/431994/2007, London, 17 December.
4. ICH Topic S2A. 1995. Genotoxicity: Guidance on specific aspects of regulatory genotoxicity tests for pharmaceuticals. *International Conference on Harmonisation of Technical Requirements for Registration of Pharmaceuticals for Human Use, Geneva*.
5. ICH Topic S2B. 1997. Genotoxicity: A standard battery for genotoxicity testing of pharmaceuticals. *International Conference on Harmonisation of Technical Requirements for Registration of Pharmaceuticals for Human Use, Geneva*.
6. Auerbach C, Robson JM. 1947. The production of mutations by chemical substances. *Proc. R. Soc. Edinb. Biol.* 62:271–283.
7. Auerbach C, Robson JM. 1947. Tests of chemical substances for mutagenic action. *Proc. R. Soc. Edinb. Biol.* 62:284–291.
8. Ames BN, Durston WE, Yamasaki E, Lee FD. 1973. Carcinogens are mutagens: A simple system combining liver homogenates for activation and bacteria for detection. *Proc. Natl. Acad. Sci. USA* 72:2423–2427.
9. Lijinsky W. 1979. A view of the relationship between mutagenesis and carcinogenesis. *Environ. Molec. Mutagen.* 14(Suppl. 16):78–84.
10. Grover PL, Sims P. 1968. Enzyme catalysed reactions of polycyclic aromatic hydrocarbons with deoxyribonucleic acid and protein in vitro. *Biochem. J.* 110:159–160.
11. Gelboin HV. 1969. A microsome-dependent binding of benzo[a]pyrene to DNA. *Cancer Res.* 29:1272–1276.
12. Ames BN, McCann J, Yamasaki E. 1975. Methods for detecting carcinogens and mutagens with the *Salmonella*/mammalian microsome mutagenicity test. *Mutat. Res.* 31:347–364.
13. Green MHL, Muriel WJ. 1976. Mutagen testing using TRP⁺ reversion in *Escherichia coli*. *Mutat. Res.* 38:3–32.
14. Matsushim T, Sawamura M, Hara K, Sugimura T. 1976. A safe substitute for polychlorinated biphenyls as an inducer of metabolic activation systems. In: *In Vitro Metabolic Activation in Mutagenesis Testing*, edited by FJ De Serres, JR Fouts, JR Bens, RM Philpot. Elsevier/North Holland, Amsterdam, pp. 85–88.
15. Ong T-M, Mukhtar M, Wolf CR, Zeiger E. 1980. Differential effects of cytochrome p450 inducers on promutagen activation capabilities and enzymatic activities of S9 from rat liver. *J. Environ. Pathol. Toxicol.* 4:55–65.
16. Maron DM, Ames BN. 1983. Revised methods for the *Salmonella* mutagenicity test. *Mutat. Res.* 113:173–215.
17. Mortelmans K, Zeiger E. 2000. The Ames *Salmonella*/microsome mutagenicity assay. *Mutat. Res.* 455:29–60.
18. Mortelmans K, Riccio ES. 2000. The bacterial tryptophan reverse mutation assay with *Eschericia coli* WP2. *Mutat. Res.* 455:61–69.
19. Organisation for Economic Cooperation and Development, Paris. 1997. *Bacterial Reverse Mutation Test*. Guideline for the Testing of Chemicals No. 471.
20. Maron D, Katzenellbogen J, Ames BN. 1981. Compatibility of organic solvents with the *Salmonella*/ microsome test. *Mutat. Res.* 88:343–350.
21. Bonneau D, Thybaud V, Melcion C, et al. 1991. Optimum associations of tester strains for maximum detection of mutagenic compounds in the Ames test. *Mutat. Res.* 252:269–279.
22. Herbold BA. 1983. Preliminary results of an international survey on sensitivity of *S. typhimurium* strains in the Ames test. *Toxicol. Lett.* 15:89–93.

23. Prival MJ, Zeiger E. 1998. Chemicals mutagenic in *Salmonella typhimurium* strain TA1535 but not in TA100. *Mutat. Res.* 412:251–260.

24. O'Donovan MR. 1990. The comparative responses of *Salmonella typhimurium* TA1537 and TA97a to a range of reference mutagens and novel compounds. *Mutagenesis* 5:267–274.

25. Dyrby T, Ingvardsen P. 1983. Sensitivity of different *E. coli* and *Salmonella* strains in mutagenicity testing calculated on the basis of selected literature. *Mutat. Res.* 123:47–60.

26. Brooks TM. 1995. The use of a streamlined bacterial mutagenicity assay, the MINISCREEN. *Mutagenesis* 10:447–448.

27. Luria SE, Delbruck M. 1943. Mutations of bacteria from virus-sensitivity to virus resistance. *Genetics* 28:491–511.

28. Gatehouse D. 1978. Detection of mutagenic derivatives of cyclophosphamide and a variety of other mutagens in a "microtitre" fluctuation test without microsomal activation. *Mutat. Res.* 53:289–296.

29. Gatehouse D, Delow G. 1979. The development of a "Microtitre[R]" fluctuation test for the detection of indirect mutagens, and its use in the evaluation of mixed enzyme induction of the liver. *Mutat. Res.* 60:239–252.

30. Reifferscheid G, Heil J. 1996. Validation of the SOS/*umu* test results of 486 chemicals and comparison with the Ames test and carcinogenicity data. *Mutat. Res.* 369:129–145.

31. Yasunaga K, Kiyonari A, Oikawa Y, et al. 2004. Evaluation of the *Salmonella* umu test with 83 NTP chemicals. *Environ. Molec. Mutagen.* 44:329–334.

32. Schmid C, Reifferscheid G, Zahn RK, Bachmann M. 1997. Increase of sensitivity and validity of the SOS/*umu* test after replacement of the β-galactosidase reporter gene with luciferase. *Mutat. Res.* 394:9–16.

33. Ptitsyn LR, Horneck G, Komova O, et al. 1997. A biosensor for environmental genotoxin screening based on an SOS *lux* assay in recombinant Escherichia coli cells. *Appl. Environ. Microbiol.* 63:4377–4384.

34. Quillardet P, Hoffnung M. 1993. The SOS chromotest: A review. *Mutat. Res.* 297:235–279.

35. Gee P, Sommers CH, Melick AS, et al. 1998. Comparison of responses of base-specific *Salmonella* tester strains with the traditional strains for identifying mutagens: The results of a validation study. *Mutat. Res.* 412:115–130.

36. Fluckiger-Isler S, Baumeister M, Braun K, et al. 2004. Assessment of the performance of the AmesII™ assay: A collaborative study with 19 coded compounds. *Mutat. Res.* 558:181–197.

37. Aubrecht J, Osowski JJ, Persaud P, et al. 2007. Bioluminescent *Salmonella* reverse mutation assay: A screen for detecting mutagenicity with high throughput attributes. *Mutagenesis* 22:335–342.

38. Moore MM, Clive D, Hozier JC, et al. 1985. Analysis of trifluorothymidine-resistant (TFTr) mutants of L5178Y/ TK+/− mouse lymphoma cells. *Mutat. Res.* 151:161–174.

39. Doerr CL, Harrington-Brock K, Moore MM. 1989. Micronucleus, chromosome aberration and small-colony TK mutant analysis to quantitate chromosomal damage in L5178Y mouse lymphoma cells. *Mutat. Res.* 222:191–203.

40. Hozier J, Applegate M, Moore MM. 1992. In vitro mammalian muatagenesis as a model for genetic lesions in human cancer. *Mutat. Res.* 270:201–209.

41. Clive 41D, Johnson KO, Spector JFS, et al. 1979. Validation and characterisation of the L5178Y TK +/− mouse lymphoma mutagen assay system. *Mutat. Res.* 59:61–108.

42. Cole J, Arlett CF, Green MHL, et al. 1983. A comparison of the agar cloning and microtitration techniques for assaying cell survival and mutation frequency in L5178Y mouse lymphoma cells. *Mutat. Res.* 111:371–386.

43. Clements J. 2000. The mouse lymphoma assay. *Mutat. Res.* 455:97–110.

44. Organisation for Economic Cooperation and Development, Paris. 1997. *In vitro Mammalian Cell Gene Mutation Test*. Guideline for the Testing of Chemicals No. 476.

45. Evans HJ. 1976. Cytological methods for detecting chemical mutagens. In: *Chemical Mutagens, Principles and Methods for Their Detection*, Vol. 4, edited by A Hollaender. Plenum Press, New York and London, pp. 1–29.

46. Scott D, Danford ND, Dean BJ, Kirkland DJ. 1990. Metaphase chromosome aberration assays in vitro. In: *Basic Mutagenicity Tests: UKEMS Recommended Procedures*, UKEMS Sub-Committee on

Guidelines for Mutagenicity Testing. Report Part I revised, edited by DJ Kirkland. Cambridge University Press, Cambridge, UK, pp. 62–86.

47. Kirkland DJ, Garner RC. 1987. Testing for genotoxicity—Chromosomal aberrations in vitro—CHO cells or human lymphocytes? *Mutat. Res.* 189:186–187.

48. Ishidate M, Harnois MC. 1987. The clastogenicity of chemicals in mammalian cells. Letter to the editor. *Mutagenesis* 2:240–243.

49. Ishidate 49M, Harnois MC, Sofuni T. 1988. A comparative analysis of data on the clastogenicity of 951 chemical substances tested in mammalian cell cultures. *Mutat. Res.* 195:151–213.

50. Hilliard C, Hill R, Armstrong M, et al. 2007. Chromosome aberrations in Chinese hamster and human cells: A comparison using compounds with various genotoxicity profiles. *Mutat. Res.* 616:103–118.

51. Greenwood SK, Hill RB, Sun JT, et al. 2004. Population doubling: A simple and more accurate estimation of growth suppression in the in vitro assay for chromosomal aberrations that reduces false positive results. *Environ. Molec. Mutagen.* 43:36–44.

52. Organisation for Economic Cooperation and Development, Paris. 1997. *In Vitro Mammalian Chromosome Aberration Test.* Guideline for the Testing of Chemicals No. 473.

53. Schmid W. 1975. The micronucleus test. *Mutat. Res.* 31:9–15.

54. Pascoe S, Gatehouse D. 1986. The use of a simple haemotoxylin and eosin staining procedure to demonstrate micronuclei within rodent bone-marrow. *Mutat. Res.* 164:237–243.

55. Hayashi M, Sofuni T, Ishidate M. 1983. An application of acridine orange fluorescent staining to the micronucleus test. *Mutat. Res.* 120:241–247.

56. Organisation for Economic Cooperation and Development, Paris. 1997. *Mammalian Erythrocyte Micronucleus Test.* Guideline for the Testing of Chemicals No. 474.

57. ICH Topic S2(R1). 2008. Genotoxicity: Testing and Data Interpretation for Pharmaceuticals Intended for Human Use. Step 2 Document. *International Conference on Harmonisation of Technical Requirements for Registration of Pharmaceuticals for Human Use, Geneva.*

58. Wakata A, Miyamae Y, Sato S, et al. 1998. Evaluation of the rat micronucleus test with bone marrow and peripheral blood: Summary of the 9th Collaborative Study by CSGMT/JEMS.MMS. *Environ. Molec. Mutagen.* 32:84–100.

59. Hamada S, Sutou S, Morita T, et al. 2002. Evaluation of the rodent micronucleus assay by a 28-day treatment protocol: Summary of the 13th collaborative study by the collaborative study group for the micronucleus test (CSGMT)/Environmental Mutagen Society of Japan (JEMS)—Mammalian Mutagenicity Study Group (MMS). *Environ. Molec. Mutagen.* 37:93–110.

60. Hayashi M, MacGregor JT, Gatehouse DG, et al. 2007. In vivo rodent erythrocyte micronucleus assay. III. Validation and regulatory acceptance of automated scoring and the use of rat peripheral blood reticulocytes with discussion of non-hematopoietic cells and a single dose-level limit test. *Mutat. Res.* 627:10–30.

61. MacGregor JT, Bishop ME, McNamee JP, et al. 2006. Flow cytometric analysis of micronuclei in peripheral blood reticulocytes. II. An efficient method of monitoring chromosomal damage in the rat. *Toxicol. Sci.* 94:92–107.

62. Kissling GE, Dertinger SD, Hayashi M, MacGregor JT. 2007. Sensitivity of the erythrocyte micronucleus assay: Dependence on number of cells scored and inter-animal variability. *Mutat. Res.* 634:235–240.

63. Hayashi M, MacGregor JT, Gatehouse DG, et al. 2000. In vivo rodent erythrocyte micronucleus assay. II. Some aspects of protocol design included repeated treatments, integrationwith toxicity testing and automated scoring. *Environ. Molec. Mutagen.* 35:234–252.

64. Singh NP, McCoy MT, Tice RR, Schneider EL. 1988. A simple technique for quantitation of low levels of DNA damage in individual cells. *Exp. Cell Res.* 175:184–191.

65. Ostling 65O, Johnson KL. 1984. Microelectrophoretic study of radiation-induced DNA damage in individual mammalian cells. *Biochem. Biophys. Res. Commun.* 175:184–191.

66. McKelvey-Martin VJ, Green MHL, Schmezer P, et al. 1993. The single cell gel electrophoresis assay (Comet assay): A European review. *Mutat. Res.* 288:47–63.

67. Brendler-Schwaab S, Hartmann A, Pfuhler S, Speit G. 2005. The *in vivo* comet assay: Use and status in genotoxicity testing. *Mutagenesis* 20:245–254.

68. Tice RR, Andrews PW, Hirai O, Singh NP. 1991. The single cell gel (SCG) assay: An electrophoretic technique for the detection of DNA damage in individual cells. In: *Biological Reactive Intermediates*

IV, Molecular and Cellular Effects and Their Impact on Human Health, edited by CR Witmer, RR Snyder, DJ Jollow, GF Kalf, JJ Kocsis, IG Sipes. Plenum Press, New York, pp. 157–164.

69. Singh NP, Tice RR, Schneider EL. 1991. A microgel electrophoresis technique for the direct quantitation of DNA damage and repair in individual fibroblasts cultured on microscope slides. *Mutat. Res.* 252:289–296.

70. Tice RR, Strauss GHS, Peters WP. 1992. High-dose combination alkylating agents with autologous bone marrow support in patients with breast cancer: Preliminary assessment of DNA damage in individual peripheral blood lymphocytes. *Mutat. Res.* 271:101–113.

71. Williams GM. 1976. Carcinogen-induced DNA repair in primary rat liver cell cultures; a possible screen for chemical carcinogens. *Cancer Lett.* 1:231–236.

72. Mirsalis JC, Butterworth BE. 1980. Detection of unscheduled DNA synthesis in hepatocytes from rats treated with genotoxic agents: An *in vivo—in vitro* assay for potential carcinogens and mutagens. *Carcinogenesis* 1:621–625.

73. Mirsalis JC, Tyson CK, Butterworth BE. 1982. Detection of genotoxic carcinogens in the *in vivo—in vitro* hepatocyte DNA repair assay. *Environ. Mutagen.* 4:553–562.

74. Organisation for Economic Cooperation and Development, Paris. 1997. *Unscheduled DNA Synthesis (UDS) Test with Mammalian Liver Cells In Vivo.* Guideline for the Testing of Chemicals No. 486.

75. Himmelstein MW, Boogaard PJ, Cadet J, et al. 2009. Creating context for the use of DNA adduct data in cancer risk assessment: II. Overview of methods of identification and quantitation of DNA damage. *Crit. Rev. Toxicol.* 39:679–694.

76. Randerath K, Reddy MV, Gupta RC. 1981. ^{32}P-labelling test for DNA damage. *Proc. Natl. Acad. Sci. USA* 78:6126–6129.

77. Reddy MV, Randerath K. 1986. Nuclease P1-mediated enhancement of sensitivity of ^{32}P-postlabelling test for structurally diverse DNA adducts. *Carcinogenesis* 7:1543–1551.

78. Phillips DH, Castegnaro M. 1993. Results of an interlaboratory trial of ^{32}P-postlabelling. In: *Postalabelling Methods for Detection of DNA Damage*, edited by DH Phillips, M Castegnaro, H Bartsch. IARC, Lyon, France, pp. 35–490.

79. Phillips DH, Castegnaro M. 1999. Standardisation and validation of DNA adduct postlabelling methods: Report of interlaboratory trials and production of recommended protocols. *Mutagenesis* 14:301–315.

80. Phillips DH, Arlt VM. 2007. The ^{32}P-postlabelling assay for DNA adducts. *Nat. Protoc.* 2:2772–2781.

81. Riley RT, Kemppainen BW, Norred WP. 1988. Quantitative tritium exchange of [^{3}H] aflatoxin B$_1$ during penetration through isolated human skin. *Biochem. Biophys. Res. Commun.* 153:395–401.

82. Phillips DH, Farmer PB, Beland FA. 2000. Methods of DNA adduct determination and their application to testing compounds for genotoxicity. *Environ. Molec. Mutagen.* 35:222–233.

83. McCann J, Choi E, Yamaski E, Ames BN. 1975. Detection of carcinogens as mutagens in the *Salmonella*/microsome test: Assay of 300 chemicals. *Proc. Natl. Acad. Sci. USA* 72:5135–5139.

84. Nagao M, Sugimura T, Matsushima T. 1978. Environmental mutagens and carcinogens. *Annu. Rev. Genet.* 12:117–159.

85. Bartsch H, Malaveille C, Camus AM, et al. 1980. Validation and comparative studies on 180 chemicals with *S. typhimurium* strains and V79 Chinese hamster cells in the presence of various metabolizing systems. *Mutat. Res.* 76:1–50.

86. Kirkland D, Aardema M, Henderson L, Muller L. 2005. Evaluation of the ability of a battery of three in vitro genotoxicity tests to discriminate rodent carcinogens and non-carcinogens. 1. Sensitivity, specificity and relative predictivity. *Mutat. Res.* 584:1–256.

87. Gocke E, Albertini S. 1996. Synergistic/co-mutagenic action in the Ames test as an indication of irrelevant positive findings. *Mutat. Res.* 350:51–59.

88. Muller L, Kasper P. 2000. Human biological relevance and the use of threshold arguments in regulatory genotoxicity assessment: Experience with pharmaceuticals. *Mutat. Res.* 464:19–34.

89. Snyder RD. 2009. An update on the genotoxicity and carcinogenicity of marketed pharmaceuticals with reference to in silico predictivity. *Environ. Molec. Mutagen.* 50:435–450.

90. Muller L, Mauthe RJ, Riley CM, et al. 2006. A rationale for determining, testing and controlling specific impurities in pharmaceuticals that possess potential for genotoxicity. *Regul. Toxicol. Pharmacol.* 44:198–211.

91. ICH Topic Q3C. 1997. Impurities: Residual solvents. *International Conference on Harmonisation of Technical Requirements for Registration of Pharmaceuticals for Human Use, Geneva.*

92. Kenyon MO, Cheung JR, Dobo KL, Ku WW. 2007. An evaluation of the sensitivity of the Ames assay to discern low-level mutagenic impurities. *Regul. Toxicol. Pharmacol.* 48:75–86.

93. Arenaz P, Hallberg L, Mancillas F, et al. 1989. Sodium azide mutagenesis: Inability of mammalian cells to convert azide to a mutagenic intermediate. *Mutat. Res.* 227:63–67.

94. Müller L, Gocke E, Lavé T, Pfister T. 2009. Ethyl methanesulfonate toxicity in Viracept—A comprehensive human risk assessment based on threshold data for genotoxicity. *Toxcol. Lett.* 190:317–329.

CHAPTER 4

USE OF STRUCTURE ACTIVITY RELATIONSHIP (SAR) EVALUATION AS A CRITICAL TOOL IN THE EVALUATION OF THE GENOTOXIC POTENTIAL OF IMPURITIES

Susanne Glowienke
Catrin Hasselgren

4.1 INTRODUCTION

Structure-activity relationships (SAR), that is the relationship between a chemical structure and a certain biological.activity, can be applied to predict the possible toxicological profile of a potential drug candidate[1-4] Due to the health implications, there has always been particular interest in the prediction of potential mutagenic and carcinogenic effects.[5] Structural groups linked to such effects were first identified by Ashby and Tennant;[6-9] these have since become standard "structural alerts." Indeed, many of these are incorporated into the software systems described later in this chapter. These have subsequently been augmented by a further series of alerts published by Kazius et al.[10]

A report examining the correlation between structural features and the outcomes of various genetic toxicity tests was also published recently.[11]This report highlighted how the various genetic toxicity tests correlate with one another based on structural features. The investigation highlighted specifically how intelligent testing strategies can be designed, based on the structural features present within a particular compound, and that this can be used as an effective alternative to the application of standard toxicity tests.

Due to the introduction of the new EMEA guideline covering limits for genotoxic impurities[12] and the related FDA draft guidance,[13] the prediction of mutagenic effects, in particular in the Ames test, has gained even more importance. Critically,

Genotoxic Impurities: Strategies for Identification and Control, Edited by Andrew Teasdale
Copyright © 2010 by John Wiley & Sons, Inc.

the guidelines explicitly mention that SAR methods can be applied to detect structural alerts for genotoxicity, and thus such systems can make an important contribution to the identification of potential genotoxic impurities in a pharmaceutical candidate.

The following chapter examines in detail the practical use of *in silico* (Q)SAR and SAR systems, evaluating those systems commonly used for such purposes, in each case detailing the basis upon which such predictions are made.

4.2 METHODOLOGY

The most common computerized systems used to predict the potential genotoxic effects of molecules are Derek for Windows (DfW; Lhasa Ltd., Leeds, UK) and MultiCase (MultiCase, Inc., Cleveland, OH, USA). Both systems are examined in detail. While a variety of other systems such as TOPKAT (Accelrys Inc.) are also used in certain organizations, they are not as widespread in their application. Also described within this chapter is Vitic (Lhasa Ltd.), a toxicity database and management system, used by a number of organizations, often in parallel to Derek for Windows.

In addition to commercial systems, many organizations, including Novartis and AZ, have developed their own internal *in silico* systems. These look to utilize propriety data to improve predictivity, especially of in-house compounds. Such a system, the AstraZeneca "Genetox Warning System," is described later in this chapter.

4.2.1 Derek for Windows (DfW)

Derek stands for Deductive Estimation of Risk from Existing Knowledge. It is a computerized expert system that uses a knowledge base approach to predict the toxicological hazard of molecules. Thus, it contains expert knowledge rules derived from the known relationship of a given substructure and a toxicological effect of the molecule and applies these rules to predict potential toxicological effects of compounds for which usually no experimental data exists.[14-16]

The vendor of DfW is Lhasa Limited.[17] The Lhasa history goes back to 1980, where the LHASA synthesis planning software (Logic and Heuristics Applied to Synthetic Analysis) was brought from the Harvard University to the University of Leeds. LHASA UK (which went on to become Lhasa Limited) was established in 1983 as a not-for-profit company and educational charity. Since that time, the interest in the LHASA system has diminished, and the current membership of Lhasa Limited almost exclusively supports the development and refinement of the DfW system, as well as other related applications, for example Meteor, Vitic, and Zeneth.

The Derek software was originally created by Schering Agrochemicals adapting the LHASA source code and then donated to Lhasa Limited, allowing toxicologists and chemists from other companies to use Derek and to contribute data and knowledge. The Derek system was later rewritten by Lhasa Limited to enable it to run on the Microsoft Windows operating system, at which point it was renamed Derek for Windows.

In principle, Lhasa Limited is owned and controlled by its members (commercial, educational, and nonprofit organizations) who license the software applications and contribute to their development by contributing data or knowledge on SARs. Exchange of knowledge takes place via several routes, including International Collaborative Group Meetings (ICGM), visits and contact made by Lhasa Limited staff to members, surveys, research initiatives, and the Lhasa Forum. Contribution of knowledge may also result from individual data donations that fall under separate secrecy agreements. Such contributions are used to both refine existing rules and to define new rules. To protect these data, no propriety structures are disclosed.

DfW contains many rules covering a broad range of toxicological endpoints. In the context of genotoxic impurities, the endpoints mutagenicity, genotoxicity, and chromosome damage are of particular interest. Mutagenicity was one of the first endpoints that the system was used to predict,[18] and remains one of its main prediction strengths.

Figure 4.1 shows a molecule processed through DfW v. 11.0. The system compares structural features of the target compound with those of the toxophore (i.e. the substructure that is thought to be responsible for the toxic effect) described in its knowledge base. An alert is activated when the toxophore it describes is found to be present in the structure under question.

The result of the DfW prediction is a list of alerts (Lhasa predictions) obtained for the compound under evaluation. The alerting substructure is identified and highlighted. For structures that fire more than alert (rule), each toxophore is shown sequentially with its associated hazard. If no alerting substructure is found, then

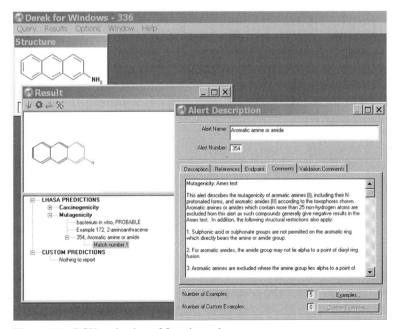

Figure 4.1   DfW evaluation of 2-aminoanthracene.

DfW reports that no toxophore has been identified in the structure. The description tab describes the structural elements that trigger the alert, while under the comment tab, information on the reaction mechanisms of the compound class is provided. Recently, validation comments have also been incorporated into the output. These display the validation data associated with a particular alert when it is activated by a queried compound. Such data are designed to assist the user in understanding the reliability of an alert and contribute to compliance with the Organisation for Economic Cooperation and Development (OECD Principles) for (Q)SAR valida-tion.[19,20] When some alerts are triggered, the system provides actual examples of compounds possessing the alerting structure concerned. It also informs the user when the queried compound has already been experimentally tested and is part of the knowledge base. Literature references are also included, again to enable the user to assess the relevance of the structural alert to the structure under evaluation.

For each prediction, DfW provides reasoning on the likelihood of a compound being active; Figure 4.2 illustrates that, for example, substituted vinyl ketones are not expected to show mutagenicity in the Ames test. The reasoning rules within the knowledge base, however, associate the presence of this alert with chromosome damage, to which a "plausible" level of likelihood is assigned. The current version of DfW (11.0) contains 74 alerts for chromosome damage, 4 alerts for genotoxicity, and 87 alerts for mutagenicity.

Another important feature of DfW is the alert editor. This allows the user to add their own rules to the knowledge base. If those rules are applicable to a queried compound, they are shown under "custom predictions." Usually, the basis of a new

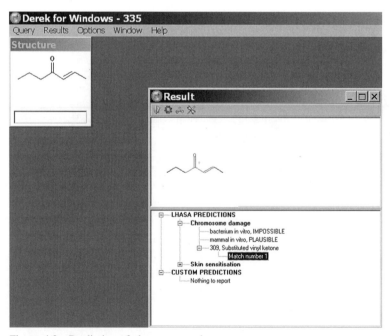

Figure 4.2   Prediction of chromosome damage.

custom alert is the knowledge of structure activity relationships created from internal (propriety) test data. These rules are not part of the commercial knowledge base, and thus, internally modified knowledge bases have to be merged with every updated commercial one in order not to lose information. The default alert set provided by Lhasa Limited cannot be modified by the user, although certain rules can be disabled.

A key strength of DfW is that it provides an easy-to-use interface with comprehensive alert explanations. It is also flexible, the editor allowing implementation of internal rules based on propriety data, providing the opportunity to improve predictivity of the system, certainly in relation to internal compounds. Another strength is that it is possible for members to influence the future development of the system through the routes described earlier.

A limitation of DfW is that no information on the structural coverage of the molecule within the knowledge base is given, which would provide information on the quality of the prediction (prediction accuracy). Attempts have been made, however, to introduce factors into the alerts and the reasoning rules, which take into account the physiochemical properties of a molecule.[21]

4.2.2 Vitic

Vitic is another part of the Lhasa Limited software portfolio.[17] It was developed as a result of the International Toxicology Information Centre (ITIC) research project, carried out at the Health and Environmental Sciences Institute (HESI), itself part of the International Life Sciences Institute (ILSI). Vitic is a structure searchable database that has been developed for the purpose of data mining and SAR analysis.[22] Originally, this database project aimed to promote the idea of data sharing. However, while the benefit of data sharing is obvious, various difficulties were encountered: these included confidentiality issues and issue relating to equality in the value of the data provided. Thus, the database was mainly populated from public sources (International Uniform Chemical Information Database [IUCLID] and National Toxicology Program [NTP] data, data from toxicology journals, Gold carcinogenicity database, etc.), and is continually updated by Lhasa Limited. More recently, data from publications cited in DfW, in particular for the mutagenicity and chromosome damage, endpoints have been incorporated in Vitic.[21]

Vitic uses a client server architecture and database server components that are either hosted on a machine at Lhasa Limited or installed locally on-site. To conduct chemical structure queries, ISISDraw, ChemDraw, or a similar package is needed. A query is started by selecting the appropriate table for the "Available Folders" window. A dialogue box appears, which prompts the user to define the search criteria using a drop-down list. For chemical structure searches, it is possible to conduct similarity, as well as exact match and substructure searches. Figure 4.3 shows an example of a structure search. Data related to a queried compound is not automatically retrieved during a search. To view data for a processed substance, the respective table containing the desired data is selected in the "Available Folders" list.

The Vitic information management system (Data Entry Client) allows the user to store in-house toxicology data electronically in a searchable format. Thus, data

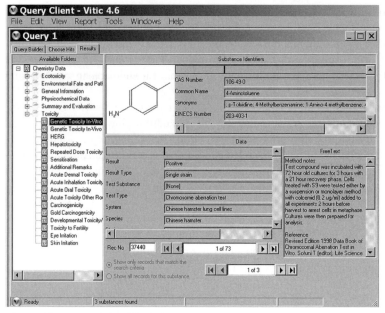

Figure 4.3   A search in Vitic 4.6.

from paper records can be transferred to a structure-searchable database that enhances data analysis and extraction of previously unknown (Q)SARs.

One of the first areas where Vitic was used related to the sharing of mutagenicity data for impurities and intermediates. In this context, Ames test data on intermediates and impurities, which are usually of low commercial sensitivity, were provided by participating companies and imported into Vitic by Lhasa Limited. A prerequisite to the incorporation of data into Vitic was that a full five-strain Ames test must have been performed with and without metabolic activation, and that the test was conducted as a plate incorporation method.

Any data entered into a Vitic format database can only be accessed by those who are part of the Vitic initiative (data sharing group). New contributors can join, the only prerequisite being that they must donate data for 50 chemicals.

4.2.3   MCASE

Multi-Computer Automated Structure Evaluation, MCASE MC4PC, is supplied by MultiCASE Inc., a software company started in Cleveland, Ohio in 1996.[23] The MCASE program was originally developed as an alpha/open VMX version, but is now available for PC/Window platforms (i.e. MC4PC) using the same program logic and algorithms as for bioactivity predictions. It is based on a hierarchical statistical analysis of a database (called the training set) containing a number of molecules and their associated biological activity data. MCASE is the successor of the CASE program. The major algorithmic difference between the two systems is the use of hierarchy in the selection of descriptors by MCASE.[24] CASE is based on the concept of identifying structural attributes of activity (or inactivity) from a learning set of noncongeneric molecules that best discriminate between active and inactive molecules.[25] Once the molecules of a learning set have been entered and processed through the program, CASE automatically fragments each molecular structure into its subunits (descriptors). Chemical structures can be entered using KLN or SMILES line notations,[26] or from three types of structure files, including MDL MOL file. The activity of each molecule in the training set is classified according to a linear scale of CASE units. Values of between 10 and 19 are associated with inactive compounds; those with CASE unit values of 20–29 are regarded as marginally active, and those with values of 30–99 are considered active to extremely active.

The main prerequisite for the molecules within the training set is that the associated data is consistent and obtained under a similar protocol. The generated descriptors are normally linearly connected strings of atoms from 2 to 10 heavy (nonhydrogen) atoms. Most of the generated fragments are completely unrelated to the observed activity. Thus, a statistical analysis is performed to select only those fragments that are significant. A binominal distribution is assumed, and a fragment is considered irrelevant if it appears randomly in both active and inactive molecules. A significant deviation, however, from the random distribution among active and inactive classes of molecules is indicative of potential significance to the biological activity. Fragments are either classified as biophore or biophobes, depending whether they are associated with activity or inactivity. CASE is also capable of applying linear regression techniques involving physiochemical properties (quantum-mechanical indices, partition coefficients, water solubility etc.) in an attempt to perform a quantitative estimation of the potency.

In contrast to CASE, MultiCASE relies on a hierarchical algorithm that breaks the learning set into logical subsets. Thus, it is capable of dealing with conflicting substituent effects and of differentiating between the fragments responsible for activity and those influencing the activity. MCASE starts by identifying the statistically most significant substructure within the learning set and labels it as the top biophore responsible for the activity of the largest possible number of active molecules. In the next step, molecules containing this biophore are removed from the database. A new analysis leading to the identification of the next biophore is performed with this reduced dataset. This procedure is repeated until either the activity of all the molecules in the learning set have been accounted for or no additional statistically significant substructure can be found (MULTIple CASE analysis). Within the subset of congeneric molecules, the program additionally identifies those fragments and physical–chemical parameters that play a role in modulating the activity of the respective biophore. Modulators can be certain substructures or calculated parameters, such as highest occupied molecular orbital (HOMO) and lowest unoccupied molecular orbital (LUMO) energies, octanol–water partition coefficient, etc.

After training of the program with a particular training set database is completed, query compounds can be submitted for assessment (calculation). An unknown molecule submitted for calculation is divided into fragments that are then compared with the previously identified biophores and biophobes. MCASE predicts the probability of activity or lack thereof on the basis of the presence or absence of these descriptors. Separate modules for the prediction of a variety of toxicological endpoints can be purchased within the MCASE program. Modules include, for example:

- Databases for the prediction of rodent carcinogenicity based upon proprietary data submitted to the FDA,[27] constructed at the FDA Center for Drug Evaluation and Research (CDER).
- Databases for the prediction of liver toxicity, the source of which are adverse drug reaction reports included in the FDA's spontaneous reporting system;[28] and
- Several databases for mutagenicity and clastogenicity endpoints (data mainly obtained from the U.S. Environmental Protection Agency [EPA] database) used as surrogate endpoints to predict outcome of carcinogenicity studies.[29]

Of particular interest is a database (AZ2) constructed through collaboration between pharmaceutical companies. This database contains mutagenicity data relating to impurities donated by the companies involved. The main goal of this project was to develop a database with balanced representations of mutagens and nonmutagens and enhanced coverage through the inclusion of data from across as wide a chemical space as possible. A comparison of the public domain data module A2H[23] with this module AZ2 (updated version AZ3)[30] has shown the predictivity of the system to be enhanced through the inclusion of propriety data. It should be noted that AZ2 and AZ3 are, however, only available to participating companies.

The output from MCASE, MC4PC, is provided in a textual format. This describes the physico-chemical properties calculated for the query, the presence of both activating (biophores) and deactivating (biophobes) fragments, inactivating modulators, and any finally unknown fragments present in the queried compound. An example output is provided in Figure 4.4.

The contributions of the different parameters to the QSAR calculation are given, and the final activity is determined and described in terms of CASE units. The underlying principle of the MCASE system is that a queried compound might either:

1. show no increases in the revertant number (be inactive);
2. show dose-dependent increases but reach no doubling (be marginally active); or
3. reach at least doubling in the revertant number (be active).

Moreover, a probability for activity is presented to the user.

Thus, the final probability that a compound will be experimentally active is defined based on the concomitant presence or absence of various descriptors. Table 4.1 illustrates a modified ICSAS method for structural warnings used to present the outcome of the calculated prediction.

Depending on their occurrence in a prediction, the queried compound is assessed to have:

- a high likelihood to be active;
- to be inactive; or
- the prediction is regarded to be inconclusive or uncertain.

```
VERSION 2.000
------------


-------------------------------------------------------------------------------
AZ3- mutagenic    - all classes, salmo.typh.overall assa- multicase#7075 1.70
-------------------------------------------------------------------------------
MC calculated Water Solubility is: 1.44 [in log(mol/m**3)]
MC calculated Log(Octanol/Water) Partition Coef.is: 0.94
Molecule satisfies the rule of 5 (bioavailable)
MC Calculated Human Intestinal Absorption is: 47.3%
** WARNING ** The following functionalities are UNKNOWN to me:
       *** NH2-CH -C  =

MULTICASE-3 Prediction
----------------------
 The molecule contains the Biophore   (nr.occ.= 2):
              NH2-c  =c  -cH =                    <3-NH2>
     The ICSAS Alert Index for this Biophore is  407
*** 10 out of the known  11 molecules ( 91%) containing such Biophore
           are  mutagenic    with an average activity of  37. (conf.level= 98%)
*** QSAR Contribution :                           Constant is    39.00
                                                                 ------
             ** Total projected QSAR activity (in CASE units) is equal to    39.00
  ** The results are QUESTIONABLE due to the
                presence of UNKNOWN functionalities **

  CONCLUSIONS:
  -----------
  ** The projected  mutagenic    activity is   39.0    CASE units **
  ** The activity is predicted to be MODERATE **
  ** The probability that this molecule is  mutagenic    is    91%   **-
```

HHHHHHHHHHHHHHHHHHHHHHHHHHHHHHHHHHHHHHHHHHHHHHHHHHHHHHHHHHHHHHHHHHHHHHHHHHHHHHHHHH

Figure 4.4   Prediction of a molecule to be active in the Ames test.

TABLE 4.1   ICSAS Method for Structural Alerts (Modified)

Symbol	Explanation
B	Significant biophore
b	Nonsignificant biophore
D	Significant deactivating fragment (biophobe)
d	Nonsignificant deactivating fragment
A	Experimentally active
M	Marginal experimental activity
I	Experimentally inactive
w	Unknown fragment warning
+	Predicted to be active
+?	Possibly active/inconclusive
−	Predicted to be inactive
*	Not covered (≥2 fragments)

With regard to acceptable coverage in a database, a substance is evaluated as covered if it contains less than two unknown fragments.[31] Queried compounds that are not covered (≥2 unknown fragments) are evaluated as having unreliable MCASE predictions. In the above example (Fig. 4.4), full coverage is assumed, and the presence of a significant biophore (amino-group $-NH_2$) results in a positive prediction for the queried molecule. A biophore identified in a test compound is evaluated as either significant, possibly significant, or not significant, depending on its statistical significance (frequency of appearance in active molecules that form part of the database) and the biologic potency (CASE unit activity).

In addition, MCASE assesses whether the queried compound's biophore has a local molecular environment that is similar or significantly different from that of mutagens within the database itself. Results from a test are labeled inconclusive (or molecule is assessed to be possibly active) if the molecule contains a biophore that is not statistically significant or exists in a significantly different environment to that of the mutagen within the database. Usually, the absolute number of biophores identified in a queried compound is not important in the evaluation of its activity, that is it is considered to have a positive prediction if at least one significant biophore is determined. The MCASE program also recognizes molecular fragments or QSAR molecular descriptors (e.g. log-P, HOMO/LUMO constants), which modulate the activity of a biophore. They include both activating and inactivating modulators, which either enhance or inhibit the mutagenic activity of a queried molecule. The result of a prediction is considered to be inconclusive (or the molecule is assessed to be possibly active) if a deactivating fragment is detected concomitantly to a biophore. Finally, a molecule is predicted to be inactive if no (significant) biophore occurs. A negative prediction may be supported by the presence of deactivating fragments.

As might be expected, there is a strong correlation between important biophores identified within MCASE and those identified as structural alerts using knowledge base systems.[32] Examples include aromatic amines, aromatic and aliphatic nitro compounds, alkylating agents (chloro- and bromomethyl subgroups), and epoxides. For these biophores, the associated mechanism of action is usually published in the literature. However, for other, less common biophores (usually supported by a smaller number of active molecules in the database), this may not be available.

Once a biophore is detected in a molecule, it is possible to query the database for the presence of active molecules upon which the prediction is based. If the database was built using proprietary data, which is, for example the case for databases constructed in a collaborative effort, or FDA databases, molecules will be displayed as removed (Fig. 4.5).

With MCASE, it is also possible to generate your own prediction models from internal test data. This can be done by either adding data to existing modules or by the generation of a completely new database, as shown in Figure 4.6.

The requirement for building a new database or adding data to existing modules is that the data are structured according to the MCASE format with structural information, and that appropriate activity is assigned to each compound. Criteria for how the database should be built, such as fragment size, also need to be entered.

```
The·Molecules·containing·fragment·:¶
·SO2-O···-CH2-CH3¶
···are·:¶
··1·in·molecule···94·(0.90)·Ethyl·methanesulfonate·········of·activity··39¶
··2·in·molecule··106·(1.00)·Diethyl·Sulfate················of·activity··39¶
··1·in·molecule··228·(0.99)·Ethyl·p-Toluenesulfonate·······of·activity··39¶
··1·in·molecule·2200·(1.00)·ethyl·ethylaminosulfonate······of·activity··39¶
··1·in·molecule·2201·(0.98)·Et-n-diMelaminosulfonate·······of·activity··39¶
··1·in·molecule·2583·(0.60)·REMOVED·······················of·activity··10¶
```

Figure 4.5   Active molecules in database containing a certain biophore.

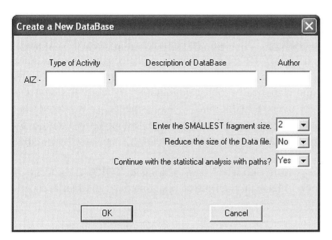

Figure 4.6   Details of the newly generated database.

MCASE is capable of performing a program-internal validation of the newly constructed database. To accomplish this, a certain percentage of molecules, which can be freely selected (default is 10%), are removed from the database (either randomly or by using an equal ratio of active and inactive compounds, or by maintaining the ratio of active and inactive compounds as it is present in the database). In addition, the number of validations can be selected. A model is then created using the remaining 90% of molecules. The resultant model is then used to predict the activity of the 10% molecules that were removed. The process is repeated up to 10 times per validation. Finally, the program calculates concordance, sensitivity, and specificity of each validation.

A key strength of MCASE is that predictions can be performed without knowledge of the mechanism of action of the molecules used to generate the training set. Furthermore the applicability of MCASE to certain predictions has been increased substantially by the input of data provided by the FDA. Its limitations include that the result of a prediction has to be deduced from the textual information. Hence, there is the risk of alternative interpretations that may lead to conflicting final conclusions for a prediction. Moreover, in order to obtain high quality predictions, modules are required that contain toxicity data from several hundreds of molecules. These data must be generated using a similar test protocol. The burden associated with this potentially inhibits the generation of modules, specifically those containing propriety data.

Given the potential difficulties associated with interpreting the textual output, AstraZenenca (AZ) take the prediction from MCASE and export it into an excel file after the molecule has been processed by MCASE expert rules. The prediction is then simply assigned a positive or negative value; thus the end user does not need to interpret the results.

4.2.4   TOPKAT

Arguably, the only other system commonly used is TOPKAT (Toxicity Prediction by Komputer Assisted Technology). This is a correlative SAR system developed by Accelrys Inc. (San Diego, CA).[33] TOPKAT uses Kier & Hall electrotopological states (E-states), as well as shape, symmetry, MW, and logP as descriptors of all possible two atom fragments to build statistically robust quantitative structure toxicity relationship (QSTR) models for over 18 endpoints.[34,35] Assessments are validated via a univariate analysis of the descriptors, a patented multivariate analysis of the fit of the query structure in optimum prediction space, and by similarity searching in descriptor space.

Unfortunately, there is little published data relating to TOPKAT in terms of its predicitivity, upon which to base any definitive assessment of the merits or otherwise of the system.

4.2.5   Propriety Systems

Many organizations, including AZ and Novartis, have looked to further improve predictivity through the development of in-house databases that are able to utilize the internal datasets established within their organizations. These are typically used in tandem with the commercial DBs, normally DEREK and/or MCASE. The format/development of one such system, the AZ Genetox Warning System (GWS), is described below.

4.2.5.1   Genetox Warning System (GWS)   The GWS, built for internal use at AstraZeneca is based on a database comprising both internal and external Ames mutagenenicity data. The number of a data points are currently ca. 2200 (AZ propriety), 7300 (MCASE datasets), and 3000 CCRIS/GeneTox data licensed from the National Library of Medicine (NLM).

4.2.5.2   Overview of the GWS   The GWS is accessed within AZ via a web interface. Any molecule submitted to the GWS is passed through a series of steps that are illustrated in Figure 4.7.

The algorithm used within the GWS is outlined below:

Is there an exact match to query compound in the database of experimental results?

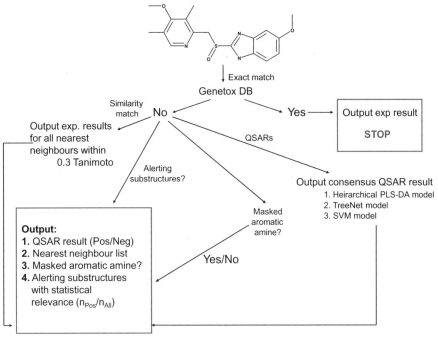

Figure 4.7   Schematic representation of the GWS workflow.

- *Yes:* output the experimental result/s to the user.
- *No:* pass the query molecule through the evaluation procedure and output the results to the user.

The results provided include:

1. a consensus QSAR result;
2. the experimental results of the structural nearest neighbours;
3. presence of a masked or free aromatic amine; and
4. substructural alerts.

The first operation performed within the system is to check if the compound that is being assessed has been experimentally tested. If there are any existing results in terms of safety data, these are returned to the user. Results from different databases are listed separately. If there are no reports, a full evaluation of the impurity is initiated.

A consensus QSAR result will be calculated for the query compound. This consists of three independent models, a partial least squares discriminant analysis (PLS-DA) model, a support vector machine (SVM) model, and a TreeNet model, which are combined in a simple majority-voting scheme. The models are built using a number of different descriptors. The SVM model uses only structural "signature" descriptors,[11] which are substructural fragments. The PLS-DA and TreeNet models use both signature descriptors and a number of physico-chemical descriptors such as pKa, HOMO–LUMO energies, polar surface area, etc. All three models were built using 80% of the available dataset, containing both internal AstraZeneca compounds and public compounds, and evaluated using the 20% of the dataset that were excluded from the model building.

The three models perform within a similar range of 76%–88% accuracy on the test set. The PLS-DA and the SVM models were found to perform slightly better in terms of the prediction of inactive compounds, whereas the TreeNet model proved slightly more accurate when assessing active compounds. The rationale for using a consensus model is that the consensus model is more stable, and coverage is more general than it would be if one of the individual models were used alone. It was seen when analyzing the individual predictions for each compound that the three models cover different chemical spaces, a desirable feature when building a global model that is to be used to predict a wide range of structures.

In addition to the consensus QSAR result, other information may be available for the compound. The system also provides information relating to structural near neighbors that have been tested, as these may have similar structural fragments and can give information on the likelihood that the impurity will be active. Compounds in the database that have a structural Tanimoto similarity score of over 0.7 to the query compound are extracted and displayed together with their activities.

The system also checks if there are any structural alerts present within the query compound and if so, what is the prevalence of the particular alert in the database. That is, how many compounds in the database contain this alert and how many of those are active. This gives an indication of the relevance of the alert. The user can, if desired, search for the compounds containing the alert to determine if they are structurally similar to the query compound. There are currently ca. 100 alerts for mutagenicity in the system originating from a number of published sources,[6–11] as well as internally identified structural moieties.

4.3   VALIDATION

Key to the application of systems like DfW and MCASE MC4PC is an understanding of their performance. To evaluate this, it is necessary to examine the predictivity of the systems in relation to the assessment of genotoxic impurities. Predictivity of such systems is often defined in terms of:

- Sensitivity: this is defined in terms of how many experimentally active compounds are predicted to be active.
- Specificity: how many compounds predicted to be active are found to be active when actually tested.

Such an exercise is now explored. A validation set comprising of 280 synthetic starting materials and intermediates was used by Novartis to assess both the sensitivity and specificity of DfW, version 11.0 and MCASE MC4PC version 2.0 (using the AZ3 version 1.9 database). In addition, comparative evaluations were made with two propriety datasets and with VITIC. The outcomes of these evaluations are described below.

The 280 impurities were tested in a five strain Ames test using Salmonella strains TA98, TA100, TA1535, TA97a, and TA102 both in the presence and absence of metabolic activation (S9 from Arcolor pretreated rats) following the recommendations of ICH and OECD guidelines. Tests were carried out as plate incorporation only and in a non-GLP mode. The highest dose was 5 mg/plate, or that determined by precipitation or bacteriotoxicity of the test compound. A compound was considered as mutagenic if at least a doubling in the revertant number was achieved in one strain (except strain TA102, which has a comparably high spontaneous mutation rate and therefore a factor of 1.5 is considered as a positive result). Initial testing was performed using two strains, TA98 and TA100, only. These strains detect most mutagens. If a substance turned out to be active in at least one of these two strains, it was considered as active and testing in the other three strains was therefore not required.

The results of the Ames tests of the 280 impurities yielded 95 positive substances, of which 75 were positive in at least strain TA98 or TA100, 18 were positive in strain TA1535 only, and 2 showed mutagenicity in strain TA97a only. One hundred seventy-eight substances did not show evidence of a mutagenic potential in the Ames test, and 7 were marginally active. It should be noted that a weak positive result can, in some instances, be related to the presence of an impurity (in the impurity) rather than to the test compound itself.

4.3.1   DfW Version 11.0

DfW version 11.0 was used to predict mutagenicity of the 280 molecules studied. Of the 7 weakly positive compounds, 5 did not fire an alert for mutagenicity, and 2 were predicted to be active based on the aromatic amine moiety. In view of absence of any alert for mutagenicity for the majority of the weakly positive molecules, further testing of the purified material was considered. For the present validation exercise, the weakly positive substances were not taken into account.

For the 95 active molecules, the following alerts were obtained (Table 4.2).

Table 4.3 illustrates the alerts occurring for the 178 negative impurities submitted to calculation.

For the active and inactive molecules of this evaluation, in total, 23 different types of alerts were identified out of a total of 87 mutagenicity alerts present in the DfW v. 11.0 database (i.e. 26% of knowledge base alerts found for queried compounds).

The overall results of the DfW prediction are given in Table 4.4.

4.3.1.1   *Nature of the Alerts*   The most prominent alerts were 027 (alkylating agent), 329 (aromatic nitro compound) and 351, 352, 353, and 354 (aromatic amine or amide), which is in concordance with Dobo et al.,[36] and represents well the kind of alerting structures likely to be encountered when examining the types of reagents/intermediates encountered in the synthesis of pharmaceuticals.

Alkylating Agents   The alert for alkylating agents (DfW alert 027) describes the genotoxicity of alkyl halides, where the functional group is attached to a primary or secondary alkyl carbon atom. This alert also includes alkyl sulfinates, sulfonates, and sulfates lacking a hydroxyl group directly bound to the sulfur (DfW v. 11.0

TABLE 4.2 Prevalence of Structural Alerts among Ames Positive Compounds

Structural alert	Number of molecules firing the alert
No alert found	17
Nitro group on aliphatic ring (alert 002)	1
Alpha-chloro-ether (alert 015)	1
Allyl halide (alert 022)	1
Hydrazine or monoacyl- or monosulphonyl-hydrazine (alert 033)	1
N-Aminoheterocycle (alert 491)	1
Azirine or aziridine (alert 051)	1
Alkyl aldehyde or precursor (alert 306)	1
gem-dihalide (alert 326)	1
Arylhydrazine (alert 039)	2
Carboxylic acid halide (alert 315)	2
Azide, hydrazoic acid or azide salt	3
Alkylating agent (alert 027)	14
Aromatic nitro compound (alert 329)	24
Aromatic amine (or amide) (alerts 351, 352, 353 and 354)	25

TABLE 4.3 Prevalence of Structural Alerts among Ames Negative Compounds

Structural alert	Number of molecules firing the alert
No alert found	83
N-Haloamine (alert 026)	1
Alkyl ester of phosphoric or phosphonic acid (alert 305)	1
Hydrazine or monoacyl- or monosulphonyl-hydrazine (alert 033)	1
Halogenated alkene (alert 331)	1
Benzimidazole (alert 583)	1
Azide, hydrazoic acid or azide salt	1
Alkyl aldehyde or precursor (alert 306)	2
Carboxylic acid halide (alert 315)	2
Isocyanate or isothiocyanate (alert 304)	5
Halogenated aromatic heterocycle (alert 492)	14
Aromatic nitro compound (alert 329)	19
Aromatic amine (or amide) (alerts 352 and 353)	18
Alkylating agent (alert 027)	29

TABLE 4.4 Predictivity of DfW

Parameter	Value (%)
Sensitivity (Correctly predicted positives/experimentally positives)	$78/95 \times 100 = 82\%$
Specificity (Correctly predicted negatives/experimentally negatives)	$83/178 \times 100 = 47\%$
Concordance	$(78+83)/273 \times 100 = 59\%$

knowledge base). Alkyl halides are electrophilic and are thus capable of directly alkylating DNA. In terms of the Ames test, activity may be seen both in the presence and absence of metabolic activation, notably in *Salmonella typhimurium* strains TA100 and TA1535.

Within the dataset examined, this alert was triggered for 43 compounds, of which 33% (positive predictivity) were experimentally active. Evaluation of the same data using two proprietary datasets showed positive predictivity results of 47% and 38%, respectively, similar to what was obtained in the present validation exercise. Interestingly, according to the DfW validation comments, the positive predictivity of this alert within the Vitic v. 4.0 database was 75% (65 substances reported active out of 87 activating this alert), indicating for this specific alert, at least the use of Vitic can enhance the specificity of the prediction. In general, these results would seem to indicate that this alert is highly sensitive, but not specific, and hence where encountered, it would seem advisable to perform an Ames test to determine whether or not the compound in question is genuinely genotoxic.

Aromatic Nitro Compounds Aromatic nitro compounds (alert 329), where active, are reported to be mutagenic almost exclusively in *S. typhimurium* strains TA98 and TA100. Due to their mechanism of action, which in the first step involves reduction by bacterial nitroreductases to the hydroxylamine, activity is thought to occur in the absence of S9 (DfW v. 11.0 knowledge base). However, for the impurities under question, activity was seen both in the presence and absence of S9. The resulting hydroxylamine is then esterified (O-esterification), which then further converts to a reactive nitrenium ion. It is the latter that is believed to bind to DNA.

As well as activity in the Ames test, aromatic nitro compounds have a mixed response in the *in vitro* chromosome aberration test, with an inconsistent requirement for S9 mix. This could be explained by the fact that the mechanism of action requires nitroreductase, which occurs in mammalian cells at varying levels or is oxygen-labile.[37]

In relation to the Ames test, a positive predictivity of 56% (24 out of 43 substances) was observed for the dataset examined. This was again compared with proprietary data sets, where again a comparable value was observed. For the two proprietary datasets, the positive predictivity values were 57% (21 compounds activated the alert, of which 12 are reported positive), and 60% (5 compounds activated the alert of which 3 are reported positive). Interestingly again, the positive predictivity of this alert within the Vitic v. 4.0 database was significantly higher, 82% (107 of 130 compounds of the Vitic v. 4.0 database activating this alert of which 107 are reported positive in the Ames test).

With regard to chromosome damage, DfW reported a high positive predictivity of 86% (18 reported active compounds out of 21 firing the alert). However, test data on a limited number of aromatic nitro compounds showed absence of a positive response in micronucleus test in vitro (using TK6 cells) (Novartis unpublished test data, July 2009).

Aromatic Amines and Amides Aromatic amines and amides following certain structural patterns activate the alerts 351, 352, 353, and 354 within Derek. Aromatic amines are expected to show mutagenicity, notably in *S. typhimurium* strains TA98 and TA100 in the presence, but not in the absence, of S9. Surprisingly, a number of the compounds tested as part of this exercise were found to be mutagenic in these strains in the absence of S9. The mechanism of action is generally considered to involve N-hydroxylation, typically mediated by cytochrome P450 1A2. Subsequently, O-esterification takes place, and the resulting esterified product again (analogous to nitro compounds) forms a reactive nitrenium ion, which is capable of binding to DNA. Aromatic amides are in general less mutagenic than their corresponding primary aromatic amines, possibly due to N-deacylation, which has to occur prior to N-hydroxylation. In this validation, only one aromatic amide activated alert 352. This compound was shown to be negative in the Ames test.

The four alerts for aromatic amines differ with regard to the type of aromatic amines by which they are activated. In principle, alert 351 is structurally restricted to ortho, para-, and meta-monosubstituted anilines with certain permitted substituents. For the impurities submitted to the validation, this alert was seen only twice, and both compounds were demonstrated to be mutagenic (100% predictivity). Alert 352 was the most prominent alert for aromatic amines and amides with regard to the frequency it was activated. This alert is associated with polysubstituted aniline rings, excluding specific substituents, for example halogen and/or trifluoromethyl substituents on the aromatic ring. Twelve of the queried compounds displaying this alert were negative, and 10 were positive in the Ames test resulting in a positive predictivity of 46%. Evaluation with propriety datasets provided similar figures. However, again, DfW, using the Vitic v. 4.0 database, reports a positive predictivity of 93%.

Aromatic heterocycles that are not part of a polycyclic aromatic ring system and have at least one substituent activate Alert 353. This alert was again seen among the negative (five molecules) and positive (one molecule) queried compounds, resulting in a positive predictivity of 17%. A value of 33% was achieved when a propriety dataset was used. DfW reports 100% using the Vitic v. 4.0 database.

Alert 354 is structurally restricted to defined polycyclic aromatic ring systems. All 12 of aromatic amines of the present validation set that activated this alert were shown to be mutagenic (100% positive predictivity), whereas using the Vitic v. 4.0 database a 78% value was achieved. The proprietary datasets yielded positive predictions of 50% and 63%.

The four alerts may also be triggered for secondary and tertiary amines if the substituents on the nitrogen are certain selected small substituents like methyl, ethyl, or vinyl.

On average, the positive predictivity for all four aromatic amine alerts of DfW was 66%.

Apart from these three major structural classes (alkylating agents, aromatic nitro compounds and aromatic amines), several other alerts were activated; however, these were generally restricted to a small number of compounds (usually only one molecule). The exception was alert 492 for halogenated aromatic heterocycles, which was seen for a number of compounds in the dataset. Substances belonging to this compound class are thought to undergo nucleophilic displacement of halogen and thus have the potential to alkylate DNA. However, the 14 molecules queried in DfW where all found to yield negative Ames test results.

Overall, the sensitivity of DfW in predicting mutagenicity of impurities was high (82%), whereas the specificity was found to be only 47%. In contrast, Snyder[38] has reported a sensitivity of 61.5% and a specificity of 88.2% for the prediction of mutagenicity in the Ames test of marketed pharmaceuticals. While this may seem problematic, the results from this exercise match exactly with the requirements of a SAR process, that is while specificity is important, by far, the most important factor is sensitivity. These results show DfW to show a high level of sensitivity for all of the major alert classes described.

It is interesting though to compare the results from this exercise with the specificity seen within Vitic. The validation data for Vitic apparently showing far great specificity in relation to the main alerts studied.

4.3.2   MCASE, MC4PC, v. 2.0

MCASE MC4PC v. 2.0, using the AZ3 database, was used to predict the potential mutagenicity of the 280 impurities studied. The seven weakly positive molecules were again omitted from the validation results. Results for the MCASE prediction of the 95 positive and 178 negative compounds are displayed in Tables 4.5 and 4.6.

MCASE, MC4PC, v. 2.0 obtained an overall predictivity as detailed in Table 4.7. Inconclusive and not covered molecules were disregarded from the considerations.

TABLE 4.5   MCASE Prediction for Ames Positive Intermediates

Number of molecules	Result	Comment[a]
41	– (inactive)	No B detected, ≤2w (fully covered), D detected for 3 compounds
2	+ (active)	A (compounds shown to be experimentally active)
1	– (inactive)	No B detected, ≥2w (not covered)
3	– (inactive)	B detected but calculated activity reduced due to I
3	+? (inconclusive)	b detected, or B and D detected concomitantly
44	+ (active)	At least one B, ≤2w (fully covered)
1	+ (active)	At least one B, ≥2w (not covered)

[a] See Table 4.1 for details of the ICSAS alerts.

TABLE 4.6   MCASE Prediction for Ames Negative Intermediates[a]

Number of molecules	Result	Comment
129	– (inactive)	No B detected, ≤2w (fully covered), D detected for 24 compounds
2	– (inactive)	I (compounds shown to be experimentally inactive)
3	– (inactive)	No B detected, ≥2w (not covered)
3	– (inactive)	B detected but calculated activity reduced due to I
6	+? (inconclusive)	b detected, or B and D detected concomitantly
35	+ (active)	at least one B, ≤2w (fully covered)

[a] See Table 4.1 for details of the ICSAS alerts.

TABLE 4.7 Predictivity of MCASE

Parameter	Value (%)
Sensitivity	$46^a/95 \times 100 = 48\%$
(Correctly predicted positives/experimentally positives)	
Specificity	$134^b/178 \times 100 = 75\%$
(Correctly predicted negatives/experimentally negatives)	
Concordance	$(46+134)/273 \times 100 = 66\%$

[a] Fully covered active compound (44)+compounds shown to be experimentally active (2).
[b] Fully covered inactive compounds (129)+compounds shown to be experimentally (2)+compounds the activity of which is reduced due to inactivating modulator (3).

In general, the number of uncovered molecules, that is queried compounds containing more or equal to two unknown fragments, was low, indicating that the database occupied a broad chemical space. Moreover, only a few inconclusive predictions were obtained, e.g. for compounds containing a biophore and a deactivating fragment. As a result, a high proportion of the compounds examined could be used to identify sensitivity and specificity.

4.3.2.1 Data Evaluation   Similar to the DfW predictions, aromatic amine, nitro compounds, and alkylating agents were the most frequent alerting moieties found.

Alkylating Agent   MCASE detected a biophore that was located in the alkylating moiety for six molecules of the validation set. Two compounds showing a biophore for alkylating agent turned out to be nonmutagenic when tested experimentally, resulting in a positive predictivity of 66%. Interestingly, this represented a much smaller dataset than was seen within DfW relating to the same alert.

Nitro Compounds   Among the correctly predicted positive compounds, 23 showed a biophore that was located in the aromatic nitro moiety. For two of these, an additional biophore was found, this being an aromatic amine moiety. Seventeen molecules showing the aromatic nitro biophore were identified, which were negative in the Ames test. Again, two of these had an additional biophore located in the aromatic amine moiety. Thus, the positive predictivity for aromatic nitro compounds was 58%, which is similar to what was obtained using the DfW system.

Aromatic Amines   For 10 mutagenic substances within the validation set, a biophore was identified, which was present in the aromatic amine substructure (two of them, as already mentioned above, contained in addition an aromatic nitro fragment). Among the Ames negative query molecules, six showed a biophore for aromatic amines (two of them as already mentioned above showed additionally a biophore for aromatic nitro compounds). The positive predictivity for aromatic amines was 63%; this again was comparable to the value obtained by DfW.

Other biophores detected by MCASE for the queried molecules were located in substructural moieties, like azide or carboxylic acid halide functionalities.

However, some biophores identified could not be directly assigned to substructures, which are known to be involved in a certain mechanism of action leading to DNA reactivity. These included, for example, biophores located in heterocylces, and they occurred more frequently in molecules shown to be inactive in the Ames test.

Overall, the sensitivity of MCASE in the prediction of molecules yielding positive Ames test results (48%) was significantly lower than DfW (82%), whereas the specificity was higher (75% by MCASE versus 47% by DfW). The sensitivity of MCASE in this validation exercise was similar to what has been reported for marketed pharmaceuticals (44.7%). The specificity, however, compared with marketed pharmaceuticals (97.1%), was lower.[36]

4.3.3 Combined DfW (v. 11.0) and MCASE (v. 2.0, AZ3 Database) Prediction

An investigation of the 273 experimentally positive and negative impurities of the validation exercise was performed to determine whether or not a combined DfW and MCASE prediction would lead to an improved predictivity. An overview of the results is given in Table 4.8.

Under the assumption that at least one positive prediction result either from DfW or MCASE would have led to the performance of an Ames test in order to verify or reject the prediction, the specificity of the combined prediction is $68/178 \times 100 = 38\%$. This is significantly lower than the value obtained for the individual validations. Correspondingly, the sensitivity is $80/95 \times 100 = 84\%$, and, hence, higher than what was seen with DfW and MCASE in isolation. However, since the sensitivity of DfW was 82%, the added value of the MCASE prediction was only 2%. The probability that a molecule with both a positive DfW and positive MCASE prediction, is experimentally positive is $44/95 \times 100 = 46\%$, and thus higher than its probability not to be mutagenic ($25/178 \times 100 = 14\%$).

TABLE 4.8   Combined DfW and MCASE Prediction

Computer system	Predicted result	Experimental result	Number of molecules
DfW	Negative	Negative	83
MCASE	Negative	Negative	134
DfW + MCASE[a]	Negative	Negative	68
DfW	Positive	Positive	78
MCASE	Positive	Positive	46
DfW + MCASE[b]	Positive	Positive	44
DfW + MCASE[c]	Positive	Positive	80
DfW + MCASE[d]	Positive	Negative	25

Remarks for Table 4.8:
[a] Negative prediction had to be obtained by DfW and MCASE.
[b] Positive prediction had to be obtained by DfW and MCASE.
[c] Positive prediction had to be obtained by either DfW or MCASE.
[d] Positive prediction had to be obtained by DfW and MCASE.

4.4 CONCLUSION

From this investigation, it can be concluded that the *in silico* determination of structural liabilities for mutagenicity provides a highly sensitive and conservative method for identification of potentially genotoxic impurities. This is precisely what is required of such systems. Furthermore, the use of internal computerized prediction systems or alerts developed on the basis of in-house knowledge may contribute to an even higher sensitivity and improved specificity.

Another important point to make is that this exercise illustrates that both DfW and MCASE reasonably well cover the scope of compounds that are typically encountered within synthetic processes. This is illustrated by the fact that only a very small number of molecules were considered uncovered (containing more than or equal to two unknown fragments) within MCASE. Predictivity, especially for more uncommon types of structures, can, however, be enhanced by incorporation of internal data.

Perhaps surprisingly, the combination of both systems seem to offer little benefit in terms of sensitivity; however, there are other advantages in combining them in terms of gaining an overall view with regards to the potential mutagenicity of a compound. For example, DfW will definitively describe the nature of any alert; this can then be augmented by the MCASE prediction, which will give an indication of probability. The combination of such factors should assist in the evaluation of the molecule and any decision as to whether testing is required.

A further conclusion that can be drawn from this and other published validation exercises is that the predictivity of such SAR systems can vary significantly depending on the nature of your test set, specifically the chemical classes contained within it. This is exemplified by the data described here relating to aromatic amines and/or nitro compounds. Within this specific class, DfW has a higher predictivity (82% sensitivity) than MCASE (48% sensitivity) does. Therefore, wherever possible, the dataset used within such validation exercises should contain as balanced a dataset as possible in terms of active and inactive molecules and in terms of the numbers of different chemical classes and the number of examples within each chemical class. This, of course, needs to be balanced against the potentially conflicting desire to ensure the dataset used is representative of the chemical classes actually practically encountered.

In conclusion, *in silico* predictive tools such as DfW/MCASE, augmented by propriety data, play a vital role in the evaluation of genotoxic potential within unknown compounds.

REFERENCES

1. Benigni A, Richard A. 1998. Quantitative structure-based modeling applied to characterization and prediction of chemical toxicity. *Methods Enzymol.* 14:264–276.
2. Greene N. 2002. Computer systems for the prediction of toxicity: An update. *Adv. Drug Deliv. Rev.* 54(3):417–431.
3. Dearden JC. 2003. In silico prediction of drug toxicity. *J. Comput. Aided Mol. Des.* 17(2–4): 119–127.

4. McKinney JD, Richard A, Waller C, et al. 2000. The practice of structure activity relationships (SAR) in toxicology. *Toxicol. Sci.* 56(1):8–17.

5. Benigni R, ed. 2003. *Quantitative Structure-Activity Relationship (QSAR) Models of Mutagens and Carcinogens*. CRC Press, Boca Raton, FL.

6. Ashby J. 1985. Fundamental structural alerts to potential carcinogenicity or noncarcinogenicity. *Environ. Mutagen.* 7:919–921.

7. Ashby J, Tennant RW. 1988. Chemical structure, Salmonella mutagenicity and extent of carcinogenicity as indicators of genotoxic carcinogenesis among 222 chemicals tested in rodents by the U.S. NCI/NTP. *Mutat. Res.* 204:17–115.

8. Tennant RW, Ashby J. 1991. Classification according to chemical structure, mutagenicity to Salmonella and level of carcinogenicity of a further 39 chemicals tested for carcinogenicity by the U.S. National Toxicology Program. *Mutat. Res.* 257:209–227.

9. Ashby J, Tennant RW. Definitive relationships among chemical structure, carcinogenicity and mutagenicity for 301 chemicals tested by the U.S. NTP. *Mutat. Res.* 257:229–306.

10. Kazius J, McGuire R, Bursi R. 2005. Derivation and validation of toxicophores for mutagenicity prediction. *J. Med. Chem.* 48:312–320.

11. Yang C, Hasselgren C, Boyer S, Arvidson K, Aveston S, Dierkes P, Benigni R, Benz RD, Contrera J, Kruhlak NL, Matthews EJ, Han X, Jaworska J, Kemper RA, Rathman JF, Richard AM. 2008. Understanding genetic toxicity through data mining: the process of building knowledge by integrating multiple genetic toxicity databases. *Toxicol. Mech. Methods* 18(2–3):277–295.

12. EMA. 2007. *Guideline on the Limits of Genotoxic Impurities*, CPMP/SWP/5199/02, EMEA/CHMP/QWP/251344/2006. Jan.

13. FDA. 2008. *FDA Draft Guidance, Guidance for Industry, Genotoxic and Carcinogenic Impurities in Drug Substances and Products: Recommended Approaches*, posted December 2008.

14. Greene N, Judson PN, Langowski JJ, Marchant CA. 1999. Knowledge-based expert systems for toxicity and metabolism prediction: DEREK, StAR, and METEOR. *SAR QSAR Environ. Res.* 10:299–313.

15. Sanderson DM, Earnshaw CG. 1991. Computer prediction of possible toxic action from chemical structure: The DEREK system. *Hum. Exp. Toxicol.* 10:261–273.

16. Ridings JE, Barratt MD, Cary R, et al. 1996. Computer prediction of possible toxic action from chemical structure: An update on the DEREK system. *Toxicology* 106:267–279.

17. LHASA Website. Available at http://www.lhasalimited.org (accessed September 20, 2010).

18. Long A, Combes RD. 1995. Using DEREK to predict the activity of some carcinogens and mutagens found in foods. *Toxicol. in Vitro* 9:563–569.

19. Williams RV, Marchant CA, Covey-Crump EM, et al. 2008. *Validating alerts in Derek for Windows presented at SCARLET Workshop on In Silico Methods for Carcinogenicity & Mutagenicity*. April 2–4, 2008, Milan, Italy.

20. Marchant CA, Covey-Crump EM, Elizabeth M, et al. 2008. *Validating Alerts for the Prediction of Mutagenicity Presented at SOT 47th Annual Meeting. 16th–20th March 2008, Washington, USA*.

21. Marchant CA, Briggs K, Long A. 2008. In Silico tools for sharing data and knowledge on toxicity and metabolism: Derek for Windows, Meteor, and Vitic. *Toxicol. Mechan. Methods.* 18(2 & 3):177–187.

22. Judson PN, Cooke PA, Doerrer NG, et al. 2005. Towards the creation of an international toxicology information centre. *Toxicology* 213(1–2):117–128.

23. MCASE website. Available at http://www.multicase.com (accessed September 20, 2010).

24. Klopmann G. 1992. MULTICASE. 1. A hierarchical computer automated structure evaluation program. *Quant. Struct. Act. Relat.* 11:176–184.

25. Klopmann G. 1984. Artificial intelligence approach to structure-activity studies, computer automated structure evaluation of biological activity of organic molecules. *J. Am. Chem. Soc.* 106:7315–7320.

26. Klopman G, Mc Gonigal MJ. 1981. Computer simulation of physical-chemical properties of organic molecules 1. Molecular system identification. *Chem. Inf. Comput. Sci.* 21:48.

27. Matthews EJ, Contrera JF. 1998. A new highly specific method for predicting the carcinogenic potential of pharmaceuticals in rodents using enhanced MCASE QSAR-ES software. *Regul. Toxicol. Pharmacol.* 28:242–264.

28. Matthews EJ, Kruhlak NL, Weaver JL, et al. 2004. Assessment of the health effects of chemicals in humans: II. Construction of an adverse effects database for QSAR modeling. *Curr. Drug Discov. Technol.* 1(4):243–254.

29. Matthews EJ, Kruhlak N, Cimino MC, et al. 2006. An analysis of genetic toxicity, reproductive and developmental toxicity, and carcinogenicity data: I. Identification of carcinogens using surrogate endpoints. *Regul. Toxicol. Pharmacol.* 44(2):83–96.

30. Email communication from MCASE as of May 18, 2004.

31. Matthews EJ, Contrera JF. 1998. A new highly specific method for predicting the carcinogenic potential of pharmaceuticals in rodents using enhanced MCASE QSAR-ES software. *Regul. Toxicol. Pharmacol.* 28(3):242–264.

32. Klopman G, Zhu H, Fuller MA, Saiakhov RD. 2004. Searching for an enhanced predictive tool for mutagenicity. *SAR QSAR Environ. Res.* 15(4):251–263.

33. Accelrys website. Available at http://accelrys.com/ (accessed September 20, 2010).

34. Kier LB. 1986. Shape indices of orders one and three from molecular graphs. *Quant. Struct. Activ. Relat.* 5:1–7.

35. Hall LH, Mohney B, Kier LB. 1991. The electrotopological state: Structure information at the atomic level. *J. Chem. Inf. Comput. Sci.* 31:76–82.

36. Dobo K, Greene W, Cyr MO, et al. 2006. The application of structure-based assessment to support safety and chemistry diligence to manage genotoxic impurities in active pharmaceutical ingredients during drug development. *Regul. Toxicol. Pharmacol.* 44:282–293.

37. Kirkland DL, Muller L. 2000. Interpretation of the biological relevance of genotoxicity test results: The importance of thresholds. *Mutat. Res.* 464:137–147.

38. Synder R. 2009. An update on the genotoxicity and carcinogenicity of marketed pharmaceuticals with reference to in silico predictivity. *Environ. Molec. Mutagen.* 50(6):435–450.

CHAPTER 5

COMPOUND-SPECIFIC RISK ASSESSMENTS FOR GENOTOXIC IMPURITIES: EXAMPLES AND ISSUES

Andrew Teasdale
Charles Humfrey

5.1 INTRODUCTION

The purpose of this chapter is to describe a number of compound-specific genotoxic impurity (GI) cancer risk assessments using a series of commonly used compounds as examples. The rationale for conducting a compound-specific assessment rather than relying on a generic application of the TTC is highlighted in the EMEA Guideline on the Limits of Genotoxic Impurities[1]:

> *The TTC concept should not be applied to carcinogens where adequate toxicity data (long-term studies) are available and allow for a compound-specific risk assessment.*

The FDA draft guideline[2] indicates support for such an approach, and indeed goes further by indicating that the use of risk assessments based on structural similarity to known carcinogens may also be appropriate to establish appropriate limits:

> *When a significant structural similarity to a known carcinogen is identified, the drug substance and drug product acceptance criteria can be set at a level that is commensurate with the risk assessment specific to that of the known compound.*

It is clear, therefore, from both EMEA and FDA guidelines, that compound-specific assessments are recommended, where they can be supported by scientific justification and data. However, it is also recognized that such approaches are complex, with more than one assessment possible for the same compound, depending on the data used. This in turn may lead to risks regarding regulatory acceptance of what may be entirely justifiable assessment methods, leading to delays to drug development or registration until a commonly agreed assessment is reached.

The variability in data and potentially conflicting findings are exemplified in some of the examples given in this chapter. In these situations, conclusions based on a weight of evidence are required rather than those based entirely on consistent data.

Nevertheless, as long as a coherent and robust process of data evaluation is followed, it is possible to reach conclusions that are scientifically justifiable in many cases.

While not intended to be a fully comprehensive evaluation of all possible approaches to compound-specific cancer risk assessments, this chapter first highlights some of the sources of data from which such assessments can be made, and thereafter outlines a number of methods appropriate to the estimation of dose levels of genotoxic impurities having an acceptable risk.

Aniline is used as an example to show how such an assessment can be made. Following this, there is a short section highlighting how permitted daily exposures (PDEs) were generated for a number of genotoxic and carcinogenic substances in the ICH Q3C Guideline, and how these figures compare with other cancer risk assessment approaches. The Appendix to this chapter highlights further compound-specific risk assessments for several more chemicals relevant to pharmaceutical drug synthesis.

5.2 EVALUATION PROCESS

5.2.1 Sources of Data

A number of sources were used to obtain data on which the assessments described are based. Most were accessed through ToxNet (TOXicology Data NETwork), a free to use service provided through the U.S. National Library of Medicine (NLM). This provides simple access to a range of databases, allowing a user the ability to simultaneously search for data across multiple databases. The following databases proved to be the most useful for the purpose of GI cancer risk assessment:

1. CCRIS (Chemical Carcinogenesis Research Information System): CCRIS is maintained by the National Cancer Institute (NCI) and provides access to results from both mutagenicity and carcinogenicity studies, derived from published studies and NCI reports. Importantly, the data reported in CCRIS are subject to peer-review by experts within the carcinogenesis and mutagenesis fields.

2. IRIS: the Integrated Risk Information System is maintained by the U.S. Environmental Protection Agency (EPA), and provides both carcinogenic and noncarcinogenic risk assessments. Although comparatively small in size, containing data for only approximately 500 compounds (largely restricted to those relevant to potential environmental risk), it nevertheless covers many of the common reagents used in the synthesis of pharmaceuticals and is thus a valuable tool in the risk analysis of specific compounds. The data contained in IRIS are reviewed in depth by EPA scientists before publication, and conclusions are believed to represent the consensus view of the agency.

3. CPDB (Carcinogenicity Potency Database): this database was co-developed by the University of California and the Lawrence Berkeley Laboratory, and provides a comprehensive record of the results of animal carcinogenicity studies performed since the 1950s with data on over 1500 chemicals.[3] The

database summarizes literature data, and gives quantitative analyses of both positive and negative studies using a standardized approach. Importantly, the database includes reference to carcinogenic potency, expressed in numerical terms as the TD_{50}; this provides a standardized, quantitative measure useful for comparisons and analyses, and is defined as the daily dose rate in mg/kg/body weight per day, which, if administered chronically for the standard lifespan of the species, will halve the probability of remaining tumor-free throughout that period. The database is available at: http://potency.berkeley.edu/cpdb.html.

4. As part of its implementation of the Safe Drinking Water and Toxic Enforcement Act (Proposition 65),[4] the Californian EPA publishes on its website a list of no significant risk levels (NSRLs) for carcinogens. NSRLs are stated as daily intake levels calculated to result in a 1 in 100,000 lifetime cancer risk, the same as that on which the TTC is based. Thus, these published values represent compound-specific assessments that may be considered in the setting of acceptable risk limits.

5. Hazardous Substances Data Bank (HSDB): The HSDB provides toxicity data for over 5000 hazardous chemicals, and includes data relating to human effects and exposure, where available.

In addition to the sources above, other useful information is contained in the ICH Q3C(R4) Guideline for limits of residual solvents. This guideline, together with its appendices, lists over 50 chemicals used as solvents in pharmaceutical drug syntheses, some of which are carcinogenic in animals, and summarizes key toxicological data from which acceptable limits or PDEs are determined. The method by which PDEs are derived is explained in detail in the next section, and an assessment of the Q3C PDE values is given later in this chapter.

Having identified some of the useful sources of literature relevant to the risk assessment of GIs, let us now review some examples of methods used to derive acceptable doses for GIs.

5.2.2 Methods to Estimate Acceptable Risk Dose Levels for GIs

Numerous approaches are available to calculate acceptable dose levels for genotoxic and/or carcinogenic chemicals. Based on the data sources described above, three example approaches are outlined in brief below:

1. the use and derivation of a PDE as outlined in the ICH Q3C(R4) residual solvents guideline;

2. computer-based modeling of animal carcinogenicity data as used in the EPA IRIS database; and

3. simple extrapolation from the TD_{50}.

Following this, the example of aniline is used to compare each approach, based on the available data for this chemical.

5.2.2.1   PDE Calculation   In principle, a PDE can be calculated for any chemical for which animal data are available. However, this is generally limited to those chemicals known to be Ames negative, that is not DNA reactive, as the current regulatory view is that there are no safe thresholds for DNA-reactive chemicals. The calculation is outlined in ICH Q3C (R4) and is as follows:

$$\text{PDE (mg/day)} = \frac{NOEL \times weight\ adjustment\ (kg)}{F1 \times F2 \times F3 \times F4 \times F5}$$

Where the NOEL is the no observed effect level in the most relevant animal study (e.g. the NOEL for increase in tumor incidence in a carcinogenicity study); a lowest observed effect level (LOEL) can also be used with an additional safety factor ($F5$) of 10. The weight adjustment is 50 kg based on an arbitrary human bodyweight for either sex.

- $F1$ is a factor to account for extrapolation between species (varies from 2 [for dog to human extrapolation] to 12 [from mice to human]).
- $F2$ is a factor of 10 to account for inter-individual variation.
- $F3$ is a variable factor to account for toxicity studies of short-term exposure (varies from 1 [for studies lasting at least 50% of lifetime and reproductive toxicity studies covering all organogenesis] to 10 [studies shorter than 3 months in rodents, 2 years in nonrodents].
- $F4$ is a factor to cover severe toxicity, including nongenotoxic carcinogenicity, neurotoxicity, or teratogenicity. For reproductive toxicity studies, this ranges from 1 (for fetal toxicity associated with maternal toxicity) to 10 (for a teratogenic effect without maternal toxicity).
- $F5$, as highlighted above, is used when only a LOEL is available. The factor varies up to 10 depending on severity of the toxicity.

As an example, consider the PDE derived for chlorobenzene that is based on a 13-week oral toxicity study in mice, in which a NOEL of 60 mg/kg was identified. The compound was administered once daily for 5 days/week over the 13 weeks, and so a correction was made for continuous dosing to give a NOEL dose level of 43 mg/kg/day. The PDE was calculated thus:

$$\text{PDE} = \frac{43 \times 50}{12 \times 10 \times 5 \times 1 \times 1} = 3.58 \text{ mg/day}$$

Where $F1$ was 12, as mice were used in the study, $F2$ was a default of 10, $F3$ was given a value of 5 to account for the 13 week study duration, $F4$ was 1 as no severe toxicity (as defined above) was observed, and $F5$ was 1 as a NOEL was determined.

5.2.2.2   IRIS Linear Extrapolation   In addition to the description of oral reference doses and inhalation reference concentrations for the chronic noncancer health effects of selected chemicals, the IRIS website lists quantitative estimates of cancer risk from exposure to carcinogenic or potentially carcinogenic substances, where data permit such assessments. Quantitative cancer risk assessments are presented in three ways:

1. *Slope factor:* An upper bound limit that represents the increased cancer risk associated with lifetime exposure to the agent concerned. It is represented in units of proportion of the population affected per mg/kg/day.

2. *Unit risk:* The quantitative estimate of risk per μg of agent present/L of drinking water (in the case of oral exposure) or per m^3 air (in the case of inhalation exposure).

3. *Drinking water concentration at specified risk levels:* This represents the concentration of the agent in μg/L terms representing a specified risk level. For the purposes of these assessments, the value equating to a 1 in 100,000 risk level has been used due to its direct correlation with the risk level used for the TTC in the European Medicines Evaluation Agency (EMEA) Guideline on Limits for Genotoxic Impurities.[2]

5.2.2.3   TD$_{50}$ Calculation   Where data exist to define the TD$_{50}$ for a chemical, such as in the CPDB referred to previously, it is possible to calculate from this a dose level associated with not a 50% incidence of cancer, but a 1 in 100,000 or 0.001% incidence. Clearly, this is a highly simplistic approach based on a linear dose response. Nevertheless, it is another approach that can be used to estimate doses associated with low levels of risk.

Having identified a number of relevant sources of information relevant to the setting of acceptable risk levels for both genotoxic and carcinogenic chemicals, the next section highlights how this information can be used, using aniline as an example.

5.3   ANILINE (CAS NO. 62-53-3)

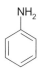

Historically, aniline has had widespread use in the dye industry, and has some limited use in drug syntheses. Aniline has been tested in a number of genotoxicity and carcinogenicity studies, a summary of which are presented below:

5.3.1   Genotoxicity Studies

5.3.1.1   Ames Test   Results for several studies are described in both the CCRIS and IRIS databases, and show aniline to be negative in all five standard strains. Two tests performed pre-1980 showed a positive response, but both were performed in the presence of the comutagen norharman (a β-carboline alkaloid), and the positive findings are considered to be a result of the formation of a mutagenic compound, aminophenylnorharman from the two components.[5] From these results, it is concluded that aniline is nonmutagenic.

Mechanism of Action   The observed genotoxicity associated with aromatic amines and also nitro compounds is related to the generation of an electrophilic nitrenium ion. See Figure 5.1.

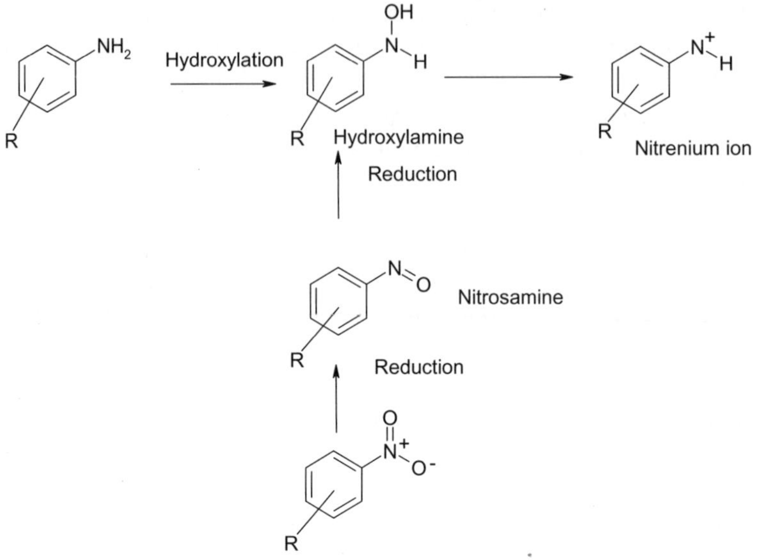

Figure 5.1 Mechanism for generation of nitrenium ions for both aromatic amine and nitro compounds.

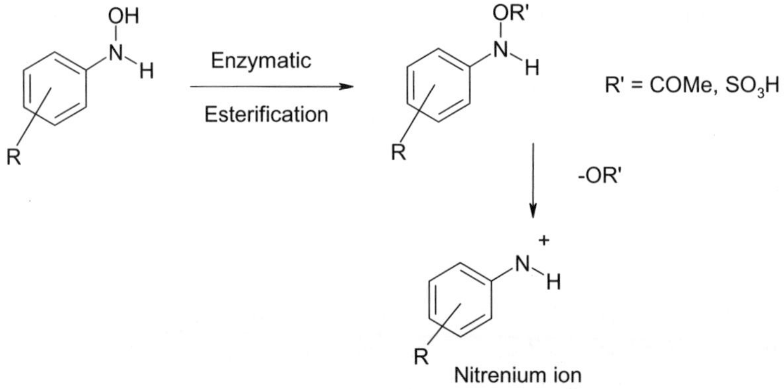

Figure 5.2 Generation of activated electrostatic complex through N-hydroxylamine esterification.

The mechanism is complex: the first step, hydroxylation, occurs as a result of enzymatic metabolic activation involving cytochrome P450 and yields the N-hydroxyl intermediate. This can then undergo N-O bond cleavage to produce the active arylnitrenium ion species. However, further activation can also occur[6] to yield an electrostatic complex in the form of either an N-acetoxy or N-sulfate ester, these permitting more facile N-O bond cleavage, Figure 5.2.

Although rat liver S9 fractions contain the necessary cytosolic enzymes, the standard S9 mix used in the Ames test does not allow esterification to occur because it is not routinely supplemented with the necessary cofactors. However, supplementation of the S9 mix with acetyl CoA has been shown to enhance the mutagenicity of benzidine.[7] Further, the bacterial strains themselves possess *O*-acetyltransferase activity and strains genetically modified to overexpress it show increased sensitivity to a range of nitroarenes and aromatic amines.[8] Sulfation of the hydroxylamine is also known to be important in the activation of some aromatic amines, but bacterial strains have little sulfotransferase (SULT) activity, and strains have also been engineered to express the relevant SULT.[9]

5.3.1.2   Other Genotoxicity Studies   As described, aniline itself is considered to be Ames negative. However, positive results have been reported for aniline in the mouse lymphoma TK assay; in addition, both negative and positive results have been observed in Chinese hamster embryo cells. From these results is concluded that aniline should be classified as clastogenic, and this is further supported by positive *in vivo* mouse micronucleus data.

5.3.2   Carcinogenicity Studies

An assessment of the carcinogenicity of aniline by the International Agency for Research on Cancer (IARC) has concluded that the evidence for carcinogenicity to humans is inadequate, and there is only limited evidence of carcinogenicity in animals.[10]

A summary of the conclusions is described:

Human data: there is inadequate evidence of carcinogenicity to humans.[10] Investigations relating to the incidence of bladder cancer among workers in the dye industry were carried out during the 1950s. However, the individuals studied were exposed to a number of aromatic amines, and it was therefore not possible to ascribe any increase in incidence of cancer specifically to aniline.

Animal Studies: there is limited evidence of carcinogenicity to rodents.[10] A number of animal studies have been performed for aniline (in the form of aniline hydrochloride), two of which are highlighted in the IRIS database. The first is a 2-year study performed by the Chemical Industry Institute of Toxicology (CIIT)[11] in rats, and this showed an increased incidence of splenic sarcomas in male rats associated with the highest dose (2000 ppm).

A similar U.S. National Cancer Institute (NCI)[12] study conducted using a different strain of rats also showed a dose-related increase in male rats, again primarily associated with the spleen. Other studies have concluded this to be linked to the accumulation of aniline within the spleen at high doses (>10 mg/kg). The mechanism has been postulated to relate to aniline binding preferentially to red blood cells, with damaged cells accumulating in the spleen; cell debris results in hemosiderosis, which induces a fibrotic response in the spleen, leading ultimately to sarcoma formation. A recent publication[13] further supports this assessment.

Based on the data above, which indicates aniline to be clastogenic but not mutagenic, combined together with the postulated mechanism regarding carcinogenicity, it is considered probable that the carcinogenic response is related to a thresholded mechanism.

Aniline has actually been administered to humans—single doses up to 65 mg have been given in studying methaemoglobinaemia.[14] A single dose NOEL of 15 mg was reported.

5.3.3   Aniline Risk Assessments

Given the safety profile of aniline, clastogenic but nonmutagenic, and the likely nongenotoxic, and thus thresholded, mechanism of carcinogenicity in animals, it is considered that adoption of the TTC concept to determine acceptable limits would be unnecessarily conservative. In this example, four different sources of information relevant to the risk assessment of aniline are considered.

1. The U.S. EPA IRIS database outlines a quantitative cancer risk assessment for aniline based on use of a linearized multistage procedure.[15] The dose associated with a 1 in 100,000 lifetime cancer risk (equal to risk level of the TTC) is 120 μg/day. However, the assessment states that this procedure may not be the most appropriate method for the derivation of the slope factor as aniline accumulation in the spleen is nonlinear.[16] Minimal accumulation of aniline and no hemosiderosis is observed at doses below 10 mg/kg, and as already described, hemosiderosis may be important in the induction of the splenic tumors observed in rats.

The postulated mechanism and the link between observed carcinogenicity and methaemoglobinaemia provides support for the existence of a threshold, and supports the use of the process defined in ICH Q3C for deriving a Permitted Daily Exposure limit (PDE) for residual solvents based on animal data.

2. The PDE calculation is: $(NOEL \times$ body weight adjustment $(kg))/F1 \times F2 \times F3 \times F4 \times F5$

The following safety factors as outlined in ICH Q3C have been applied to determine a PDE for aniline; these are:

$F1 = 10$ (rat to man)

$F2 = 10$ (inter-individual variability)

$F3 = 1$ (study duration at least half lifetime)

$F4 = 10$ (severe toxicity)

$F5 = 1$ (using a NOEL)

Data derived from the CIIT 2-year rat carcinogenicity study[11] have been used to derive risk-based dose levels. Dose levels were 200, 600, and 2000 ppm aniline hydrochloride in the diet, equivalent to dose levels of aniline of 7.2, 22, and 72 mg/kg/day. Tumors were observed in high dose animals, and one stromal sarcoma of the spleen was identified at 22 mg/kg/day. Based on these data, the lowest dose of 10 mg/kg/day has been used to define the NOEL.

On this basis, the PDE was calculated as follows:

$$PDE = 7.2 \times 50 \text{ kg}/(5 \times 10 \times 1 \times 10 \times 1) = 720 \text{ μg/day}$$

3. In the CPDB (http://potency.berkeley.edu/cpdb.html), the harmonic mean $TD_{50}{}^*$ for aniline hydrochloride is 269 mg/kg/day. Extrapolation from this dose

---

* A summary measure that accounts for all positive results of a chemical in each species, from experiments that may differ, for example, in animal strain, route of administration, dose levels tested and duration of experiment.

level giving a 50% incidence of tumors to one giving 1 case in 100,000 (0.001%) gives a dose of 0.0054 mg/kg/day, which equates to a PDE dose of 269 μg/day for a 50 kg individual.

4. The Californian EPA NSRL for aniline is 100 μg/day.

5.3.4 Aniline Summary

From the assessments presented above, an acceptable risk dose limit for aniline ranges from 100 to 720 μg/day, with less than one order of magnitude separating the lowest and highest values derived from these different approaches. Which value should be used in the risk assessment? Is any one of these approaches more valid than the others? Although there are limitations to each approach, it is considered that they are all valid, and therefore effective arguments could be constructed for the use of any of the data described to justify a limit for aniline. However, while it may provide the greatest flexibility to adopt the upper limit of 720 μg/day, automatic selection of the highest value is not necessarily recommended, as other factors, including the ease of control of aniline levels in drug substance, should be taken into account in line with the principle of as low as reasonably practicable (ALARP).

Further examples of chemicals relevant to pharmaceutical drug syntheses and their risk assessments are included in the appendix.

5.4 COMPARISON OF PERMITTED DAILY EXPOSURES (PDE) LIMITS DESCRIBED IN INTERNATIONAL CONFERENCE ON HARMONISATION (ICH) Q3C GUIDELINE AND QUANTITATIVE CANCER RISK ESTIMATES

The ICH Q3C Guideline for residual solvents, most recently updated as version R4,[17] lists recommended acceptable amounts for solvent residues in pharmaceuticals based on toxicological risk assessments. Solvents are divided into three classes based on toxicity:

Class 1 solvents are those to be avoided, and include known human carcinogens such as benzene.

Class 2 solvents are those to be limited, and include nongenotoxic carcinogens, such as acetonitrile and 1,4-dioxane.

Class 3 solvents are considered to have low toxic potential and have PDE levels of 50 mg/day or more. Examples of compounds in this class include acetone and ethanol.

Of the 30 solvents included in Classes 1 and 2, a total of 12 compounds have PDE limits established on the basis of carcinogenicity studies (see Table 5.1), and this includes PDEs for four of the five solvents in Class 1. As described above, the PDE approach is generally applied to compounds that are not considered to be DNA reactive, and thus would be negative in the Ames test. In the case of 1,1-dichloroethene, a compound reported to be positive in the Ames test but to be negative in various

TABLE 5.1 Selected Solvents from ICH Q3C: Derivation of PDE Values Based on Carcinogenicity Studies

Chemical	PDE (μg/day)	Ames (ICH Q3C)	IARC classification	Evidence of carcinogenicity	Basis for derivation of PDE
Benzene	20	−ve	1	yes	U.S. EPA IRIS quantitative cancer risk estimate for 1 in 10^5 lifetime risk.
Carbon tetrachloride	40	−ve	2B	yes	Mice aged 3 months at study start, dosed with up to 80 mg/kg/day for 120 days and examined for hepatomas at 8 months old. PDE based on NOEL at 10 mg/kg/day.
1,2-dichloroethane	50	—	2B	yes	Data not specified. Limit based on 1 in 10^5 excess cancer risk based on hemangiosarcoma using a linearized multistage model without body surface correction.
1,1-dichloroethene	80	+ve	3	Yes (inhalation)	Mice dosed by inhalation for 52 weeks with 25 ppm for 4 h/day, 5 days/week, retained until 98 weeks; showed increased incidence of renal adenocarcinomas, mainly in males. *PDE based on effect level.*
Acetonitrile	4100	−ve	Not evaluated	Yes (inhalation)	Rats dosed by inhalation of up to 400 ppm for 6 h/day, 5 days/week for 2 years; slight increase in hepatocellular adenoma or carcinoma (combined) in high dose males. PDE based on NOEL at 200 ppm.
Chloroform	600	−ve	2B	Yes	Male mice dosed by oral gavage of 17 or 60 mg/kg, 6 days/week for 80 weeks followed by 16-week observation period; increases in liver and kidney tumors at high dose. PDE based on NOEL of 17 mg/kg.
Dichloromethane	6000	+ve	2B	Yes	Mice exposed by inhalation to 2000 or 4000 ppm, 6 h/day, 5 days/week for 2 years showed increases in lung and hepatocellular carcinomas at both dose levels. PDE based on NOEL (6 mg/kg) from rat study dosed at up to 250 mg/kg in drinking water for 2 years; fatty liver changes and areas of foci but no neoplastic changes in any tissues.

Compound					Comments
N,N-dimethylacetamide	10,900	–ve	Not evaluated	No	Rats dosed by inhalation with up to 350 ppm for 6 h/day, 5 days/week for 2 years; no increases in tumor incidence. PDE based on NOEL for increased liver weights and liver histopathology of 25 ppm.
1,4-dioxane	3800	–ve	2B	Yes	Mice treated with 0.5 or 1% in drinking water for 90 weeks; increased liver tumors. *PDE based on effect level.*
Nitro methane	500	–ve	2B	Yes	Mice dosed by inhalation with 188 to 750 ppm for 6 h/day, 5 days/week for 2 years; increases in various tumors at all dose levels, including hepatocellular adenoma and adenoma or carcinoma combined in low dose females. *PDE based on effect level* (188 ppm).
Tetrahydrofuran	7200	–ve	Not evaluated	Yes	Rats dosed by inhalation to 200 to 1800 ppm for 6 h/day, 5 days/week for 105 weeks; increased incidences of kidney adenoma or carcinoma (combined) in males and of hepatocellular adenomas and carcinomas in females. PDE based on low dose (200 ppm).
1,1,2-trichloroethene	800	–ve	2A	Yes	Rats dosed by inhalation to 100–600 ppm for 7 h/day, 5 days/week for 2 years had dose-related increases in Leydig cell tumors and at high dose level, increase in renal tumors. *PDE based on effect level* (100 ppm).

in vivo assays for genotoxicity and to cause an increase in renal tumors in mice when dosed by inhalation (Table 5.1), the PDE was derived from an effect level for carcinogenesis as reported in Appendix 5 to ICH Q3C.[18] It is encouraging to observe that the positive Ames data appears to have been outweighed by an overall negative weight of evidence for genotoxicity. However, the derivation of a PDE based on a dose level having a carcinogenic response rather than a NOEL is surprising, and is an approach that is unlikely to receive scientific or regulatory support today. This approach was also used to set PDE values for the Class 2 solvents 1,4-dioxane, nitromethane and 1,1,2-trichloroethene. The additional safety factor ($F5$) used in the PDE calculation in these cases is 10-fold to account for a LOEL being used in lieu of a NOEL. Whether this additional factor is sufficient to account for a lack of knowledge of where the LOEL sits on the dose-response curve and how it relates to the NOEL is not known.

It is also of interest to compare the PDE values determined from animal carcinogenicity studies using the formula outlined earlier in this chapter, with acceptable risk dose levels published elsewhere or calculated in other ways. Table 5.2

TABLE 5.2 Selected Solvents from ICH Q3C: Comparison of PDE Values with Acceptable Lifetime Excess Cancer Risk Estimates

Chemical	ICH Q3C PDE (µg/day)	Dose level (µg/day) associated with 1 in 10^5 excess lifetime cancer risk		
		From CPDB TD_{50}[a]	From U.S. EPA IRIS[b]	From NSRL (Feb 09)[c]
Benzene	20	77.5	20	6.4 (oral) 13 (inhal)
Carbon tetrachloride	40	27.8	6	5
1,2-Dichloroethane	50	14.6	8	10
1,1-Dichloroethene	80	34.6	—[d]	Not reported
Acetonitrile	4100	All studies negative	No quantitative estimate	Not reported
Chloroform	600	111	500	20 (oral) 40 (inhal)
Dichloromethane	6000	724	100	200 (inhal) 50
N,N-Dimethylacetamide	10,900	All studies negative	Not evaluated	Not reported
1,4-dioxane	3800	204	60	30
Nitromethane	500	40.4	Not evaluated	39
Tetrahydrofuran	7200	407	Not evaluated	Not reported
1,1,2-Trichloroethene	800	343	Withdrawn	50 (oral) 80 (inhalation)

[a] Lowest harmonic mean value for rat or mouse, divided by 1000 from mg/kg/day in animals to a daily dose in a 50 kg individual.

[b] Data from oral estimates for drinking water where available, and assuming consumption of 2 L water/day.

[c] Values published as Proposition 65 safe Harbor Levels—No Significant Risk Levels for Carcinogens[4].

[d] Suggestive evidence for carcinogenicity by inhalation but not sufficient to assess human carcinogenic potential; data for oral administration inadequate to assess human carcinogenic potential.

summarizes data derived from the University of Berkley CPDB, the U.S. EPA IRIS database and the Californian EPA NSRL values for the same 12 solvents considered above. Data from at least one alternative source to the PDE are available for 10 of these 12 compounds, and in all but one case (benzene), the excess cancer risk dose estimates are lower than the PDE values, in several cases by more than 10-fold, and in the case of 1,4-dioxane, by more than 100-fold.

In summarizing this analysis, it is worth reiterating a number of key points:

1. Not all solvents for which PDE calculations are based on carcinogenicity data are Ames negative; a weight of evidence approach was applied to the assessment of genotoxicity data.

2. Several solvents shown to be carcinogenic in animal studies have PDEs calculated based on effect levels for tumorigenesis rather than NOELs.

3. When compared with other assessments of acceptable risk dose levels, PDEs for solvents carcinogenic in animal studies are generally higher, and sometimes significantly so.

4. The continued updating of ICH Q3C with the most recent Step 4 version dated February 2009 demonstrates the continued support for the PDE calculation and process. Therefore, where appropriate data are available, the calculation of a PDE should form part of an overall assessment of acceptable risk levels for chemicals that are nongenotoxic animal carcinogens.

5.5   OVERALL CONCLUSIONS

It is clear from current regulatory guidance on the control of genotoxic impurities that compound-specific cancer risk assessments are recommended in preference to application of the standard TTC, where they can be supported by scientific justification and data. It should also be clear from some of the examples and issues highlighted in this chapter that such approaches are complex, and it is entirely possible to calculate more than one acceptable risk dose for the same compound. This is not unexpected, as variability may reflect biological variability and/or differences in risk assessment assumptions and modeling. However, as a result of this, the use of different approaches to compound-specific risk assessments may itself lead to risks regarding regulatory acceptance of what may be entirely justifiable methodologies, and this in turn may lead to delays to drug development or registration until a commonly agreed approach is reached.

An objective of this chapter has been to highlight the variability in data in some of the examples used, and to propose in these situations that conclusions be based on an overall weight of evidence approach. While it is not intended to be a comprehensive evaluation of all possible approaches to compound-specific cancer risk assessments, it is hoped that the reader has gained some insight into the sources of data appropriate for such assessments, and some of the methods used to estimate acceptable risk dose levels for genotoxic impurities. It should also be clear that the focus of this chapter has been on establishing limits for genotoxic impurities based on the same level of excess cancer risk as that on which the TTC is based. The primary intent in the control of genotoxic impurities in drugs is to minimize risk to patients; as part of this assessment, any final limits proposed should consider the feasibility of controlling the particular impurity in the drug substance itself or whether this might be more readily applied to an upstream intermediate at the level indicated by the risk assessment. While toxicologists usually talk in terms of dose (e.g. μg/day), synthetic chemists and analysts generally focus on concentrations (e.g. ppm or ppb); the key to bringing these two together is the daily dose of the drug, usually the maximum dose at any given time during development, or the maximum registered dose of a drug on the market. It is when the concentration limit for the impurity in the drug substance is identified that the effort required from both analytical and control perspectives and any technical feasibility issues become apparent.

The examples of assessments given in this chapter may help to form the basis of compound-specific limits to discuss with regulatory authorities. However, it is considered that publication of examples of compound-specific assessments leading to defined acceptable limits by regulatory authorities, or better internationally harmonized regulatory guidance through the vehicle of ICH, would help clarify one or more acceptable approaches. An important benefit of this would be that pharmaceutical companies could avoid potentially unacceptable approaches, leading to an improvement in the consistency of responses to regulatory submissions.

5.6 APPENDIX

5.6.1 Substituted Anilines

Substituted anilines are used in the synthesis of a large number of drugs, often as key building blocks of the parent molecule. Because of their widespread use, there is considerable interest in their potential genotoxicity. Although aniline is itself Ames negative, many substituted anilines are positive and hence considered to be mutagenic. As a result, these compounds are subject to control as defined by the EMEA guideline.[1] However, it is also true that many other substituted anilines are nongenotoxic. Current SAR tools do not allow the confident prediction of mutagenic potential of these chemicals, and so the holy grail in respect to such compounds would be to accurately predict their potential genotoxicity based on their structure through the establishment of a direct correlation between a specific property (descriptor) of the compound and a mutagenic response. A number of publications have addressed this subject: for example Brock et al.[19] studied the binding of ortho (OT) and para toluidine (PT) to rat hepatocytes, and showed no direct correlation between the extent of binding and carcinogenic potency.

Kerdar et al.[20] recognized that the ultimate reactive species was the nitrenium ion and studied the formation, reactivity, and genotoxicity of a range of arylamines and nitroarenes to explore the potential link between chemical structure and mutagenicity. Arylnitrenium ions were generated from the equivalent arylazide through photolysis, and a series of studies were performed, including ^{32}P-postlabeling DNA binding studies, Ames test, and mammalian cell assays, the latter to determine the extent of chromosomal damage. The test compounds were mostly amines that varied in their ring system, and some correlation between structure and mutagenicity was identified; the size of the aromatic ring system was shown to affect the level of mutagenicity observed, with larger ring systems being more potent. However, this is of little practical application in the context of drug-related syntheses, where substituted phenyl derivatives and hetero-aromatic amines are more prevalent. Some tentative correlation between the position of methyl and chloro substituents was reported, along with other correlations linked to planarity of structure and ring position of the nitrenium ion. It was concluded that the most likely explanation related to stability of the nitrenium ion. Where this could be stabilized, as a result of charge delocalization, then the level of the observed mutagenic response was greater.

Aβmann et al. 1997[21] studied a range of nitro and aminobenzenes, and showed a correlation between substitution pattern and genotoxic potential. Where aniline or nitrobenzene incorporated an additional nitro group in the either the meta or para position, the resultant derivative was uniformally genotoxic. In contrast, aniline and nitrobenzene are nongenotoxic, as were their ortho derivatives. This indicates that both electronic and steric factors are influential in determining genotoxicity.

Chung et al.[22] studied a series of benzidine analogues to evaluate structure-activity relationships between physico-chemical parameters and mutagenic activity, assessed by a two-strain (TA100 and TA98) Ames test. A range of parameters was studied, including oxidation potentials, energy differences between highest occupied and lowest unoccupied orbitals (HOMO and LUMOs), ionization potential, dipole moments, partition coefficients, and basicity; no correlations were established. It was concluded that principal component analysis may help establish a correlation, but no analysis was reported.

In an extensive study of over 80 aromatic and hetero-aromatic amines, Hatch et al.[23] attempted to correlate observed mutagenic response to a particular molecular property, using the complex multivariate analysis suggested by Chung et al.[22] It was concluded that although the stability of the nitrenium ion was a contributory factor, the main determinant was the extent of the aromatic π electron system. The most interesting aspect was the proposed link between aromaticity, essentially the size of the ring system, and the role of cytochrome P-450 1A in the oxidation of the amine.

A recent paper published by Borosky[24] has returned to the potential correlation between the nitrenium ion stability and genotoxic potency. Density formation theory (DFT) was employed to study the formation of the nitrenium ion from the associated electrophilic precursors. Borosky studied not only the N-O bond dissociation within N-hydroxyl derivatives of aniline, but also that of its N-acetoxy and N-sulfate esters. These investigations showed the N-sulfate ester to be the most facile and thus the most likely reactive precursor to the nitrenium ion. Studies carried out on a series of N-acetoxy esters also established a correlation between mutagenic potency and the charge density of the nitrogen within the nitrenium ion, when the anilines in question were classified into aromatic, imidazo-carboxylic, and imidazo-heterocyclic classes. The need to subcategorize the compounds into these classes showed that mutagenic potency was clearly influenced by the ring system involved, indicating a further factor in determining mutagenicity. This correlates with the earlier findings of Hatch et al.[23]

A recent paper by Leach et al.[25] specifically focused on the dissociation energy of the N-acetoxy intermediate. In general, active compounds were found to possess lower activation energies. This was postulated to be related to the need for a weak bond to facilitate generation of a nitrenium ion. It was also postulated that steric factors were important, regarding the ability to access the heme portion of the CYP1A2 and bind effectively. The *in silico* model used showed a clear correlation between dissociation energy and genotoxicity, although some outliers were observed. Most compellingly of all was that when the outliers were examined, they related to compounds shown to demonstrate an atypical genotoxic profile, that is the outliers were found to correlate with those that were active without S9 activation. The paper also examined the potential correlation between other factors, such as secondary oxidation and nitroso reactivity and mutagenic activity. No correlation between either of these factors and activity was observed.

It is clear from this review that mutagenicity is likely to be linked to a number of factors, prime among them are the size and shape of the aromatic ring and stability of the nitrenium ion. Also apparently critical is the substitution pattern and nature of the substituents. However, at present, the data falls short of explaining in full how each of these factors are interrelated, and as a result, it is not possible to predict with a high level of confidence whether an aniline derivative will be genotoxic purely from its structure. With this current level of uncertainty, it is recommended that any novel aniline or hetero-aromatic amine is evaluated in an Ames test.

5.6.2   Hydrazine (CAS No. 302-01-2)

NH_2-NH_2

Hydrazine has a variety of uses synthetically both as a reducing agent and also in the formation of hydrazides. As a result, it is used in the synthesis of a number of drugs, such as the tuberculosis treatments Isoniazid/Hydralazine and Iproniazid. Hydrazine itself, in the form of its sulphate salt, has been used therapeutically to treat TB and sickle cell anaemia.[26]

5.6.2.1   Genotoxicity Studies   A review of the wealth of data reported in both IRIS and CCRIS demonstrates hydrazine to be unequivocally mutagenic, with positive responses in various *S. typhimurium* and *E. coli* strains. CCRIS reports the results of a chromosomal aberration test conducted with hydrazine showing clear structural changes both with and without S9 activation.

In addition to *in vitro* studies, IRIS reports the results from a radio-labeled binding study performed with hydrazine and radio-labeled methionine showing that hydrazine mediates the indirect alkylation of DNA.[27] Similar results showing the generation of methyl adducts have been reported by Parodi et al.[28] and Zeilmaker et al.[29]

5.6.2.2   Carcinogenicity Studies   Several carcinogenicity studies have been carried out on hydrazine, many of which are described in CCRIS and the IRIS databases, and demonstrate tumor formation at multiple sites with evidence of a dose-related response in some of studies. While according to IRIS and the ATSDR

(Agency for Toxic Substances and Disease Registry) (1997), hydrazine is classified by the EPA as a class B2 carcinogen (a probable human carcinogen), the IARC has classified hydrazine in Group 2B (possibly carcinogenic to humans).[30]

Most of the data on hydrazine relates to studies performed on hydrazine sulphate rather than hydrazine itself, due to the impracticality of performing studies with such a reactive substance. Although there is little doubt that hydrazine is responsible for the observed tumorigenic response, it is noted in the IRIS database that bioavailability of the two compounds is likely to be different, and thus results derived from hydrazine sulphate may not be totally representative of hydrazine itself, even when molecular weight and concentration differences are taken into account.

5.6.2.3 Calculation of Limits The drinking water concentration at the 1 in 100,000 risk level is 0.1 μg/L (IRIS). Adjusting this to reflect typical daily consumption of 2 L per day gives an intake of 0.2 μg/day. In contrast, the Cal EPA NSRL for hydrazine is 5-fold lower at 0.04 μg/day.

The CPDB reports values for rat/mice and hamster studies. Of these, the lowest TD_{50} value originates from rat studies, and the harmonic mean TD_{50} value is 0.613 mg/kg/day, although considerable variability (greater than 10-fold) is noted in the database. When converted to a dose representing a 1 in 100,000 risk by simple linear extrapolation, this equates to a dose of 0.61 μg/day.

Recently, a paper published by Miller et al. in PharmEuropa, 2006[31] highlighted further safety studies, including results from a study conducted by Delft et al.[32] This study, focused on induction of *in vivo* N7 and O6 methyl guanine (adduct formation in rat liver), and reported a NOEL of 0.1 mg/kg, converted by the authors to a PDE of 1 μg/day.

Another important source of data is the paper by Kroes et al.,[33] in which data that formed the basis of the TTC were further evaluated and divided into specific chemical classes. Of the 57 hydrazines studied, only 2 were found to represent a risk greater than 1 in 1,000,000 at the 0.15 μg level. As a result of this, hydrazines were not considered to be part of the subset that were defined as unusually toxic and thus outside of the scope of the TTC.

Considering these different evaluations, and given the high level of variability seen in the carcinogenicity study data, the conservative approach taken in extrapolating such data to low doses, and that much of the data relates to hydrazine sulphate rather than hydrazine, the use of the default TTC limit of 1.5 μg/day in the case of hydrazine would seem appropriate.

5.6.3 Pyridine (CAS No. 110-86-1)

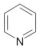

5.6.3.1 Background Synthetically, pyridine is often employed as a base in reactions such a tosylations. Although generally now replaced by less toxic bases such as triethylamine, it is still used, often where other bases prove unsuitable.

5.6.3.2 Genotoxicity Studies Data cited in CCRIS indicate pyridine is Ames negative in all tested strains (both *S. typhimurium* and *E. coli* strains). Negative results are reported for the mouse lymphoma assay, both with and without S9 activation and for a UDS assay in mouse hepatocytes.

5.6.3.3 Carcinogenicity Studies In CCRIS, several results are reported from oral studies conducted using multiple doses of pyridine in drinking water. These rodent studies (both mouse and rat) show a positive carcinogenic response.

5.6.3.4 Calculation of Limits The IRIS risk assessment for pyridine indicates that it has not been assessed under the EPA risk evaluation program, and hence no data are presented, although an oral reference dose of 1 µg/kg/day (equivalent to a daily dose of 50 µg/day for a 50 kg individual) is listed for noncancer health effects.

In the CPDB, a mean TD_{50} value of 24.4 mg/kg/day is reported for mice, with a higher mean of 67.3 mg/kg/day in rats. Linear extrapolation from the mouse TD_{50} to a 1 in 100,000 risk level gives a daily dose of approximately 25 µg/day. In the absence of any evidence of mutagenicity or clastogenicity, it is likely that the mechanism of carcinogenicity of pyridine is not directly related to interaction with DNA, and hence is likely to be subject to a threshold. Indeed, this is indirectly supported by the fact that ICH Q3C lists a PDE for pyridine of 2 mg/day, although this is based not on carcinogenicity data but on a 90-day toxicity study in rats. A study by Mason et al.[34] cited in PharmEuropa 1997 under carcinogenicity that involved twice weekly subcutaneous injections of pyridine in rats for 1 year only led to a higher PDE (derived from the NOEL) at 2.86 mg/day.

In this case, the ICH PDE for pyridine of 2 mg/day is 80-fold higher than the dose derived from simple linear extrapolation from the most sensitive animal carcinogenicity TD_{50} value, and is over 1300-fold higher than the TTC limit.

5.6.4 Ethylene Oxide (CAS No. 75-21-8)

Ethylene oxide is used synthetically in the manufacture of polyethylene glycol (PEG) and nonionic surfactants. It is also widely used as a sterilizing agent for instruments in hospitals. Indeed, its use as a sterilizing agent is linked to its effectiveness in damaging bacterial DNA. The inherent strain and polarity of the C-O bond make it very susceptible to nucleophilic attack.

5.6.4.1 Genotoxicity Studies Several reported positive Ames results are reported in CCRIS in both TA1535 and TA100 strains. Positive results for the rat micronucleus test are also reported in CCRIS.

Based on these data, ethylene oxide should be considered to be both mutagenic and clastogenic.

5.6.4.2 Carcinogenicity Studies

Animal Studies Results of gavage and inhalation carcinogenicity studies in both rats and mice are reported in CCRIS, all of which are positive. Based on these data, it is concluded that ethylene oxide is an animal carcinogen.

Human Data A series of epidemiological studies exploring instances of human cancer associated with ethylene oxide exposure has been conducted.[35–37] These are linked to two groups, those exposed industrially through:

1. exposure associated with manufacture and/or use of ethylene oxide; and
2. those exposed through its use as a sterilization agent.

The IARC assessment[37] stated that the most informative of the studies carried out involved investigation of sterilization personnel in the United States. This study was reported to have found small but significant increases in incidence of lymphatic leukemia and non-Hodgkin's lymphoma. Associated mortality rates were reported as being only marginally increased. Other smaller studies conducted in the United Kingdom and Sweden reported similar but nonsignificant increases in lymphatic and hematopoietic cancer.

The IARC assessment also reported that these studies included data showing that ethylene oxide readily forms adducts with proteins and DNA. For protein adducts, hemoglobin was used as a biomarker, and a correlation was demonstrated between exposure to ethylene oxide and the level of N-terminal hydroxyl-ethyl valine in the hemoglobin of exposed workers. A correlation was also observed between the number of DNA adducts and level of exposure. Interestingly, both hemoglobin and DNA adducts of ethylene oxide were measurable in individuals classified as not exposed.

In addition to adduct formation, the IARC assessment also reported that chromosomal damage was also consistently observed in the lymphocytes of workers exposed to ethylene oxide; both chromosomal aberrations and micronuclei were seen.

Based on the mutagenicity and clastogenicity data, together with the animal and human carcinogenicity data, ethylene oxide has been classified by the IARC as a known human carcinogen (Group 1).

5.6.4.3 *Other Data* In spite of the compelling data referred to above, the formation of low level adducts to DNA and hemoglobin even in the absence of exposure to ethylene oxide requires closer examination. Bolt et al.[38] explored the hydroxyethylation of hemoglobin and of guanine (component of DNA) in both humans and animals, and reported that this was linked to endogenous formation of ethylene oxide, several sources of which were reported. Primary among these are lipid peroxidation, through metabolism of unsaturated lipids, and production of ethylene in the gut linked to bacteria, followed by subsequent peroxidation to yield ethylene oxide.

The authors reported the outcome of a series of studies focused on the level of endogenously formed N7-(2-hydroxyethyl) guanine. Each of the studies reported adduct levels at around 2 pmole/mg DNA independent of the animals studied, the method used, and tissue type, and clearly indicated a consistent level of background exposure to endogenous ethylene oxide.

5.6.4.4 *Metabolism of Ethylene Oxide* Two principal pathways have been identified that are associated with ethylene oxide metabolism:

1. hydration—epoxide hydrolase (EH); and
2. glutathione conjugation.

Of these, it is believed that EH enzyme-promoted hydration is the major pathway, resulting in the formation of ethylene diol. It is highly probable that this efficient system has evolved as a direct result of the endogenous exposure described. Like all enzyme systems, this can become overwhelmed at high exposure levels, potentially explaining the animal carcinogenicity data, where the doses involved were well in excess of any likely threshold levels.

5.6.4.5 *Calculation of Limits*   As already outlined, the toxicological profile of ethylene oxide is complex. There is clear evidence of both mutagenicity and carcinogenicity, resulting in classification as a human carcinogen. However, there is also evidence of significant endogenous production of ethylene oxide, together with well-stablished metabolic pathways to address endogenous generation, both of which indicate a threshold is likely to exist, below which ethylene oxide is efficiently detoxified.

The IRIS database does not include a cancer risk assessment for ethylene oxide, although an assessment of the closely related propylene oxide is available, indicating the 1 in 100,000 lifetime cancer risk dose to be 2 µg/day. Interestingly, this same dose level is quoted by the Cal EPA as the NSRL for ethylene oxide itself. In addition, the CPDB lists mean TD_{50} values in the rat and mouse of 21.3 and 63.7 mg/kg/day, respectively. Based on the lower of these figures, a limit of 21 µg/day would be associated with a 1 in 100,000 risk level derived through simple linear extrapolation. In the absence of any other relevant data, it is suggested that the latter figure would be justifiable as a limit for ethylene oxide, particularly considering the likely existence of a threshold linked to endogenous exposure. However, it is recommended that further evaluation of the data is needed together, with additional research to enable a true assessment of the risk to be determined.

5.6.5 Formaldehyde (CAS No. 50-00-0)

Formaldehyde has a number of uses, including industrial use, primarily to manufacture resins, and also as a synthetic reagent in the manufacture of pharmaceuticals. Also, as for ethylene oxide above, formaldehyde is produced endogenously in the human body and can be found in air, food, and drinking water. With regard to its use in pharmaceutical manufacturing, there is a need to assess the risk to patients in the context of the mutagenic and carcinogenic studies highlighted below.

5.6.5.1 *Genotoxicity*   Formaldehyde is widely reported as mutagenic in the Ames test, showing a positive response in several strains, most clearly using the preincubation protocol. Although some negative results have been reported, these tend to relate to early studies and are potentially linked to evaporation of formaldehyde using the standard plate-incorporation method. It has also been shown to cause chromosomal damage and a variety of other mutagenic endpoints *in vitro* and *in vivo*. Based on this evidence, formaldehyde is considered to be mutagenic and clastogenic.

5.6.5.2 Carcinogenicity A number of animal studies, particularly rodent inhalation studies, have shown a clear correlation between exposure to formaldehyde and tumorigenesis, particularly squamous cell carcinomas of the nasal cavity. This is also accompanied by significant increases in mortality at higher doses.

Only a limited number of studies have assessed the carcinogenic potential of formaldehyde by the oral route of exposure. The most recent evaluation by the IARC cites four carcinogenicity studies in which formaldehyde was administered in drinking water to rats.[39] One study, in males only, showed an increased incidence of forestomach papillomas following treatment with the carcinogen N-methyl-N-nitro-nitrosoguanidine (MNNG)[40] A second study in male and female rats[41] reported statistically significant increases in the incidence of gastrointestinal leiomyosarcomas in females and in both sexes combined. These rats were the offspring of breeders (males and females) that had received formaldehyde in drinking water for life, and they themselves also received formaldehyde in drinking water from gestation onwards. A third study by Soffritti et al.[42], again in both sexes, reported an increase in the number of males that developed malignant tumors and the incidences of hemolymphoreticular tumors (lymphomas and leukaemias) and testicular interstitial-cell adenomas in males. However, a fourth study by Til et al.[43] showed no evidence of a formaldehyde-related tumor response when given for 104 weeks at mean dose levels of up to 82 mg/kg/day in males and 109 mg/kg/day in females.

In addition to animal studies, IRIS details a number of epidemiological studies focused on industrial workers exposed to formaldehyde and products containing formaldehyde, in particular those working in the resin manufacturing industry. The two largest studies conducted[44,45] both showed a significant increase in incidence of lung and nasopharyngeal cancer deaths, although no correlation was seen between level of exposure and incidence rates.

Based on these data, the IARC has classified formaldehyde as a known human carcinogen (Group 1[39]) while in the United States, it (specifically as formaldehyde gas) is classified as reasonably anticipated to be a human carcinogen by the NTP.

5.6.5.3 Sources of Exposure For decades, concerns have existed over exposure to formaldehyde, particularly formaldehyde vapor. These concerns apparently supported by the rodent carcinogenicity studies, and epidemiological studies reported above have led to legislation to tightly control exposure to formaldehyde by many regulatory authorities, with stringent standards being established for both air quality and drinking water.

To understand and assess the risk of exposure to formaldehyde, it is important to consider the total level of exposure to formaldehyde that occurs through a variety of routes, including inhalation, drinking, and through the diet. In relation to food, formaldehyde is a natural component present in many different food types, with levels varying significantly (see Table 5.3). It has been estimated that through the diet alone, the daily intake of formaldehyde is between 1.5–14 mg/day.[46]

TABLE 5.3 Formaldehyde Concentration in Various Food Groups[43]

Food type	Formaldehyde level (mg/kg)
Meat	5.7–20
Fish	6.4–293
Fruit/vegetables	1–98
Coffee	3.4–16

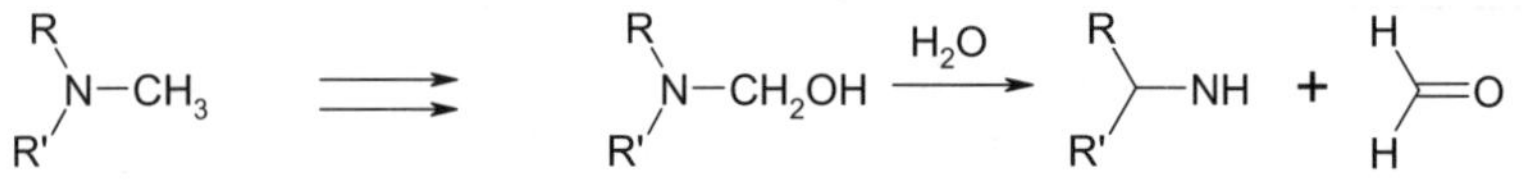

cP450 Mediated C-hydroxylation

Figure 5.3   Simplified mechanistic scheme of cytochrome P450-catalysed N-dimethylation.

Exogenous exposure to formaldehyde, however, represents only a small fraction of total human exposure; endogenous formation in animals and humans occurs as an integral part of the one-carbon metabolic process. It is estimated that turnover is of the order of 30–60 g per day.[45] Studies have shown that exogenous exposure has no impact on levels of formaldehyde within the body, with typical blood levels being around 2.5 ppm.[47] The half-life of formaldehyde is reported to be approximately 1.5 min, based on animal studies, due to metabolism to formic acid, and, ultimately, carbon dioxide.

Another potential source of exposure to formaldehyde can arise from pharmaceuticals, not through low-level chemical residues, but as a result of metabolism. N-demethylation (see Fig. 5.3) is a common metabolic pathway in humans and is catalyzed by cytochrome P450.[48] cP450 mediated C-hydroxylation results in generation of an unstable carbinolamine that undergoes rapid hydrolysis, forming the demethylated amine and formaldehyde.

Although less common, O-dealkylation can also occur in relation to aryl alkyl ethers.[48] In this instance, an unstable hemi-acetal is generated, which rapidly hydrolyses, yielding the corresponding alcohol and formaldehyde. As a practical example, this is the route by which codeine is activated to yield morphine.

5.6.5.4 Calculation of Limits   For inhalation exposure, the cancer risk assessment in the IRIS monograph indicates that the dose associated with a 1 in 100,000 lifetime cancer risk is $0.8 \mu g/m^3$, equating to a daily dose of $16 \mu g/day$ (assuming inhalation of $20 m^3$ air/day). Similarly, the Cal EPA has published a NSRL for formaldehyde gas of $40 \mu g/day$.

Regarding oral exposure to formaldehyde, a recent evaluation by WHO concluded that: "On the basis of studies in which humans and experimental animals were exposed to formaldehyde by inhalation, IARC…has classified formaldehyde in Group 1 (carcinogenic to humans). The weight of evidence indicates that formaldehyde is not carcinogenic by the oral route." This is supported by previous reviews by Restani and Galli[49] and IPCS[50], which concluded that formaldehyde is a normal mammalian metabolite and is not carcinogenic at low levels of exposure.

Furthermore, WHO commented that "Owing to formaldehyde's high reactivity, effects in the tissue of first contact following ingestion are more likely to be related to the concentration of the formaldehyde consumed than to its total intake. IPCS[50] has established a tolerable concentration of 2.6 mg/litre for ingested formaldehyde based on the NOEL of 260 mg/L for histopathological effects in the oral and gastric mucosa of rats administered formaldehyde in their drinking water for 2 years,[43] and using an uncertainty factor of 100 (for inter- and intraspecies variation)."

Based on this evaluation, the WHO did not consider it necessary to set a formal guideline value for formaldehyde as a result of the significant difference between the expected concentrations of formaldehyde in drinking water and the tolerable concentration. This conclusion appears to supersede a previous guideline value of 900 µg/L for formaldehyde in drinking water, published by the WHO in 1996 and derived from the same Til et al. paper.[43] A NOAEL of 15 mg/kg/day in this 2-year rat study was divided by a 100-fold uncertainty factor to account for inter- and intraspecies variation, and a body weight of 60 kg was used to derive a tolerable daily intake of 9 mg/day. From this, 20% (1.8 mg/day) was allocated to exposure from drinking water and using an assumed consumption value of 2 L drinking water/day, resulted in the guideline value of 900 µg/L.

It is interesting to observe that while the IRIS monograph has no cancer risk assessment for oral exposure to formaldehyde, it does list an oral RfD of 0.2 mg/kg/day that equates to a total dose of 14 mg/day (using the EPA default value of 70 kg body weight), a value very similar to the WHO TDI.

In summary, based on the different levels of concern and risk assessments related to inhalation and oral exposure for formaldehyde, it is appropriate to consider separate limits for these different routes of exposure. For drug substances administered by the inhalation route, the Cal EPA limit of 40 µg/day for formaldehyde can be justified and used to establish a concentration limit, based on the maximum therapeutic dose of the drug. For drugs administered by the oral route, guidance can be taken from the drinking water and other relevant evaluations in which intakes of 9–10 mg/day are considered to be tolerable. As described above, there are multiple potential sources of exposure to formaldehyde, and, as a result, it is appropriate to set a limit for potential exposure from pharmaceuticals as a fraction of the total acceptable limit. In this regard, the former WHO limit used 20% of the TDI, and so a limit from pharmaceutical sources of 10%–20% would seem justifiable and appropriate; giving rise to an oral dose limit of approximately 1–2 mg/day.

5.6.6 Alkyl Halides

Alkyl halides are widely used in synthetic chemistry as a means of incorporating alkyl groups into a molecule and thus are arguably the single largest class of alkylating agents encountered in synthetic chemistry. Due to their electrophilic nature, they are highly susceptible to nucleophilic attack from a range of nucleophiles, including natural bases, for example DNA. They are thus, as a class, potentially genotoxic, although in reality, their alkylating potential varies significantly and hence their genotoxicity also varies considerably. Within this subsection, three example alkyl halides are considered in more detail.

5.6.6.1 Methyl Iodide (CAS No. 74-88-4)

Methyl iodide (iodomethane) is perhaps the most classical example of an alkylating agent. It is commonly used to introduce methyl groups into a molecule, and is an excellent reagent for this purpose, as a result of its sterically unhindered structure and excellent leaving group in the form of iodide, making it a versatile reagent in SN_2 substitution reactions.

Genotoxicity Data CCRIS reports that methyl iodide shows a positive response with the *S. typhimurium* TA 100 strain, which is sensitive to the induction of point mutations. Both positive and negative results are reported for TA 1535. Great care is required for such tests due to the high volatility of methyl iodide and sealed systems need to be employed to avoid significant loss of compound during the test. Certainly, some results may be affected by such physical loss.

CCRIS also reports positive results in the mouse lymphoma test.

Based on these, data methyl iodide should be considered to be both mutagenic and clastogenic.

Carcinogenicity Studies

Animal Studies CCRIS contains two references to animal studies conducted on rats and mice. Both are reported to show positive findings.[51]

Human Data There are no reported human epidemiological studies of methyl iodide. Due to the lack of data, methyl iodide is classified as a class 3 substance (unclassifiable as to its carcinogenicity toward humans).[52] Furthermore, there are no reported data in the carcinogenicity potency database.[3]

This absence of data correlates with the investigations into the carcinogenicity database conducted by Delaney[53] that commented on the poor coverage in the database of reagents commonly used in synthetic processes. It was highlighted that as a result of the CPDB's origin, the database, and, certainly, the TTC concept derived from it, are skewed based on molecules more typically associated with the food arena than synthetic pharmaceutical manufacturing processes.

Calculation of Limits Due to the absence of any significant safety data upon which to base a quantitative cancer risk assessment, there is little option in the case of methyl iodide but to apply the standard TTC limit of 1.5 μg/day.

5.6.6.2 Benzyl Chloride (CAS No. 100-44-7)

Benzyl chloride is widely used in synthetic processes as a means to incorporate a benzyl protecting group into a molecule, usually to protect an alcohol. Such groups are typically removed through hydrogenation.

Genotoxicity Studies CCRIS reports that benzyl chloride shows a positive response with the *S. typhimurium* TA100 strain that is sensitive to the induction of point mutations. A positive response with *E. coli* WP2 uvrA(pKM101) is also reported. However, it has been suggested that benzyl chloride was generally not mutagenic in *in vivo* systems.[54]

Despite the equivocal findings in *in vivo* systems, based on a weight of evidence approach benzyl chloride is considered to be mutagenic.

Carcinogenicity Data

Animal Data   The data in the IRIS database for benzyl chloride include conclusions from a small number of rodent studies. The studies conducted vary from 2-year oral gavage rodent bioassay studies (benzyl chloride administered in corn oil) to skin studies aimed at assessing the potential of benzyl chloride to be a skin tumor initiator. The overall conclusion is that benzyl chloride is an animal carcinogen, based on a significant increase in both benign and malignant tumors at multiple sites in both male and female mice, and an increase in incidence of thyroid tumors in female rats.

Human Data   The IRIS database assessment reports the findings from a number of studies linked to occupational exposure to benzyl chloride. Although these appear to suggest increased incidences of some tumor types, the studies were considered inconclusive due to the fact that exposure was not limited to benzyl chloride, but was confounded by exposure to a number of other chlorinated compounds. Furthermore, no controls were in place in terms of smoking within the study population.

Calculation of Limits   The IRIS monograph on benzyl chloride gives a drinking water concentration at the 1 in 100,000 lifetime cancer risk level of $2\mu g/L$, which, adjusting to reflect typical daily water consumption of $2L$ per day, gives an intake of $4\mu g/day$.

The CPDB reports values for rat, mice, and hamster studies. Interestingly, it reports that there are no positive results for rats, including the study by Lijinsky,[55] which in the IRIS monograph is summarized as showing a significant treatment-related increase in thyroid C-cell adenoma/carcinoma in the female high-dose group. For mice, the CPDB reports a harmonic mean TD_{50} value of $61.5\,mg/kg/day$, but considerable variability (>10-fold) was noted. When converted to a dose representing a 1 in 100,000 risk by simple linear extrapolation, this equates to an acceptable risk dose of $62\mu g/day$, a figure significantly higher than both the standard TTC limit, and also the limit defined by the EPA IRIS risk assessment.

5.6.6.3   *n-Butyl Chloride (CAS No. 109-69-3)*

The IRIS risk assessment for n-butyl chloride includes references to a series of rodent carcinogenicity studies. These studies, oral gavage studies in rats and mice, were all reported to be negative. Furthermore, n-butyl chloride is also reported to be negative in all standard Ames test strains, in CHO cell *in vitro* chromosomal aberration tests, both with and without S9 activation. A review of the CPDB also shows that there are no positive findings in any rodent studies and thus no TD_{50} is reported.

Based on these data, it would seem appropriate to conclude that n-butyl chloride is both nongenotoxic and noncarcinogenic.

The three alkyl halides chosen for inclusion in this dataset were selected to illustrate the point that despite all belonging to the same class of potential genotoxins, that is alkyl halides, there is a significant difference in their actual activity. Indeed, n-butyl chloride is clearly nongenotoxic. It also illustrates the point that simple application of the TTC to all genotoxins, even those within the same class, without taking into account the nature of the agent in question, is a crude approach to assessment of risk.

5.6.6.4 *Common Nongenotoxic Reagents*

This final section highlights two reagents that have been subject to regulatory scrutiny based on purported genotoxicity. As a result of regulatory challenge, applicants have been asked to control both on the basis of assumed genotoxicity, and hence both have been, on occasion, subject to unnecessary measures and potential restrictions. This is despite, as illustrated below, no evidence that the reagents in question are genotoxic. Indeed evidence exists in both cases to support both being classified as nongenotoxic.

Carbon Disulfide (CAS No. 75-15-0) A detailed evaluation of both the genotoxicity and carcinogenicity of CS_2 was published by WHO.[56] This evaluation, performed by Environment Canada and Health Canada, concluded that the weight of evidence for both carcinogenicity and genotoxicity is considered inadequate. Specifically, this reported that in several studies in bacteria, carbon disulfide did not induce point mutations in *S. typhimurium* or in *E. coli*, both with and without metabolic activation. Evidence derived from in vitro studies performed using mammalian cells exposed to carbon disulfide was also equivocal.

The HSDB similarly reports that carbon disulphide shows no clear evidence of genotoxicity, although there is some evidence of weak and or no equivocal clastogenicity *in vitro* or *in vivo*. This dataset, albeit incomplete, does not appear to support a regulatory concern regarding the control of carbon disulphide as a genotoxic impurity.

Mesityl Oxide (CAS No. 141-79-7) Mesityl oxide, a potential impurity formed as a result of self-condensation of acetone, has been subjected to numerous genotoxicity assessments. Data published in the U.S. Federal Register indicate that when tested in an Ames test at up to 5000 µg/plate, the compound was negative for mutagenic activity (57 FR 29319, July 1, 1992). This negative finding in the Ames test has also been confirmed by Bingham et al. (2001),[57] and these authors provided additional data indicating mesityl oxide was also negative in a mouse micronucleus assay.

Further support for this originates from Cheh[58] who used *Salmonella* strain TA100 to show that mesityl oxide was nonmutagenic, but chlorinated mesityl oxide (mesityl chloride formed *in situ* from mesityl oxide added to pH buffered media containing sodium hypochlorite), formed in substantial amounts in the pH range 7.5 to 9.5 in chlorinated wastewater polluted with mesityl oxide, was mutagenic.

No other *in vivo* genotoxicity or carcinogenicity data relating to mesityl oxide were identified during the course of the construction of this chapter, and therefore the cause of the regulatory concern, beyond suspicion based on structure alone, remains unclear.

REFERENCES

1. EMEA. 2008. *Guideline on the limits of genotoxic impurities.* EMEA/CHMP/QWP/251344/2006.
2. Center for Drug Evaluation and Research (CDER). 2008, December. *Guidance for industry genotoxic and carcinogenic impurities in drug substances and products: Recommended approaches Draft.*
3. CPDB. 2007. *Summary Table by Chemical of Carcinogenicity Results in CPDB on 1547 Chemicals.* The Carcinogenic Potency Project of the University of California at Berkley, California, USA. Available at http://potency.berkeley.edu/cpdb.html (accessed September 2010).
4. Cal EPA. 2009. *Proposition 65 Safe Harbor Levels: No Significant Risk Levels for Carcinogens and Maximum Allowable Dose Levels for Chemicals Causing Reproductive Toxicity.* Reproductive and Cancer Hazard Assessment Branch, Office of Environmental Health Hazard Assessment, California Environmental Protection Agency. February 2009. Available at http://oehha.ca.gov/prop65.html (accessed September 2010).
5. Totsuka Y, Kataoka H, Takamura-Enya T, et al. 2007. *In vitro* and *in vivo* formation of aminophenyl-norharman from norharman and aniline. *Mutation Research* 506–507:49–54.
6. Kadlubar FF, Beland FA. 1985. Chemical properties of ultimate carcinogenic metabolites of aryl amines and arylamides. In: *Polycyclic Hydrocarbons and Carcinogenesis*, edited by RG Harvey. ACS Symposium Series, pp. 283, 341–370.
7. Kennelly JC, Stanton CA, Martin CN. 1984. The effect of acetyl-CoA supplementation on the mutagenicity of benzidines in the Ames assay. *Mutation Research* 137:39–45.
8. Watanabe M, Ishidate M Jr., Nohmi T. 1990. Sensitive method for the detection of mutagenic nitroarenes and aromatic amines: New derivatives of *Salmonella typhimurium* tester strains possessing elevated O-acetyltransferase levels. *Mutation Research* 234:337–348.
9. Glatt H, Meinl S. 2005. Sulfotransferases and acetyltransferases in mutagenicity testing: Technical aspects. *Methods in Enzymology* 400:230–249.
10. IARC. 1987. *Monographs on the Evaluation of Carcinogenic Risks to Humans, Overall Evaluations of Carcinogenicity: An Updating of IARC Monographs*, Vols. 1–42, Suppl. 7, pp. 99–100. International Agency for Research on Cancer, Lyon, France.
11. CIIT (Chemical Industrial Institute of Toxicology). 1982. 104-week chronic toxicity study in rats: Aniline hydrochloride. Final report.
12. NCI (National Cancer Institute). 1978. Bio-assay for aniline hydrochloride for possible carcinogenicity. ITS Carcinogenesis Technical Report Ser No. 130. US DHEW, PHS, NIH, Bethesda, MD. DHEW Publ. No (NIH) 78-1385.
13. Jeffrey AM, Iatropoulos MJ, Williams GM. 2006. Nasal cytotoxic and carcinogenic activities of systemically distributed organic chemicals. *Toxicologic Pathology* 34:827–852.
14. Jenkins FP, Robinson JA, Gellatly JBM, et al. 1972. The no-effect dose of aniline in human subjects and a comparison of aniline toxicity in man and the rat. *Food and Cosmetics Toxicology* 10:671–679.
15. IRIS. 2008. *United States Environmental Protection Agency Integrated Risk Information System Monograph on Aniline (CAS No 62-53-3).* Available at http://www.epa.gov/ncea/iris/subst/0350.htm (Version accessed January 10, 2008).
16. Robertson O, Cox MG, Bus JS. 1983. *Response of Blood, Spleen and Liver to Aniline Hydrochloride Insult in Male and Female Fischer 344 Rats and in Male B6C3F1 Mice.* (Cited in CIIT Activities publication).
17. ICH Q3C(R4). (2009). ICH harmonised tripartite guideline. Impurities: Guideline for residual solvents. *International Conference on Harmonisation of Technical Requirements for Registration of Pharmaceuticals for Human Use.* Current Step 4 version dated February 2009. Available at http://www.ich.org/LOB/media/MEDIA5254.pdf (accessed September 2010).
18. PharmEuropa. 1997. ICH Guideline: Residual Solvents. Toxicity data assessment extracted from ICH residual solvents guideline (step 2), Appendices 5 (toxicological data for class 1 solvents), 6 (toxicological data for class 2 solvents) and 7 (toxicological data for class 3 solvents). *PharmEuropa* 9(Suppl. 1):S5–S68.
19. Brock WJ, Hundley G, Lieder PH. 1990. Hepatic macromolecular binding and tissue distribution of ortho and para-toluidine in rats. *Toxicology Letters* 54(2–3):317–325.

20. Kerdar RS, Dehner D, Wild D. 1993. Reactivity and genotoxicity of aryl nitrenium ions in bacterial and mammalian cells. *Toxicology Letters* 67(1–3):73–85.

21. Aβmann N, Emmrich M, Kampf G, et al. 1997. Genotoxic activity of important nitrobenzenes and nitroanilines in the Ames test and their structure activity relationship. *Mutation Research* 395(2–3):139–144.

22. Chung K-T, Chen S-C, Wong TY, et al. 2000. Studies of Benzidine and its analogs: Structure-Activity relationships. *Toxicological Sciences* 56(2):351–356.

23. Hatch FT, Knize MG, Colvin ME. 2001. Extended quantitative structure-activity relationships for 80 aromatic and hetero-aromatic amines: Structural, electronic and hydropathic factors affecting mutagenic potency. *Environmental and Molecular Mutagenesis* 38(4):268–291.

24. Borosky GL. 2007. Ultimate carcinogenic metabolites from aromatic and heterocyclic aromatic amines: A computational study in relation to their mutagenic potency. *Chemical Research in Toxicology* 20(2):171–180.

25. Leach AG, Cann R, Tomasi S. 2009. Reaction energies computed with density functional theory correspond with a whole organism effect; modelling the Ames test for mutagenicity. *Chemical Communications* 9:1094–1096.

26. Von Burg R, Stout T. 1991. Hydrazine. *Journal of Applied Toxicology* 11:447–450.

27. Quintero-Ruiz A, Paz-Neri LL, Villa-Trevino S. 1981. Indirect alkylation of CBA mouse live DNA and RNA by hydrazine in vivo. A possible mechanism of action as a carcinogen. *Journal of the National Cancer Institute* 67(3):613–618.

28. Parodi S, Deflora S, Cavanna M. 1981. DNA-damaging activity *in vivo* and bacterial mutagenicity of sixteen hydrazine derivatives as related quantitatively to their carcinogenicity. *Cancer Research* 41:1469–1482.

29. Zeilmaker MJ, Horsfall MJ, van Helten JB. 1991. Mutational specificities of environmental carcinogens in the *lacI* gene of *Escherichia coli* H. V: DNA sequence analysis of mutations in bacteria recovered from the liver of Swiss mice exposed to 1,2-dimethylhydrazine, azoxymethane, and methylazoxymethanolacetate. *Molecular Carcinogenesis* 4:180–188.

30. IARC. 1999. *Monographs on the Evaluation of Carcinogenic Risks to Humans. Re-Evaluation of Some Organic Chemicals, Hydrazine and Hydrogen Peroxide*, Vol. 71, pp. 991–1013. International Agency for Research on Cancer, Lyon, France.

31. Kean T, McB. Miller JH, Skellern GC, Snodin D. 2006. Acceptance criteria for levels of hydrazine in substances for pharmaceutical use and analytical methods for its determination. *PharmEuropa Scientific Note* 2:23–33.

32. van Delft JH, Steenwinkel MJ, Groot AJ, et al. 1997. Determination of N-7 and O-6 methylguanine in rat liver DNA after oral exposure to hydrazine by use if immunochemical and electrochemical detection methods. *Fundamental and Applied Toxicology* 35(1):131–137.

33. Kroes R, Renwick AG, Cheeseman M, et al. 2004. Structure based thresholds of toxicological concern (TTC): Guidance for application to substances present at low levels in the diet. *Food and Chemical Toxicology* 42:65–83.

34. Mason MM, Cate CC, Baker J. 1971. Toxicology and carcinogenesis of various chemicals used in the preparation of vaccines. *Clinical Toxicology* 4:185–204.

35. Steenland KL, Stayner A, Greife W, et al. 1991. Mortality among workers exposed to ethylene oxide. *New England Journal of Medicine* 324(20):1402–1407.

36. Teta MJ, Benson LO, Vitale JN. 1993. Mortality study of ethylene oxide workers in chemical manufacturing: A 10-year update. *British Journal of Industrial Medicine* 50(8):704–709.

37. IARC. 1994. *Some Industrial Chemicals. IARC Monographs on the Evaluation of Carcinogenic Risk of Chemical to Humans*, Vol. 60. IARC, Lyon, France.

38. Bolt H. 1996. Quantification of endogenous carcinogens—The ethylene oxide paradox. *Biochemical Pharmacology* 52:1–5.

39. IARC. 2006. *Monographs on the Evaluation of Carcinogenic Risks to Humans, Overall Evaluations of Carcinogenicity: An Updating of IARC Monographs*, Vol. 88, pp. 1–487. International Agency for Research on Cancer, Lyon, France.

40. Takahashi M, Hasegawa F, Furukawa F, et al. 1986. Effects of ethanol, potassium metabisulfite, formaldehyde and hydrogen peroxide on gastric carcinogenesis in rats after initiation with N-methyl-N'-nitro-N'-nitrosoguanidine. *Japanese Journal of Cancer Research* 77:118–124.

41. Soffritti M, Maltoni C, Maffei F, et al. 1989. Formaldehyde: An experimental multi-potential carcinogen. *Toxicology and Industrial Health* 5(5):699–730.
42. Soffritti M, Belpoggi F, Lambertini L, et al. 2002. Results of long-term experimental studies on the carcinogenicity of formaldehyde and acetaldehyde in rats. *Annals of the New York Academy of Sciences* 982:87–105.
43. Til HP, Wouterson RA, Feron VJ. 1989. Two-year drinking water study of formaldehyde in rats. *Food and Chemical Toxicology* 27(2):77–87.
44. Blair A, Stewart P, Hoover RN. 1987. Cancers of the nasopharynx and oropharynx and formaldehyde exposure. *Journal National Cancer Institute* 78(1):191–193.
45. Stayner LT, Elliot L, Blade L, et al. 1988. A retrospective cohort mortality study of workers exposed to formaldehyde in the garment industry. *American Journal of Industrial Medicine* 13(6):667–682.
46. Dhareshwar SS, Stella VJ. 2008. Your pro-drug releases formaldehyde: Should be concerned? No! *Journal of Pharmaceutical Sciences* 97(10):4184–4192.
47. Heck H, Casanova-Schmitz M, Dodd PB, et al. 1985. Formaldehyde concentrations in the blood of humans and Fischer-344 rats exposed to $CH2_O$ under controlled conditions. *American Industrial Hygiene Association Journal* 46:1–3.
48. Testa B, Caldwell J. 1995. *The Metabolism of Drugs and Other Xenobiotics—Biochemistry of Redox Reactions.* Academic Press, London, pp. 204, 236.
49. Restani P, Galli CL. 1991. Oral toxicity of formaldehyde and its derivatives. *Critical Reviews in Toxicology* 21(5):315–328.
50. IPCS. 2002. *Formaldehyde.* Concise International Chemical Assessment Document No. 40. World Health Organization, Geneva.
51. Poirier LA, Stoner DK, Shimkin M. 1975. Bioassay of alkyl halides and nucleotide base analogs by pulmonary tumor response in strain A mice. *Cancer Research* 35:1411–1415.
52. IARC. 2009. *Agents Reviewed by the IARC Monographs*, Vols. 1–100A. Available at http://monographs.iarc.fr/ENG/Monographs/vol71/mono71-106.pdf (accessed September 2010).
53. Delaney E. 2007. An impact analysis of the application of the threshold of toxicological concern concept to pharmaceuticals. *Regulatory Toxicology and Pharmacology* 49:107.
54. Scott K, Topham JC. 1982. Sperm head abnormality test. *Mutation Research* 100:345–350.
55. Lijinsky W. 1986. Chronic bio-assay of benzyl chloride in F344 rats and (C57BL/6J x BALB/c)/F1 mice. *Journal of the National Cancer Institute* 76(6):1231–1236.
56. WHO. 2002. *International Programme on Chemical Safety INCHEM.* Concise International Chemical Assessment Document No. 46: CARBON DISULFIDE. Published under the joint sponsorship of the United Nations Environment Programme, the International Labour Organization, and the World Health Organization, and produced within the framework of the Inter-Organization Programme for the Sound Management of Chemicals. World Health Organization, Geneva. Available at http://www.inchem.org/documents/cicads/cicads/cicad46.htm#8.4 (accessed September 2010).
57. Bingham E, Cohrssen B, Powell CH. 2001. *Patty's Toxicology*, Vols. 1–9, 5th ed. John Wiley & Sons, New York, NY, pp. 6, 237.
58. Cheh AM. 1986. Mutagen production by chlorination of methylated alpha, beta-unsaturated ketones. *Mutation Research* 169(1–2):1–9.

CHAPTER 6

HUMAN GENOTOXIC METABOLITES: IDENTIFICATION AND RISK MANAGEMENT

Krista Dobo
Don Walker
Andrew Teasdale

6.1 INTRODUCTION

The following chapter looks to explore the challenging and complex issue of how to assess the potential presence and risk posed by genotoxic metabolites. Within this, it will examine the way in which metabolite studies are conducted and the challenges faced in looking to examine genotoxic metabolites through such studies. It will also look to consider in practical terms how the potential risk posed by a genotoxic metabolite may be addressed should it be discovered, outlining how ADME (absorption, distribution, metabolism, and elimination) data can be used to assess the extent of the risk posed.

To examine this in full, it is important to first consider what a metabolite is. In simple terms, a metabolite is a chemical modification of the drug by the body to alter it in such a way as to render it amenable to elimination from the body. Metabolism is the body's protection against natural poisons/xenobiotics. Metabolites can take a number of forms, they can be active—that is have a similar pharmacology to the drug itself and thus be of potential benefit, increasing efficacy; however, they may also be reactive, leading to a toxic effect. This is the particular concern relating to genotoxic metabolites, reactivity relating to genotoxicity, and hence ultimately a carcinogenic risk.

In general, drug metabolism involves the introduction or exposure of polar groups, and hence metabolites are more polar than the parent drug. This assists in their elimination, either by increasing water solubility and decreasing membrane permeability, thereby reducing reabsorption in the kidney or by recognition of the polar groups by transport proteins involved in elimination. The majority of drug

Genotoxic Impurities: Strategies for Identification and Control, Edited by Andrew Teasdale
Copyright © 2010 by John Wiley & Sons, Inc.

metabolism occurs within the liver and involves a range of enzymes and enzyme families. The metabolizing processes can broadly be categorized as Phase I and Phase II as follows:

Phase I: Oxidative and hydrolytic metabolism, for example hydroxylation, N-oxidation, de-alkylation, ester hydrolysis.

Phase II: Conjugation, for example glucuronidation, sulfation, and acetylation.

In the context of genotoxic metabolites, it is Phase I metabolism involving chemical modification that is typically of most interest. By far, the most important enzymes involved in oxidative metabolism are the cytochrome P450 (CYP) family of enzymes, which are involved in the metabolism of most drug molecules. At a cellular level, CYP metabolism takes place on the endoplasmic reticulum.

Cytochrome P450 enzymes are a huge superfamily of enzymes with molecular weights ranging from 45 to 55,000 Da, and are found across virtually all life forms, for example mammals, insects, bacteria, and even plants. These are based around a central heme unit and catalyze a vast array of oxidative reactions. There are, though, considerable differences across different species in terms of the CYP enzymes present, and this can obviously impact upon the correlation between animal and human metabolite studies. Despite the recognized differences in these enzymes, the chemical structure of drugs will provide sites on the molecule that are more vulnerable to metabolic conversion, and thus there is in general a high concordance (at least qualitatively if not quantitatively) of metabolic pathways between humans and laboratory animal species,[1] and human unique metabolites are rare.[2]

Another important area to consider is the pharmacokinetics of the molecules in question. Pharmacokinetics describes the movement of a compound into, around, and out of the body. Ultimately, when considering the potential risk posed by a genotoxic metabolite, it is important to appreciate the ADME of the drug and also any metabolites. This is explored in more detail later in the chapter.

A very important and perhaps obvious point to make relating to any metabolite is that it is difficult to modify the body's reaction to a drug, and hence any effective control over metabolites has to be achieved through the design of the drug itself. Thus, the most obvious way to avoid the issue of a genotoxic metabolite is to consider this during the design of a candidate drug. A good example of this involves embedded anilines that are built into the molecular structure through potential labile bonds, for example an amide/sulfonamide bond. Such bonds are susceptible to both chemical and enzymatic cleavage, "freeing" up the aniline as a potential metabolite. Within many organizations this is addressed by avoidance of labile anilines or through prescreening of anilines via an Ames test, ensuring that the aniline selected is nongenotoxic.

Metabolites are the subject of explicit regulatory guidance, specifically the FDA: Safety Testing of Metabolites (2008), often referred to as the MIST guidelines.[3] This proposes a level for a human metabolite of AUC_{ss} (area under the concentration vs. time curve at steady state) of 10% relative to the parent, above which the metabolite must be qualified. This threshold for metabolite qualification differs from that proposed in more recent ICH guidelines,[4] where a level of 10% of the total AUC of drug related material (i.e. 10% relative to parent plus all radiolabeled metabolites) is provided as an appropriate threshold for qualification. The ICH guideline has been recognized as taking precedence over the FDA guidance.[5] In practical terms, this equates to ensuring that sufficient exposure (i.e. equivalent to human exposure or greater) is achieved within animal studies, most importantly, carcinogenicity studies, to adequately qualify the metabolite concerned. Should any human metabolite not be qualified through exposure in at least one toxicology species, then specific additional studies may be required to assess its safety. It is not the purpose of this chapter to examine the metabolite guidelines themselves; however, it is important to highlight the practical difficulties experienced when trying to link metabolite guidelines and the European Medicines Agency (EMEA) guideline addressing genotoxic impurities (GIs).[6]

6.2   PREDICTING HUMAN METABOLITES

Clearly, in the context of a genotoxic metabolite, prevention or avoidance is the simplest and best option. To do so requires an understanding of possible human drug metabolism. One option is to utilize *in silico* predictive models. This is discussed in detail in Chapter 4, and involves the use of commercial systems, such as DEREK or MCase to examine the probability of an impurity being mutagenic. This can be extended to metabolites, and a number of metabolite prediction software packages are available. Indeed, Lhasa, who developed the DEREK software, have also developed software called METEOR, which can be used to predict metabolic pathways.[7] Predicted structures can then be screened for potential mutagenicity. Caution should, however, be taken when using such tools. There is a very real risk of overpredicting the extent and number of metabolites, and it is perhaps advisable to take any such predictions and examine them in the overall context of other *in vitro* and *in vivo* data relating to metabolites before screening.

Typically, in the discovery and development of a drug, the next available information relating to metabolites arises from *in vitro* studies.

6.2.1   *In Vitro* Metabolic Studies

Such studies are typically conducted using either hepatocytes or subcellular liver fractions, for example microsomes. Each system has advantages and disadvantages. Microsomes are simpler to work with, being easier to store; however, they generally only generate Phase I metabolites (likely to be sufficient in the context of evaluation of a genotoxic metabolite), and also require the addition of co-factors. Hepatocytes, on the other hand, possess a close to full complement of drug metabolizing enzymes, and hence are often considered more biologically relevant. However, hepatocytes are less amenable to storage, and therefore generally less convenient for routine use.

These studies are generally used to qualitatively assess potential metabolic pathways; however, correlation with actual human metabolite data can be variable. A thorough investigation into the predictive capability of *in vitro* systems demonstrated that the major metabolic pathway was correctly identified up to 90% of the time; however, predicting all human metabolites was only achieved 50% of the time or less.[8]

One specific weakness of such *in vitro* systems is the virtual absence of amidases. This is particularly pertinent in the context of amide bond cleavage, where such cleavage could result in generation of an aromatic amine as a metabolite (this being a potential genotoxic metabolite). Such studies have been shown to be a poor predictor of the stability of such bonds, subsequent studies in humans showing significant cleavage as a result of the much higher prevalence of amidases.

6.2.2 Early *In Vivo* Animal and Human Studies

Drug discovery programs will typically examine the pharmacokinetics of compounds in animal species used in pharmacology and toxicology studies. These are performed in order to understand the pharmacodynamic response seen in pharmacology models, and to optimize the pharmacokinetics of selected drug candidates. As part of this process, it will also be typical to obtain information on the metabolic fate of compounds in order that this, in conjunction with *in vitro* metabolism data, may be incorporated into the compound design strategy. As candidate molecules are selected and progressed through early toxicology studies, there is also the opportunity to gain an early insight into circulating metabolites that may be of safety concern. General toxicology studies are performed in two species, a rodent (most commonly the rat) and a nonrodent (often the dog, although occasionally primates). Other species may be used if specific to the drug discovery program. Studies are generally conducted using the clinical route of administration, often supplemented with intravenous studies that will allow the pharmacokinetic parameters, clearance, volume of distribution, and bioavailability to be obtained.

Such studies provide further insight into the role of metabolism in compound clearance and the metabolic fate of the compound in an intact animal, which may be different from that seen *in vitro*. However, they again can only be used to indicate potential human metabolites, which may differ from those in animal species. Such "metabolite scouting" studies can also be performed in early phase 1 clinical studies (single or multiple escalating dose studies in healthy volunteers) to gain real information on human metabolism *in vivo*. It should always be remembered, however, that such investigations, usually performed using unlabelled compound (nonradioactive), cannot be considered definitive, as metabolite products may go undetected due to loss during sample work-up or through detector insensitivity to the analyte. These studies can only be regarded as semi-quantitative at best, unless authentic metabolite standards are available to facilitate quantitation. That said, advances in mass spectrometer sensitivity over recent years means that much useful information can be gained early in the lifetime of a drug candidate that may be used to inform the risk assessment of drug metabolites prior to definitive (and costly) metabolism studies with radiolabeled compound.[9]

6.2.3 Radiolabeled Studies

Such studies are expensive and time consuming and require very careful planning and control. Synthesizing radiolabeled drug is itself nontrivial and expensive; there are also challenges and stringent safety precautions required for safe handling of radioactive materials. Finally, any such studies in humans needs to meet stringent requirements in terms of ethical approval. As a consequence, such studies have often, historically at least, been performed late in development, typically after the drug has been proven to provide the intended pharmacological action in clinical studies. The MIST debate and guideline has, however, led to reconsiderations on this timing or increased generation and utilization of nonradiolabeled metabolism information as discussed above. Either way, it is the metabolite information generated using radiolabeled compound that is considered to be definitive, as these studies ensure that all drug derived material is tracked and identified.

In terms of the studies themselves, these involve the administration of a "hot" radiolabeled form of the drug generally by the clinical route of administration at pharmacologically (human) or toxicologically relevant (animal species) dose levels. Blood and excreta are then collected and examined for total radioactivity to establish rates of clearance of total drug derived material and routes of elimination. Subsequent profiling of selected plasma and excreta samples by extraction and gradient elution HPLC allows for a quantitative profile of metabolites to be established. Such studies are described in detail elsewhere.[10,11] Although there are a number of isotopes available to utilize in such studies, most are performed using either tritium (^{3}H) or carbon-14 (^{14}C). The main reasons for this are the presence of carbon and hydrogen in all drug molecules, and the long half-lives of both isotopes. The long half-life precludes the need for any correction of data to compensate for radioactive decay. In terms of choice between the two, both have advantages and disadvantages. Tritium is often simpler from a synthetic perspective, and activity is higher, thus increasing the sensitivity of the assay, a potentially important factor in the context of a genotoxic metabolite. However, there are significant disadvantages in using tritium, principally the lack of biological stability; the tritium label can undergo hydrogen exchange or be displaced from its position and converted into tritiated water. This water will then enter the general body pool, complicating mass balance and losing the radiolabel from drug-derived metabolites. As a consequence, ^{14}C labeling is generally preferred in ADME studies, unless the complexity of the synthesis precludes its use.

Another important factor in such studies is the position of the radiolabel. The decision as to where to incorporate the label should take into consideration not only the feasibility of the synthesis, but also potential metabolic pathways. Placing the label in a metabolically labile (e.g. N-methyl) position could render the study meaningless, particularly in the context of where there is a specific metabolite of concern, for example a potentially genotoxic metabolite.

Without question though, such studies provide a very effective means of establishing both metabolite identities and quantifying the amount of metabolite formed, the latter ultimately being critical in assessing the risk posed by a genotoxic metabolite. There is, however, one final important point for consideration when evaluating data derived from such studies, and this relates to the excretory metabolites observed in such studies. Reactive metabolites may not be themselves detected in excreta. For example, phenol metabolites may well be detected as a glucuronide conjugates and other secondary metabolites.[12] This is particularly relevant in the context of genotoxic metabolites that by their very nature are likely to be reactive. Thus, evaluation of a genotoxic metabolite may well be indirect and complex, there being the potential, for example that several metabolites may be formed from the initial transitory genotoxic metabolite.[13]

6.2.4   Extent of Metabolite Formation

The control of GIs as defined within the EMEA guideline[6] and draft FDA guideline,[14] is based on the threshold of toxicological concern (TTC) principle (see Chapters 1 and 2 for a detailed examination of this principle). Thus, the risk posed by a GI needs to be assessed quantitatively via assay of the substance concerned. It is likely that a similar logic should apply to metabolites, and hence quantitative ADME data are critical to the assessment of the risk associated with a genotoxic metabolite.

While ultimately ADME data derived from radiolabeled studies provides the most accurate assessment of metabolite exposure, it is possible to obtain some estimate from *in vitro* studies. The prediction of human pharmacokinetics for novel agents is an established practice within the pharmaceutical industry using *in vitro* metabolism data, enzyme kinetic equations, and various physiological scaling factors.[15] Clearly there are caveats associated with a specific metabolic transformation within *in vitro* studies. However, such an approach could be used during early stages of drug development to ascertain whether or not there was a significant risk associated with a genotoxic metabolite when it is observed, by providing a more quantitative assessment. Scaling to the *in vivo* situation may then permit an informed decision to be made regarding the acceptability of such a risk.

6.2.5   Limitations of Metabolite Studies in the Context of Genotoxic Metabolites

As already highlighted, metabolite identification is a multistep process involving *in silico*, *in vitro*, and *in vivo* data that leads, over the timescale of the development of the drug, to an increasing understanding of the metabolic pathways involved. The level of understanding involved is, however, framed around the requirements defined by the regulatory guidelines concerning metabolite characterization and qualification. It is impractical, if not impossible, to rely on such studies to identify all potential genotoxic metabolites, certainly not at the levels that would be commensurate with the EMEA guideline covering GIs,[6] specifically the levels defined by the TTC concept. Thus, any assessment of likely genotoxic metabolites will necessarily need to involve a predictive element based on prior understanding of the potential risk of forming a genotoxic metabolite. This is perhaps best highlighted by the case of an "embedded" aromatic aniline linked into the drug substance molecule via a potentially labile bond.

Examples of embedded anilines (Fig. 6.1) include the β-adrenoreceptor antagonist, practolol, which was withdrawn from the market due to severe skin and eye lesions in some patients. Evidence points to liberation of the aromatic aniline via hydrolysis of the amide bond.[16] Another example is the insulin secretagogue, repaglinide, where oxidation of the piperidine ring has been shown to form the phenyl aniline metabolite as a major product in man.[17]

In such instances, there are essentially two options: (1) simply assume metabolism and design out any genotoxicity associated with the aniline; or (2) deliberately study and quantify through ADME studies the extent of metabolism. The latter approach may require the synthesis of radiolabel material to enable reliable quantification.

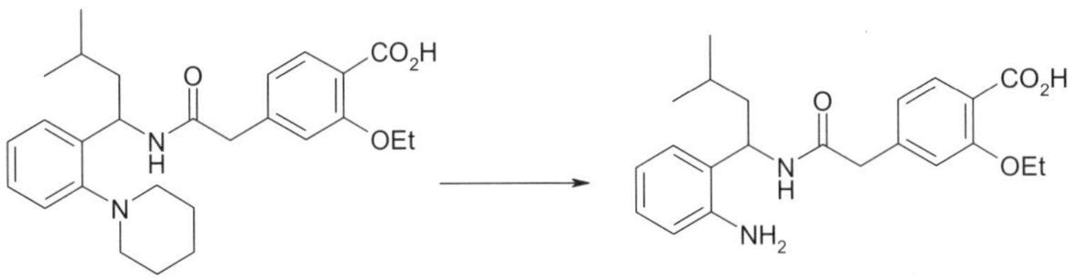

Repaglinide   Aniline metabolite

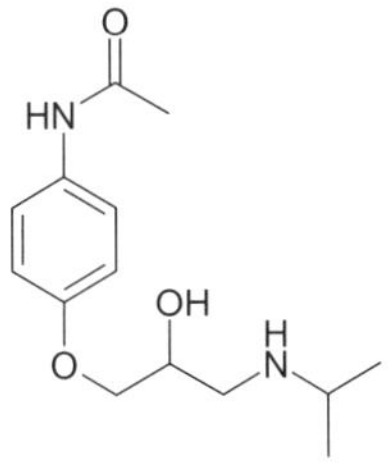

Practolol

Figure 6.1   Examples of embedded aniline structures in the insulin secretagogue, repaglinide and the β-adrenoreceptor antagonist, practolol.

As a consequence of the practical difficulties described and the increasing refinement of the knowledge surrounding metabolites, there remains the potential risk that a genotoxic metabolite may be identified during development after clinical trials have been instigated. In such a scenario, it is therefore important to understand how the risk posed by exposure to a genotoxic metabolite may be assessed. It is this scenario that is now considered in detail. This looks in particular as to how human ADME data can be correlated with animal ADME data obtained from carcinogenicity studies to provide a quantitative assessment of the cancer risk posed by exposure to the genotoxic metabolite in question.

6.3   GENOTOXIC METABOLITES DISCOVERED IN EARLY CLINICAL DEVELOPMENT

6.3.1   Background

Following the implementation of the EMEA guideline on limits for genotoxic impurities,[6] sponsors have increased scrutiny on the identification and control of GIs starting with the first human investigation. A consequence of this diligence is an increased likelihood of identifying or generating positive Ames bacterial mutation data for an intermediate, impurity, or degradant, which is also a potential human metabolite (meaning that the metabolite has been observed using *in vitro* models, but not yet confirmed to be present in humans).

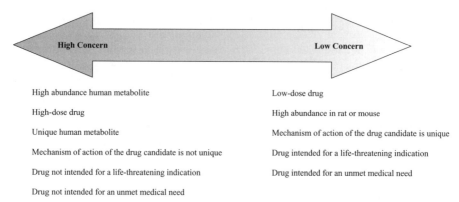

High abundance human metabolite

High-dose drug

Unique human metabolite

Mechanism of action of the drug candidate is not unique

Drug not intended for a life-threatening indication

Drug not intended for an unmet medical need

Low-dose drug

High abundance in rat or mouse

Mechanism of action of the drug candidate is unique

Drug intended for a life-threatening indication

Drug intended for an unmet medical need

Figure 6.2   Factors that influence degree of concern associated with exposure to a mutagenic metabolite during clinical development.

Discovery of a genotoxic impurity that is a potential human metabolite while preparing to initiate human clinical investigations is particularly problematic and warrants special consideration. The level of a metabolite, unlike impurities, clearly cannot be controlled via specified limits applied to the drug substance. In the case of metabolites, therefore, human investigations are needed to confirm the presence of a genotoxic metabolite and to assess the exposure and risk. For genotoxic impurities, it has been recommended that the acceptable excess cancer risk, and therefore the allowable limits in the drug product be exceptionally low because impurities impart no benefit to the patient.[6,18] In contrast, drug metabolism is associated with the intrinsic properties of the drug, such as pharmacokinetics, pharmacology, and clearance. Therefore, unlike impurities, the risk associated with exposure to a genotoxic metabolite needs to be considered on a case-by-case basis and balanced with the pharmaceutical benefit for each drug candidate. Figure 6.2 illustrates points to consider when evaluating risk associated with a genotoxic metabolite and the pharmaceutical benefit of the potential new drug.

There are some factors that differ between *in vitro* and *in vivo* genotoxicity testing, which may lead to the observation of a mutagenic response in the Ames assay that does not translate to a response *in vivo*. For example, differing metabolic pathways can exist *in vitro* and *in vivo*. Furthermore, in the intact animal, metabolic inactivation can occur, an active metabolite may not reach the target cell *in vivo*, or rapid detoxification and elimination can occur. Despite the fact that one might expect discrepancies between *in vitro* and *in vivo* test systems, developing a testing strategy to understand the risk and relevance of a mutagenic response observed in the Ames assay is a significant challenge for a drug candidate development project.

Currently, there is no guidance regarding appropriate follow-up testing strategies for understanding the risk and relevance of a mutagenic response in the Ames assay. The FDA guidance, "Recommended Approaches for Integration of Genetic Toxicology Study Results," provides general recommendations intended to support the safety of clinical study participants when genetic toxicology data suggests a potential cancer or genetic hazard exists.[19] However, this guidance is most useful when faced with a positive *in vitro* mammalian cytogenetic assay result. In general, if a drug substance tests positive in an *in vitro* genotoxicity assay, it is expected that a sponsor will provide evidence for a mechanism of action, as well as relevance of the mechanism at anticipated human exposures in order to support progression with clinical development.[19] Alternatively, a sponsor can try to rule out direct interaction with DNA. In those cases, in which the drug substance directly interacts with DNA, it is recommended that treatment be permitted for use in patients with debilitating or life-threatening diseases, such as cancer, but not be administered to healthy subjects.[19,20] The challenge with developing a testing strategy intended to understand the mechanism and relevance of a positive response in the Ames assay to subjects in a clinical investigation, is that the mechanism of action is assumed to involve direct interaction with DNA, with a linear dose response relationship, that is a "non-thresholded" mechanism. Thus, for a genotoxic metabolite suspected to be formed in human, a cautious approach to progressing with early clinical development, and, in some instances, rigorous *in vivo* genotoxicity testing, may be required to manage the safety of healthy volunteers and patients.

6.3.2 Factors for Consideration Prior to Initiation of Clinical Studies

In most cases in which a genotoxic metabolite is suspected to be formed in human, a clinical investigation involving a single dose of the drug candidate should be acceptable without the conduct of any additional genotoxicity testing. The rationale for this approach is that the duration of dosing is a key factor in the carcinogenic risk, as exemplified by Doll and Peto's[21] algorithm for the risk of carcinogenicity from tobacco smoke which factors both dose and duration. That is,

$$Risk = Dose^2 \times Duration^{4.5}$$

The algorithm shows that duration of dosing is key to the carcinogenic risk. Similarly, in deriving limits for genotoxic impurities, duration of treatment was a major factor in establishing allowable limits for clinical investigations of less than 12 months in duration.[14,18,22] The key assumption underlying the derivation of the limits is that carcinogenic risk is dependent on a stochastic mode of action (driven by total cumulative dose).[23]

Assuming the decision is taken to progress to a single-dose clinical investigation, an important objective would be to gather human metabolism data to assess exposure, as well as aid in the design of follow-up *in vivo* genotoxicity studies. First and foremost, it would be prudent to determine if the predicted human metabolite of concern is actually detected in humans. If the metabolite, and/or downstream metabolites of the predicted reactive species, are not detected, then this would significantly decrease concern about the risk posed to humans, as it indicates that the metabolite is not formed, or that it represents a pathway that is so minor that it is not detectable (thus minimizing exposure and risk). In cases where a human genotoxic metabolite is confirmed to be present in the single dose clinical investigation, a case-by-case evaluation regarding the appropriateness to progress to multidose clinical investigations would need to be conducted, taking into consideration factors such as those outlined in Figure 6.2.

Furthermore, in cases where the genotoxic metabolite is confirmed to be formed in humans, the need for additional genotoxicity testing to support multidose clinical investigations should be considered.

Ultimately, follow-up genotoxicity testing should be designed with the objective to understand the risk for a mutagenic effect *in vivo*. Although it is not possible to define a single testing strategy that would be appropriate in every case, there are a couple of major factors to consider. First and foremost, having information on exposure to the genotoxic metabolite in both human and nonclinical species is essential. This information will allow one to assess human exposure relative to achievable rodent exposures, such that the adequacy or limitations of any subsequent *in vivo* genotoxicity studies are understood. When designing *in vivo* genotoxicity tests for a metabolite of concern, ideally, the test species selected and doses administered will lead to the generation of quantities (e.g. mg/kg) that significantly exceed those formed in humans. What is considered an appropriate multiple over human exposure will need to be determined on a case-by-case basis. In general, the higher the multiple of rodent:human exposure, the greater the confidence there would be in utilizing the results to support decisions regarding continuation of human clinical investigations. Further, tissues that would be expected to be most highly exposed to the metabolite of concern should be the target of the genotoxicity assessment. For example, if the genotoxic metabolite is a circulating metabolite, blood and bone marrow may be the most appropriate tissue. In contrast, in cases where the metabolite of concern is highly reactive and rapidly conjugated, then the liver and possibly organs involved in excretion (colon and bladder) would likely be more appropriate sites of assessment. Finally, the decision as to when within the clinical development timeline to conduct follow-up studies should take into consideration that the induction of gene mutations is not a reversible event, and it has been experimentally demonstrated that chronic exposures to mutagens can lead to an accumulation of DNA damage (i.e. increased mutant frequency over time)[24-29] Therefore, in some cases, it may be prudent to conduct additional *in vivo* genotoxicity studies prior to initiating multidose clinical investigations.

6.3.3   Preclinical Testing to Support Clinical Study Progression

There are numerous *in vivo* genotoxicity assays that have been shown to be sensitive to the detection of mutations or DNA lesions. However, many *in vivo* test systems are limited, in that mutation or DNA damage can only be assessed in one or two tissues, as is the case with specific locus mutation assays using endogenous genes.[30-35] Currently, there are only a few *in vivo* assays that allow for the evaluation of mutation induction or DNA damage in all potential target tissues of interest for human genotoxic metabolites. Those which would be most broadly applicable (and subject of further description) include the *in vivo* comet assay and transgenic rodent mutation models, such as commercially available Muta™Mouse[36] and BigBlue® rat and mouse.[37] Both the *in vivo* comet assay and *in vivo* transgenic mutation assays have been the topic of international workshops, which have published guidance on general conduct of the assay, test conditions, and data interpretation.[25,38-41] Therefore, although no regulatory harmonized guidance is yet available, the proceedings of these workshops are a valuable resource for pharmaceutical sponsors interested in conducting the studies.

Introduced by Östling and Johanson,[42] the comet assay (single-cell gel electrophoresis) assesses DNA damage by placing a single cell suspension into an agarose matrix, which is then subjected to electrophoresis. DNA damage is viewed microscopically as fragments of DNA migrate away from the main nuclear region, giving the appearance of a comet. Although there are various conditions to which cells can be exposed in the conduct of the assay, the alkaline variation (pH for DNA unwinding and electrophoresis ≥ 13) developed by Singh[43] is considered the method of choice, as it can detect the broadest spectrum of DNA damage including alkaline labile sites and single strand breaks associated with incomplete excision repair both which have relevance to the induction of mutations[39,41] In the context of *in vivo* follow-up testing for a genotoxic metabolite, the major advantage of the comet assay is that DNA damage can be assessed in any tissue for which a single cell suspension can be prepared. In addition to this simple requirement, some other advantages of the comet assay include (1) sensitivity to detect low levels of DNA damage; (2) DNA fragmentation can be evaluated following an acute treatment regimen; (3) DNA damage can be rapidly quantitated using a relatively small number of cells per sample; (4) there is the potential to conduct the assay in a variety of non-clinical toxicology species (e.g. whichever affords the greatest exposure to the genotoxic metabolite of concern); and (5) the assay is relatively inexpensive and not very time consuming to conduct. The main disadvantage of the comet assay is that it detects DNA damage that may not ultimately result in mutations. It is recommended that tissues be collected 2–6h after the last treatment (in cases where test article is administered for 2 days or more), as well as at 16–24h post final treatment (in cases where a single acute treatment is administered).[39,41] The early sampling time is intended to afford sensitivity to rapidly absorbed as well as unstable or direct-acting compounds, while the later sampling time should detect compounds that are more slowly absorbed, distributed, and metabolized. However, it is possible that damage detected shortly after test article exposure may represent DNA lesions that are readily repaired and have no mutagenic consequence. Another limitation of the comet assay that is important to consider in the context of understanding the mutagenic risk associated with longer term exposure to a genotoxic metabolite, is that it would not be expected to be sensitive to the accumulation of DNA damage.

In contrast to the comet assay, *in vivo* transgenic mutation models detect the ultimate endpoint of concern, that is the potential to form fixed, heritable, mutations in DNA. Furthermore, these models have been shown to be sensitive to the detection of the accumulation of DNA damage over time,[25,40,44,45] this is particularly relevant to cases where humans are expected to be chronically exposed to a metabolite shown to be mutagenic *in vitro*. In transgenic animal models, such as MutaMouse and BigBlue® (which have been most widely utilized), all cells contain multiple tandem copies of a bacterial reporter gene (e.g. *lac Z*, *lac I*), embedded in a bacteriophage lambda shuttle vector. Therefore, the assay allows the screening of a large number of copies of the locus quickly in any tissue of interest. Determination of mutation frequency is carried out by extracting DNA from the tissue(s) of interest, packaging the lambda shuttle vector *in vitro* in lambda phage heads, infecting an appropriate bacterial strain with the phage DNA, and then testing for the presence of mutations. This is accomplished by plating the bacteria onto selective medium that effectively differentiates cells carrying wild-type and mutated reporter genes. Comprehensive recommendations for the design and conduct of transgenic studies have been reported following International Workshops on Genotoxicity Testing held in 1999 and 2001.[25,40] Although the details of these publications will not be reviewed here, it is important to note that the recommended duration of treatment is 28 days, such that even a weak mutagen would be expected to be readily detected.[40] In addition to the fact that a transgenic mutation assay requires a significant amount of time to complete, the use of transgenic animals also makes the assay costly. Despite the time and cost, transgenic animal models perhaps provide the best validated approach for investigating tissue-specific induction of mutations and the clarification of *in vitro* gene mutation findings. Therefore, for a drug candidate with a human metabolite showing evidence of mutagenicity in the Ames assay, one should consider the conduct of a transgenic assay prior to progressing into longer term multidose clinical investigations (e.g. ≥1 month).

In summary for early development, case-by-case evaluation of risk and pharmaceutical benefit should be considered when making decisions to progress with clinical investigations. In addition case-by-case consideration should be given to the design and conduct of *in vivo* genotoxicity testing intended to assess the risk and relevance of positive findings in the Ames mutation assay. Single-dose clinical investigations by the nature of the limited duration of treatment pose little risk and allow the generation of additional information on human and rodent exposures to the metabolites, which is critical in characterizing human risk, as well as facilitating the design of any *in vivo* follow-up testing. Ultimately, decisions to conduct genotoxicity assessments to better understand the risk and relevance of positive Ames results to *in vivo* situation, as well as continue to progress with clinical development, need to be made by balancing the anticipated benefit of a given drug candidate against risks to patients.

6.4 GENOTOXIC METABOLITES DISCOVERED IN LATE CLINICAL DEVELOPMENT

The conduct of genotoxicity testing for drug synthesis intermediates, often needed to comply with worker safety and transportation regulations, is typically conducted in parallel with Phase 2 and/or Phase 3 clinical investigations. In some instances, a synthetic intermediate of a drug candidate is also a known or suspected human metabolite. Consequently, there are cases in which the genotoxic potential of a human metabolite can be discovered in the later stages of clinical development.

As was suggested for early development, one could conduct acute and subchronic *in vivo* genotoxicity testing to understand the relevance of the *in vitro* finding to support important late stage development decisions (i.e. continue, delay, or discontinue clinical development). However, unlike the early stages of clinical development, in the later stages, many metabolites have been identified and quantitated in human and nonclinical toxicology species. Having this information available allows a robust assessment of human and rodent exposure to be conducted. Furthermore, if carcinogenicity testing has been conducted or is being planned, it is possible that the outcome of the rodent carcinogenicity studies can provide perspective with regards to the carcinogenic risk associated with long-term exposure to a genotoxic metabolite. Therefore, another approach to consider in the later stages of drug development is the conduct of a human carcinogenic risk assessment.

Risk-based safety assessments have been applied to manage human exposure to genotoxic/carcinogenic compounds for numerous situations. The most recent example of broad application of risk-based safety assessments within the pharmaceutical industry is establishing allowable limits of exposure to GIs present in active pharmaceutical ingredients[6,14] The same basic and highly conservative assumptions underlying the risk-based approach for impurities were used to derive a risk-based approach for assessing genotoxic metabolites of pharmaceuticals.[12] Similar to the approach that is applied to GIs, one factor that is taken into consideration is the expected human daily exposure to the genotoxic metabolite. However, unlike other risk assessments, the method proposed for genotoxic metabolites also takes advantage of the possibility that exposures in rodent carcinogenicity testing may be relatively high compared with human exposure. Thus, an additional factor, which is the total body burden of the genotoxic metabolite in rodents, is incorporated into the risk assessment framework. The intent is to determine the probability that metabolite exposure in a 2-year rat or mouse carcinogenicity assay is high enough to detect an oncogenic and/or tumorigenic signal.

Robust exposure data is essential to the conduct of the risk assessment determination for genotoxic metabolites and therefore relies on the availability of both human and rodent quantitative ADME data. More specifically, excreted drug-related material is used to quantify the total body burden to the genotoxic metabolite in both species. This quantitative data is then used to estimate the total body burden to the genotoxic metabolite in rodents at the highest dose utilized in rodent carcinogenicity test, as well as in humans at the intended efficacious concentration. The specific approach for quantifying the total body burden to a genotoxic metabolite, the method for deriving cancer risk estimates, and important underlying assumptions, are described in detail elsewhere.[12] However, a couple of key principles associated with estimating the carcinogenic risk are highlighted in Table 6.1 and are as follows. First, the probability of a favorable cancer risk assessment outcome increases as exposure in rodents' increases. For example, if the effective animal exposure to the metabolite is >10 mg/kg/day, then there is a high probability (88%–100%) of not exceeding a 10^{-5} excess cancer risk, because high rodent exposures increases detection in the carcinogenicity study. Second, the probability of not exceeding an acceptable excess cancer risk over background increases as human exposure decreases. That is, low human exposure decreases the potential effect of a genotoxic metabolite. For example, metabolite exposure of 0.00001 mg/kg or less has a high probability (93%–100%) of not exceeding an excess cancer risk of 10^{-5}. Lastly, the probability of a favorable risk assessment outcome also increases as the ratio of animal exposure over human exposure increases. For example, when the ratio is 1000× or greater, there is a high probability (92%–100%) of not exceeding a 10^{-5} excess cancer risk,

TABLE 6.1 Total Probability of Not Exceeding a 1 in 100,000 Cancer Risk for a Genotoxic Metabolite[45]

		Human exposure to metabolite (mg/kg)							
		100	10	1	0.1	0.01	0.001	0.0001	0.00001
Animal preclinical exposure to metabolite (mg/kg)	100	97%	97%	97%	97%	100%	100%	100%	100%
	10	88%	88%	88%	88%	94%	100%	100%	100%
	1	74%	74%	74%	74%	80%	92%	100%	100%
	0.1	61%	61%	61%	61%	67%	78%	93%	100%
	0.01	54%	54%	54%	54%	60%	71%	86%	97%
	0.001	51%	51%	51%	51%	57%	69%	83%	94%
	0.0001	50%	50%	50%	50%	56%	68%	83%	93%
	0.00001	50%	50%	50%	50%	56%	68%	82%	93%

1. The model was adapted from Fiori and Meyerhoff,[46] which analyzed the carcinogenic potencies of 705 animal carcinogens.

2. Animal preclinical exposure is the total body burden to the metabolite estimated in the 2 year oncogenicity study. It can be estimated by using short-term radiolabeled animal studies in the same species.

3. Human exposure is the total body burden to the metabolite estimated in humans. It can be estimated by using radiolabeled clinical studies.

4. ▭ Where the combination of exposure in animals and humans results in a probability below 85% of not exceeding a 1 in 100,000 excess risk of cancer.

with a favorable contribution from both the likelihood of detection in the rodent carcinogenicity study and low human exposure.

It is important to mention a couple of observations that were reported following the evaluation of the genotoxic metabolite risk assessment method using pharmaceutical case studies.[12] A significant conclusion from this work was that the lifetime daily limit for human exposure of 1.5 µg/day (as is used for GIs) is not a practical limit for metabolites. This is due to the fact that metabolites present at such a low total body burden would rarely, if ever, be identified and quantitated. Radiometric HPLC, which is used to quantitate metabolites, struggles to reliably quantitate metabolites that represent less than 5% of the radiolabelled material.[46] For example in the case of low dose drugs, for example 10 or 1 mg/day, the limit for quantitating metabolites would be 500 or 50 µg/day, respectively. In addition, the evaluation of case studies indicated that the total body burden to genotoxic metabolites in rodents had a greater influence on the outcome of the risk assessment than other factors. In effect, the methodology allows one to understand if the amount of metabolite formed in the rodent is sufficient to provide confidence that a negative outcome in a carcinogenicity study in essence "qualifies" the metabolite(s) of concern. Therefore, the model could also be used proactively in the selection of doses for the rodent carcinogenicity studies. That is, assuming that there is knowledge of a human metabolite of genotoxic concern prior to initiation of a 2-year bioassay, and that the metabolite is also formed in rodent, then a sponsor could consider feasibility of selecting doses that would provide confidence in metabolite qualification (e.g. ≥10 mg/kg/day exposure to metabolite or other criteria).

In applying this or any other carcinogenic risk assessment approach, an acceptable risk would need to be considered on a case-by-case basis, and would be variable depending on a number of factors. For example, an acceptable daily exposure could be adjusted upwards for those pharmaceuticals administered over a less-than-lifetime duration. In the case of GIs, it has been recommended that the duration of treatment be accounted for in establishing an allowable limit, that is higher exposure limits have been defined for short-term exposure conditions.[18,22] Similar considerations could be incorporated into the risk assessment framework for genotoxic metabolites to account for treatment scenarios that are intended for less than lifetime treatment. Also, when a metabolite is related to a drug for an unmet medical need, one must also consider the benefit of the medication when considering the risks of the metabolite. A precedent for this perspective can be found in the FDA Guidance on Safety Testing of Drug Metabolites, which exempts drugs for life-saving diseases from the proposed recommendations.[3] The patient population is another consideration, and increased or decreased conservatism may be appropriate for certain groups. For example, ICH S9 indicates that genotoxicity testing is not essential to treat patients with advanced cancer, but rather should be performed to support marketing.[47] It would seem reasonable to extend similar expectations to the characterization of metabolites, even those that show evidence of mutagenicity in the Ames assay. Ultimately, the conduct and outcome of a carcinogenic risk assessment for a human genotoxic metabolite should be considered a tool to aid in making drug development decisions. However, using this information in the context of good judgment, considerations of other existing relevant regulatory guidance, and understanding the risk/benefit of the medication is essential.

REFERENCES

1. Smith DA. 1991. Species differences in metabolism and pharmacokinetics: Are we close to an understanding? *Drug Metab. Rev.* 23:355–373.
2. Leclercq L, Cuyckens F, Mannens GSJ, et al. 2009. Which human metabolites have we MIST? Retrospective analysis, practical aspects, and perspectives for metabolite identification and quantification in pharmaceutical development. *Chem. Res. Toxicol.* 22:280–293.
3. FDA Guidance for Industry. 2008. *Safety Testing of Drug Metabolites*. Available at http://www.fda.gov/downloads/Drugs/GuidanceComplianceRegulatoryInformation/Guidances/ucm079266.pdf.
4. ICH M3 (S2). *Note for Guidance on Non-Clinical Safety Studies for the Conduct of Human Clinical Trials and Marketing Authorization for Pharmaceuticals*. Available at http://www.emea.europa.eu/pdfs/human/ich/028695en.pdf.
5. Robison TW, Jacobs A. 2009. Metabolites in safety testing. *Bioanalysis* 1:1193–1200.
6. Committee for Medicinal Products for Human Use (CHMP). 2006. *Guidelines on the limits of genotoxic impurities*. London, June 26. CPMP/SWP/5199/02.
7. Anari MR, Baillie TA. 2005. Bridging cheminformatic metabolite prediction and tandem mass spectrometry. *Drug Discov. Today* 10:711–717.
8. Dalvie D, Obach RS, Kang P, et al. 2009. Assessment of three human *in vitro* systems in the generation of major human excretory and circulating metabolites. *Chem. Res. Toxicol.* 22:357–368.

9. Walker D, Brady J, Dalvie D, et al. 2009. A holistic strategy for characterizing drug metabolites through drug discovery and development. *Chem. Res. Toxicol.* 22:1653–1662.

10. Penner N, Kluk LJ, Prakash C. 2009. Human radiolabelled mass balance studies, objectives, utilities and limitations. *Biopharm. Drug Dispos.* 30:185–203.

11. Roffey SJ, Obach RS, Gedge JI, et al. 2007. What is the objective of the mass balance study? A retrospective analysis of data in animal and human excretion studies employing radiolabelled drug. *Drug Metab. Rev.* 39:17–43.

12. Dobo KL, Obach RS, Luffer-Atlas D, et al. 2009. A strategy for the risk assessment of human genotoxic metabolites. *Chem. Res. Toxicol.* 22:348–356.

13. Smith DA, Obach RS, Williams DP, et al. 2009. Clearing the MIST (metabolites in safety testing) of time: The impact of duration of administration on drug metabolite toxicity. *Chem. Biol. Interact.* 179:60–67.

14. Center for Drug Evaluation and Research (CDER). December. 2008. *Guidance for industry genotoxic and carcinogenic impurities in drug substances and products: Recommended approaches draft.*

15. Obach RS, Baxter JG, Liston TE, et al. 1997. The prediction of human pharmacokinetic parameters from preclinical and *in vitro* metabolism data. *J. Pharmacol. Exp. Ther.* 283:46–58.

16. Nelson SD. 1982. Metabolic activation and drug toxicity. *J. Med. Chem.* 25:753–765.

17. Bidstrup TB, Bjørnsdottir I, Sidelmann UG, et al. 2003. CYP2C8 and CYP3A4 are the principal enzymes involved in the human *in vitro* biotransformation of the insulin secretagogue repaglinide. *Br. J. Clin. Pharmacol.* 56:305–314.

18. Muller L, Mauthe RJ, Riley CM, et al. 2006. A rationale for determining, testing, and controlling specific impurities in pharmaceuticals that possess potential for genotoxicity. *Regul. Toxicol. Pharmacol.* 44:198–211.

19. Center for Drug Evaluation and Research (CDER). 2006. *FDA Guidance for Industry and Review Staff: Recommended Approaches to Integration of Genetic Toxicology Study Results.* FDA, Rockville, MD.

20. International Conference on Harmonization. 1996. ICH S2A: Guideline for industry: Specific aspects of regulatory gentoxicity tests for pharmaceuticals. *International Conference on Harmonization.*

21. Doll R. 1978. An epidemiological perspective of the biology of cancer. *Cancer Res.* 38: 3573–3583.

22. European Medicines Agency. 2008. *CHMP question and answers on the CHMP guideline on the limits of genotoxic impurities.*

23. Bos PM, Baars BJ, van Raaij MT. 2004. Risk assessment of peak exposure to genotoxic carcinogens: A pragmatic approach. *Toxicol. Lett.* 151:43–50.

24. Aidoo A, Lyn-Cook LE, Heflich RH, et al. 1993. The effect of time after treatment, treatment schedule and animal age on the frequency of 6-thioguanine-resistant T-lymphocytes induced in Fischer 344 rats by N-ethyl-N-nitrosourea. *Mutat. Res.* 298:169–178.

25. Heddle JA, Dean S, Nohmi T, et al. 2000. In vivo transgenic mutation assays. *Environ. Mol. Mutagen.* 35:253–259.

26. Hitotsumachi S, Carpenter DA, Russell WL. 1985. Dose-repetition increases the mutagenic effectiveness of N-ethyl-N-nitrosourea in mouse spermatogonia. *Proc. Natl. Acad. Sci. USA* 82:6619–6621.

27. Miura D, Dobrovolsky VN, Kimoto T, et al. 2009. Accumulation and persistence of Pig-A mutant peripheral red blood cells following treatment of rats with single and split doses of N-ethyl-N-nitrosourea. *Mutat. Res.* 677:86–92.

28. Tao KS, Heddle JA. 1994. The accumulation and persistence of somatic mutations in vivo. *Mutagenesis* 9:187–191.

29. Tao KS, Urlando C, Heddle JA. 1993. Mutagenicity of methyl methanesulfonate (MMS) in vivo at the Dlb-1 native locus and a lacI transgene. *Environ. Mol. Mutagen.* 22:293–296.

30. Aidoo A, Lyn-Cook LE, Mittelstaedt RA, et al. 1991. Induction of 6-thioguanine-resistant lymphocytes in Fischer 344 rats following in vivo exposure to N-ethyl-N-nitrosourea and cyclophosphamide. *Environ. Mol. Mutagen.* 17:141–151.

31. Bryce SM, Bemis JC, Dertinger SD. 2008. In vivo mutation assay based on the endogenous Pig-a locus. *Environ. Mol. Mutagen.* 49:256–264.

32. Jones IM, Burkhart-Schultz K, Carrano AV. 1985. A method to quantify spontaneous and in vivo induced thioguanine-resistant mouse lymphocytes. *Mutat. Res.* 147:97–105.

33. Miura D, Dobrovolsky VN, Kasahara Y, et al. 2008. Development of an in vivo gene mutation assay using the endogenous Pig-A gene: I. Flow cytometric detection of CD59-negative peripheral red blood cells and CD48-negative spleen T-cells from the rat. *Environ. Mol. Mutagen.* 49:614–621.

34. Miura D, Dobrovolsky VN, Mittelstaedt RA, et al. 2008. Development of an in vivo gene mutation assay using the endogenous Pig-A gene: II. Selection of Pig-A mutant rat spleen T-cells with proaerolysin and sequencing Pig-A cDNA from the mutants. *Environ. Mol. Mutagen.* 49:622–630.

35. Winton DJ, Blount MA, Ponder BA. 1998. A clonal marker induced by mutation in mouse intestinal epithelium. *Nature* 333:463–466.

36. Gossen JA, de Leeuw WJ, Tan CH, et al. 1989. Efficient rescue of integrated shuttle vectors from transgenic mice: A model for studying mutations in vivo. *Proc. Natl. Acad. Sci. USA* 86:7971–7975.

37. Kohler SW, Provost GS, Fieck A, et al. 1991. Short spectra of spontaneous and mutagen-induced mutations in the lacI gene in transgenic mice. *Proc. Natl. Acad. Sci. USA* 88:7958–7962.

38. Burlinson B, Tice RR, Speit G, et al. 2007. Fourth International Workgroup on Genotoxicity testing: Results of the in vivo Comet assay workgroup. *Mutat. Res.* 627:31–35.

39. Hartmann A, Agurell E, Beevers C, et al. 2003. Recommendations for conducting the in vivo alkaline Comet assay. 4th International Comet Assay Workshop. *Mutagenesis* 18:45–51.

40. Thybaud V, Dean S, Nohmi T, et al. 2003. In vivo transgenic mutation assays. *Mutat. Res.* 540:141–151.

41. Tice RR, Agurell E, Anderson D, et al. 2000. Single cell gel/comet assay: Guidelines for *in vitro* and in vivo genetic toxicology testing. *Environ. Mol. Mutagen.* 35:206–221.

42. Ostling O, Johanson KJ. 1984. Microelectrophoretic study of radiation-induced DNA damages in individual mammalian cells. *Biochem. Biophys. Res. Commun.* 123:291–298.

43. Singh NP, McCoy MT, Tice RR, et al. 1988. A simple technique for quantitation of low levels of DNA damage in individual cells. *Exp. Cell Res.* 175:184–191.

44. Chen T, Mittelstaedt RA, Aidoo A, et al. 2001. Comparison of hprt and lacI mutant frequency with DNA adduct formation in N-hydroxy-2-acetylaminofluorene-treated Big Blue rats. *Environ. Mol. Mutagen.* 37:195–202.

45. Zhang XB, Felton JS, Tucker JD, et al. 1996. Intestinal mutagenicity of two carcinogenic food mutagens in transgenic mice: 2-amino-1-methyl-6-phenylimidazo[4,5-b]pyridine and amino(alpha) carboline. *Carcinogenesis* 17:2259–2265.

46. Smith DA, Obach RS. 2006. Metabolites and safety: What are the concerns, and how should we address them? *Chem. Res. Toxicol.* 19:1570–1579.

47. International Conference on Harmonization. 2010. ICH guidance for industry: S9 nonclinical evaluation for anticancer pharmaceuticals. *International Conference for Harmonization.*

PART 3

PERSPECTIVE ON RISK POSED BY GENOTOXIC IMPURITIES

CHAPTER 7

GENOTOXIC THRESHOLDS

Gareth J.S. Jenkins
George E. Johnson
James M. Parry
Shareen H. Doak

7.1 INTRODUCTION TO GENOTOXIC DOSE RESPONSES

In genetic toxicology, induced DNA damage is used as a surrogate for cancer risk, as it is well known that cancer is induced by genetic aberrations. Therefore, genetic damage (mutation) is often used as a short term biomarker of cancer risk. In terms of dose responses, while there has been linearity assigned to genotoxic dose responses (see below), the dose relationship with cancer induction is much less clear. This is partly due to the expense (and number of animals required) to investigate this aspect thoroughly. It has been suggested that cancer is induced in a nonlinear fashion, and this certainly reflects human carcinogenesis, where a number of genetic hits are known to be required to induce cancer. Indeed, linearity in the cancer response would lead to tumor formation occurring much more frequently in the human population. Therefore, it has been suggested that the dose responses for mutation and cancer differ. This has been well demonstrated by some researchers. For example, Williams et al.,[1] showed elegantly that initial DNA damage (adduct formation) was induced in a linear-like manner, whereas later neoplastic lesions (hepatocellular altered foci) and frank tumors were induced in a markedly nonlinear manner. More recently, Bailey et al.[2] demonstrated in a "mega-animal" study that cancer was induced by dibenzopyrene (DBP) in a decidedly nonlinear manner using trout as a model organism, which allowed very large animal numbers (>40,000 individual animals) to be readily studied.

7.1.1 The Linear Default Position for Genotoxic Carcinogens

Genotoxic agents that are DNA reactive and direct acting have long been assumed to display linear dose responses.[3] Genotoxic agents that require metabolic activation, while having the confounding effect of the kinetics of enzymatic activation, are still

Genotoxic Impurities: Strategies for Identification and Control, Edited by Andrew Teasdale
Copyright © 2010 by John Wiley & Sons, Inc.

also assumed to induce linear responses. However, due to this need for metabolic activation and considerable variation in metabolic enzyme levels between different organs, most research into dose response relationships for genotoxins has focused on DNA reactive genotoxins.

In the linear model, DNA damage induction is directly proportional to dose; hence, the implication is that there are no safe genotoxic doses in terms of DNA damage (and hence by extension, cancer). This linear model has been implemented partly due to the precautionary principle designed to protect human populations from exposure to potential genotoxins. This linear concept has been controversial and has recently been challenged by ourselves and others, as it assumes a binary situation where chemicals are either genotoxic or not, but does not account for the effect of dose. As pointed out by Paracelsus in the 16th century, "only the dose permits something not to be poisonous."

In the case of indirect-acting genotoxins that have non-DNA targets (aneugens targeting the mitotic spindle and agents interacting with DNA modifying enzymes), nonlinear relationships would logically be assumed to apply, and, indeed, thresholds have now been generally accepted.[4-6] Hence, the presentation of solid experimental evidence has already successfully altered the default linear position on the dose response relationship for some chemicals. However, for direct-acting DNA-damaging genotoxins, linear models are still assumed to apply. The linear model was supported by some early dose response data, which was often carried out using high doses of genotoxin. High doses of test agent have traditionally been used in genotoxicity testing (approaching or exceeding the LD_{50} values *in vivo* or *in vitro*) to ensure that DNA damaging effects are identified in the available tests (due to test sensitivity constraints). Because it has widely been assumed that genotoxic effects are induced in a linear manner, these high-dose values are then extrapolated back to the low-dose region. The implications emanating from the linear model for genotoxins can be wide reaching and can have a significant impact on the development of a new pharmaceutical. This can often lead to the need to control a genotoxic impurity down to very low (ppm) levels, and can, in some instances, even lead to clinical delays that significantly affect the development of the product concerned. Even without this, controlling such impurities down to the levels required by the application of the "threshold of toxicological concern" (TTC) can be a significant technical challenge.

7.1.2   Theoretical Evidence for Thresholded Responses

The main argument against a linear dose response for genotoxins is the presence of natural defenses, which have evolved to cope with our daily exposure to unavoidable genotoxins. Humans are constantly exposed to genotoxic substances, like cytosolic oxidative agents, sunlight, dietary amines, inhaled hydrocarbons, and many others. Low-level exposures to these genotoxins have occurred throughout evolutionary time and have led to the development of efficient homeostatic defenses to protect organisms against the deleterious mutagenic consequences. Figure 7.1 displays some of the hurdles preventing an exposure event to a genotoxin resulting in fixed DNA alterations. DNA repair is one such homeostatic defense mechanism that may impact

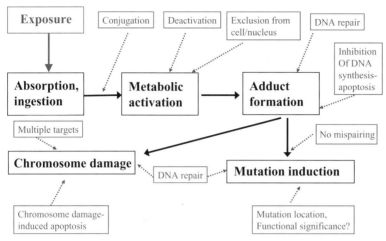

Figure 7.1   Flow chart illustrating potential mechanisms underlying genotoxic thresholds (taken from Jenkins et al.[60]).

TABLE 7.1   Potential Mechanisms that May Be Responsible for Genotoxic Thresholds

Biomolecular target/activity	Mechanism
Epithelial barriers	Prevent genotoxin entry into the body
Compartmentalization of tissues	Preventing access of genotoxins to target organs, thus reducing their availability within the body
Membranes	Shielding or exclusion of compound from cell or nucleus. Pumps can also exclude chemicals
Redundant cellular targets (e.g. microtubules)	Inactivation or damage to multiple targets before significant perturbations observed
Metabolic enzymes	Detoxification or conjugation of agents promoting excretion before they interact with biomolecular targets
DNA repair	Damage correction or removal of altered bases prior to becoming fixed as genetic aberrations
DNA redundancy	Only damage in coding or regulatory sequences lead to mutagenicity, based on current phenotypic tests
Apoptosis, autophagy, or anoikis triggers	Cell death eliminates damage; fixed DNA damage only presents when apoptosis is evaded

heavily on the outcome of genotoxin exposure. Indeed, even simple bacteria have intricate defenses (like DNA repair) against genotoxins. As multicellular organisms, humans have several tiers of protection against DNA damage induction, as shown in Table 7.1.

Hence, it is almost inconceivable that genotoxins cause DNA damage in a manner proportional only to dose. This is due in part to the failure of the genotoxin to readily access the DNA of a target tissue. Even in a simple cell culture system, it is unlikely that true linearity will be seen due to extracellular and intracellular interactions between the genotoxin and non-DNA biomolecules, as well as membrane-based exclusion. Furthermore, once in the nucleus, genotoxins must overcome the homeostatic protection afforded by DNA repair to produce permanent DNA sequence alterations resulting in phenotypic changes.

Over recent decades, DNA repair has been shown to function in a complex, and, in some cases, in an inducible manner to control the genetic stability of the host cell's genome. Several overlapping DNA repair pathways exist that are responsible for repairing specific DNA damage types (e.g. base excision repair, nucleotide excision repair, homologous recombination, mismatch repair, etc.). Hence, it is likely that DNA repair will impact directly on the linearity of genotoxic dose responses by removing DNA damage. This is particularly true at low doses of genotoxin exposure, as DNA repair has evolved to deal with constant low-level DNA damage induction. At higher doses, DNA repair may be saturated and hence may not be able to remove newly damaged DNA bases. There is some evidence that DNA adduct formation accrues in a linear fashion,[7–9] but it is likely that fixed mutations (point mutations, chromosome damage) will not. One complication with comparing the DNA adduct data to the mutation data (point mutation or chromosome mutation) is that DNA adducts can be detected to a level that is three to four orders of magnitude more sensitive than that to which DNA mutations can currently be measured. Furthermore, another complication with this comparison is that DNA mutations (point mutations in particular) are detected in specific gene sequences (hprt, tk, lacZ, lac I etc), whereas DNA adduct measurements do not define where in the genome the adducts are present. Given that cells have evolved efficient measures to keep gene coding sequences damage-free at the expense of noncoding regions,[10] it is not possible to currently say if DNA adducts accrue in a linear fashion in the coding sequences that form the basis for most genotoxicity tests. Therefore, it is not straightforward to currently compare the dose relationships between adducts and mutations.

7.1.3 *In Vitro* Experimental Evidence for Thresholds

Up until recently, most of the *in vitro* experimental evidence demonstrating nonlinear (thresholded) dose responses were available for indirect or non-DNA reactive agents. As their mechanisms of action are well understood, thresholds are now largely accepted for these compounds (Table 7.2). Indirect acting compounds generally target non-DNA biomolecules, possessing functional redundancy, and therefore these genotoxins must damage multiple targets before a significant adverse effect arises. Hence, low concentrations of these compounds can be tolerated by cells, until a critical point (the threshold) is reached, after which subsequent increases in exposure results in measurable genetic damage.

Classical examples of indirect acting (non-DNA reactive) genotoxic compounds that demonstrate *in vitro* thresholds are spindle poisons. These compounds damage tubulin monomers, which are in excess within cells. Thus, at low concentrations, although damage to these biomolecules will arise, it is not sufficient to disrupt microtubule formation, and hence chromosome segregation at mitosis. Only when a substantial degree of damage is induced will malformation of the spindle apparatus

TABLE 7.2 *In Vitro* **Studies Demonstrating Genotoxic Thresholds with Chemical Agents**

Compound(s)	Class	DNA reactivity	Damage mechanism	Test system	Reference
Disperse Red 1, Disperse Orange 1	Azo dyes	Direct	DNA adducts repaired	Micronucleus assay	Chequer et al.[16]
Rotenone, bisphenol-A	Insecticide, polycarbonate manufacture	Indirect	Disruption of mitotic spindle	Micronucleus assay	Johnson and Parry[15]
MMS, EMS	Alkylating agents	Direct	DNA adducts repaired	Micronucleus assay, HPRT forward mutation assay	Doak et al.[13]
Etoposide, doxorubicin, genistein, ciprofloxacin	Drugs (chemotherapy, antibacterial)	Indirect	Topoisomerase II inhibitors	Micronucleus assay, comet assay, γ-H2AX	Lynch et al.[5]; Smart et al.[12]
Colchicine, carbendazim, mebendazole, nocodazole	Spindle poisons	Indirect	Disruption of microtubule assembly	Micronucleus assay	Elhajouji et al.[4,11]

occur, which in turn leads to aneuploidy through missegregation of the replicated chromosomes. Using the micronucleus assay coupled to fluorescence *in situ* hybridization (FISH), thresholds have been established *in vitro* for several chemicals with this underlying biological mechanism, including the aneugens colchicine, mebendazole, carbendazim, and nocodazole[4,11] (Table 7.2). More recently, another class of indirect acting genotoxins, topoisomerase II inhibitors, have also been shown to display thresholded dose-responses *in vitro*.[5,12] Type II topoisomerase enzymes play an essential role in modulating DNA tension and topology during replication, transcription, and repair. Through transiently cutting the DNA strand, these enzymes relieve torsion at key places along the genome before the DNA is re-sealed. Agents that inhibit topoisomerase II enzyme action often lead to DNA strand breakage during DNA replication by stabilizing the DNA-topo II complex. Again, these enzymes represent a redundant target within the cells, hence low concentrations of topoisomerase II inhibitors can be tolerated by cells, as the excess type II topoisomerase molecules ensure that the required level of activity is maintained. However, at higher doses (above the threshold), a genotoxic compound will significantly disrupt topo II activity, leading to clastogenicity.

In contrast to the above examples, DNA reactive chemicals have largely been assumed to have a nonthresholded dose response as they directly induce DNA lesions that can potentially be fixed as point mutations or chromosomal aberrations. However, as mentioned earlier, homeostasis in mammalian cells allows them to adapt to environmental insults, therefore leading to a range of low doses that have a biologically insignificant effect. Nonetheless, experimental evidence for the existence of thresholds for agents that directly damage DNA is considerably more limited than for indirect acting agents, although some such studies are now starting to emerge (Table 7.2). It is important to point out that only large datasets with high-quality data can truly be used to confirm that thresholds exist. This is discussed below.

One of the first reports to comprehensively demonstrate that direct acting genotoxins could exhibit thresholds for mutation induction and chromosome breakage *in vitro* focused on a set of four well-known genotoxic and carcinogenic alkylating agents: methyl methane sulfonate (MMS), methyl nitrosourea (MNU), ethyl methanesulfonate (EMS), and ethyl nitrosourea (ENU).[13] Consistent with their more potent DNA alkylating activity, MNU and ENU displayed linear-like dose responses. However, strikingly, MMS and EMS were found to demonstrate thresholds for both chromosomal damage and mutagenicity (Fig. 7.2), which was subsequently confirmed by elaborate statistical modeling approaches.[14] Given that MMS and EMS were known carcinogens and were often used as positive controls in genotoxicity testing, this evidence clearly refuted the linear model that was assumed to apply for all direct acting genotoxins. MMS and EMS both displayed a range of low doses where no significant DNA mutation was detected relative to the untreated controls, with a lowest observable effect level (LOEL) at 0.85 μg/mL for MMS and 1.4 μg/mL for EMS for the induction of chromosomal damage, and at 1.25 μg/mL for MMS and

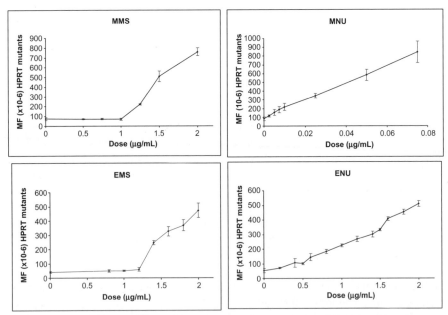

Figure 7.2 Mutation frequency dose response curves for MMS, MNU, EMS and ENU as determined using the HPRT forward mutation assay (MF; the number of 6-thioguanine resistant clones/10⁻⁶ clone-forming cells). MMS and EMS demonstrated thresholds, while MNU and ENU had linear dose-responses (taken from Doak et al.[13]).

1.4 µg/mL for EMS for point mutations (at the hprt locus). This data confirmed the greater reactivity of methylating agents, with MMS having a lower LOEL than EMS. The LOELs were not at concentrations that significantly decreased cell viability, thus the sharp increases in chromosomal damage and mutation frequencies observed were not induced via a cytotoxicity-related mechanism.[13] Furthermore, this study was followed by supporting data demonstrating a linear increase in DNA adduct formation (N7methylG) by MMS across the same dose range, thus confirming that adequate nuclear exposure was achieved with this experimental set-up.[9] Therefore, direct acting genotoxic carcinogens like EMS and MMS can display dose ranges where there is no elevation of genetic damage above background levels.

Another example of DNA reactive compounds that have non-linear dose-responses are azo dyes, a group of chemicals used in a variety of industries for their colorant properties[15] (Table 7.2). A recent study by Chequer et al.[16] indicated the possibility that these compounds may have a thresholded dose response as the lowest concentration tested in this investigation demonstrated no significant increase in micronucleus frequency, while subsequent increases in dose caused significant levels of damage for both compounds tested. However, this study was not conclusive, as only a limited dose range was assessed, and therefore a more substantial investigation of these compounds is required in order to determine if azo dyes do indeed have nonlinear curves. Some data has also been recently reported for several pro-oxidants, where nonlinear responses were reported. Unfortunately, too few cells were analyzed to confirm that the nonlinear responses were truly indicative of genotoxic thresholds.[17]

At present, only a limited amount of good quality *in vitro* evidence is available for the existence of genotoxic thresholds, and this relates to a small number of chemicals. Although thresholds are well accepted for indirect acting (non-DNA reactive) genotoxins, more evidence is required for direct-acting agents, and this data needs to be supported with a clear biological explanation for the shape of the respective dose response curve. Further investigation is therefore required on a compound-by-compound basis, at least in the short term until sufficient data across different chemical classes has been compiled.

7.1.4 *In Vivo* Evidence for Genotoxic Thresholds

Intuitively, genotoxic thresholds demonstrated to occur *in vitro* in cells cultured in the laboratory should also be present in animal tissues *in vivo*. Furthermore, due to the extra homeostatic systems in place *in vivo* (e.g. detoxification and excretion), one would even expect the thresholds to be exaggerated. Hence, it should be more difficult for a chemical to exhibit a threshold *in vitro*, as only cell-based homeostatic mechanisms would apply. There has been very little convincing threshold data generated *in vivo* due mainly to studies not being carried out in the low dose region. There is some evidence for nonlinearity of dose responses, for example for EMS-induced mutation *in vivo*,[18,19] which supports the notion of thresholds in general, but until recently, no firm evidence was available.

However, in 2009, a comprehensive analysis of the genotoxic dose responses for two alkylating agents (EMS and ENU), was reported.[20] This research was instigated as a result of the contamination of the drug Viracept (nelfinavir mesylate)® (Hoffman-La Roche, Basel, Switzerland) with EMS. This occurred as a consequence of a GMP failure that resulted in a reaction between methane sulfonic acid and ethanol inadvertently mixed in a tank used in the manufacturing process. This *in vivo* genotoxicity analysis formed the basis of an assessment of the risks posed to patients as a result of their exposure to the contaminated product. The *in vivo* data compared dose responses for both point mutation (LacZ locus in three tissues) and chromosome damage (bone marrow micronuclei) between ENU and EMS across a range of low doses, which were spaced closely together. This seminal piece of work elegantly confirmed the previous *in vitro* threshold for EMS (but not ENU) for both micronucleus induction and LacZ mutation induction *in vivo*.[20] Furthermore, through comprehensive pharmacokinetic studies, a cross species analysis allowed extrapolation from the genotoxic threshold dose observed in the mice to a corresponding threshold in humans. Hence, a threshold for EMS has been identified, providing a potential precedent for future safety assessment of other genotoxic carcinogens that may also possess thresholded dose response curves. Figure 7.3 shows some of this seminal data confirming thresholded genotoxic responses to EMS *in vivo* (Gocke et al.,[20]). In Figure 7.3, the chromosome breakage in bone marrow and mutation induction in bone marrow, gut, and liver are plotted against dose. It is clear that NOELs exist for all endpoints up to 25 mg/kg/day.

Interestingly, the *in vivo* chromosome damage data also showed a potential hormetic effect for micronucleus induction *in vivo*, suggesting homeostatic mechanisms were induced, which also removed some endogenous DNA damage.[20] Hormetic effects have never before been observed in genetic toxicology, and reinforce the concept that organisms can adapt to tolerate low levels of DNA damage, and this adaptation probably functions through upregulation of DNA repair processes. The

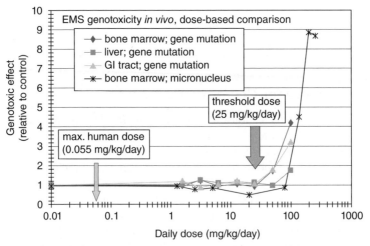

Figure 7.3   EMS induced thresholded dose responses *in vivo*. Data taken from Gocke et al.,[20] and includes both chromosome breakage data and Lac Z mutation data. Here the data are plotted on a log–linear graph to allow better visualisation of the data. In the publication by Gocke et al., linear–linear graphs are also plotted.

acceptance of hormetic effects in the low-dose region of genotoxin exposure may lead to a significant rethink in regulatory toxicology.[21] Another interesting observation from this *in vivo* study was that dose fractionation abolished the mutation induction by EMS.[20] When chronic doses (12.5 mg/kg/day × 28 days) were compared with acute doses (1 × 350 mg/kg), it was noted that animals tolerated the chronic dosing, with no increases in LacZ mutations, whereas the acute dose (which was the equivalent cumulative dose) caused increased mutagenicity. This observation reinforces the concept that homeostatic mechanisms (e.g. DNA repair) can effectively deal with low dose exposures, but become saturated at high doses leading to mutagenesis.

7.2   MECHANISMS BEHIND THRESHOLDS

It is becoming increasingly apparent that there are a number of biological explanations that argue against the assertion that all genotoxins have linear dose responses, as mammalian cells have numerous homeostatic mechanisms that provide protection. Humans are complex multicellular organisms and therefore have several tiers of protection against DNA damage, as summarized in Table 7.2 and Figure 7.1.

With regards to indirect- and direct-DNA damaging agents, assuming they are able to gain access to the cellular environment, there is a significant disparity in the potential mechanism underlying their thresholded dose responses due to the differences in their biomolecular targets. Indirect-acting genotoxins do not damage DNA directly, but instead interfere with DNA replication, transcription, or repair processes. Nuclear division is a multifactorial process involving a large number of components required for DNA synthesis, subsequent equal partitioning of the replicated chromosomes, and several signal transduction-based checkpoints to monitor the mitosis process. Indirect-acting agents may therefore target mechanical components vital for segregation of replicated chromosomes (e.g. microtubules, centrosomes), DNA replication (e.g. topoisomerase enzymes, DNA polymerases, imbalanced nucleotide pools), or DNA repair proteins (e.g. glycosylases, polymerases, endonucleases, ligases), subsequently resulting in structural and numerical chromosomal abnormalities.[22,23] Consequently, these agents have to damage multiple targets before a significant adverse biological effect occurs; a prime example being spindle poisons (e.g. nocodazole) that will only induce nondisjunction and chromosome loss at a dose that damages a sufficient number of tubulin monomers to disrupt microtubule assembly, and thus appropriate formation of the spindle apparatus.[11] Low doses of a spindle poison lead to slight damage to the microtubules, which is of no consequence in terms of mutagenesis, at higher doses modest damage, and nondisjunction occur with more serious damage, leading to chromosome loss and the formation of micronuclei at even higher doses.[4] Indirect-acting agents are therefore well accepted to have a thresholded dose response due to the redundancy of their targets.

In contrast, DNA reactive genotoxins have long been assumed to have a linear dose response because of their capacity to directly damage the macromolecule either inducing strand breakages or DNA lesions such as adducts. This linear model is still largely assumed as a precaution for these agents, and direct-acting genotoxins will only be accepted as having nonlinear dose responses if accompanying data on their mechanism of action supporting the shape of the dose response curve is available. Although data is starting to emerge indicating that not all direct acting genotoxins have linear dose responses (Table 7.2), evidence explaining the biological basis for these responses is limited. However, theoretically, DNA repair processes may be the key mechanism for low exposure doses resulting in no significant increase in mutagenic effects.

The ability of a cell to repair its DNA following damage is a vital means for maintaining the genetic stability of the cell's genome. However, at higher genotoxin doses, these DNA repair pathways may become saturated and hence be unable to efficiently remove all the damage induced. Currently, the evidence to indicate that DNA repair is indeed responsible for nonlinear dose responses following exposure to direct-acting genotoxins is limited, but data supporting this theory is starting to emerge in relation to alkylating agents. Theoretically, it is likely that DNA repair will be strongly involved in influencing the shape of the respective dose response curves in the case of alkylating agents, as N7G, N3A, and O^6G have specific repair mechanisms associated with their removal (base excision repair [BER] involving methyl purine glycosylase and methyl guanine DNA methyl transferase, respectively), while O^2T and O^4T are very poorly corrected. Table 7.3 shows DNA adduct profiles for MMS, MNU, EMS, and ENU, and Figure 7.4 shows the location of the DNA adducts coupled to DNA repair pathways involved in their correction. Consequently, at low MMS exposure levels, DNA repair is likely to be primarily responsible for the efficient removal of the N7G, N3A, and O^6G DNA adducts resulting in a NOEL, while failing

TABLE 7.3   DNA Adduct Profiles for the Alkylating Agents MMS, MNU, EMS, and ENU

Adduct	MMS	MNU	EMS	ENU
s-value	>0.83	0.42	0.67	0.26
Phosphotriesters	0.8	12–17	12–13	55–57
N7-G	81–83	65–70	58–65	11–11.5
N3-G	0.6	0.6–1.9	0.3–0.9	0.6–1.6
N7-A	1.8	0.8–2	1.1–1.9	0.3–0.6
N3-A	10.4–11.3	8–9	4.2–4.9	2.8–5.6
N3-T	0.1	0.1–0.3	Nd	0.8
N3-C	<1	0.06–0.6	0.4–0.6	0.2–0.6
O^6-G	0.3	5.9–8.2	2	7.8–9.5
O^2-T	Nd	0.1–0.3	Nd	7.4–7.8
O^4-T	Nd	0.1–0.7	Nd	1–2.5
O^2-C	Nd	0.1	0.3	2.7–2.8

Figures represent the percentages of total adducts arising at the given site—all possible adducts are not included. Nd, not detected (adapted from Beranek[52]).

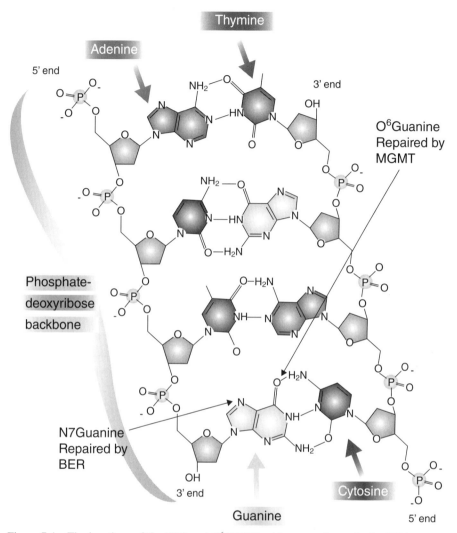

Figure 7.4   The locations of the N7G and O^6G DNA adducts are shown in the DNA structure. Note that the O^6G is directly miscoding as it interferes with Watson and Crick base pairing, whereas the N7G adduct is not miscoding as it does not interfere with DNA replication. The DNA repair pathways involved in the repair of these specific adducts are also shown.

to fully remove all the damage at higher concentrations, due to saturation of enzymatic activity, resulting in a LOEL and subsequent dose-dependent increases thereafter. With respect to the nitrosoureas, it is possible that at low exposure levels, the N7G, N3A, and O^6G may be repaired, but those at the O^2T and O^4T positions would persist, giving rise to the more linear dose-response observed.[13,24] Indeed, the importance of the thymine adducts have been shown by Guttenplan and colleagues[25] when they reported that at low ENU doses, mutations at adenine-thymine (AT) sites predominated (as a result of O^2- and O^4- ethylT), but as concentrations increased, more mutations were induced at guanine-cytosine (GC) sites due to saturation of O^6-ethylG repair.

With respect to alkyl-DNA adducts, N7-alkyl guanine lesions are usually removed and replaced by the BER pathway. BER is initiated by enzymatic hydrolysis of the N-glycosydic bond catalyzed by *N*-methylpurine-DNA glycoslase (MPG), which incises the DNA either side of the adducted base to enable its removal.[26–28] The abasic site is then further processed by apurinic endonuclease (Ape1), and the base replaced using the opposite strand as a template. Finally, the newly inserted base is ligated to seal the DNA strand. This repair process is particularly important in the correction of lesions that arise at the N7G and N3A positions, and although the MPG enzyme is most proficient at removing methyl groups, it is also capable of acting on larger adducts, albeit at a lower efficiency. Hence, BER may contribute to DNA repair-mediated thresholds for alkyating agents, such as MMS and EMS in particular, which preferentially target N7G and N3A sites. Abasic sites resulting from spontaneous loss of N7G lesions or by-products of BER can in theory induce point mutations through error-prone repair (by DNA polymerase β); however, this error rate is believed to be low, at around 1 in 10^4,[29] and so these point mutations would be induced very infrequently. Indeed, a recent thorough review of the literature on N7G DNA adducts has concluded that they pose few mutational risks due to their noncoding nature.[30] More of a concern is the role that abasic sites arising from depurination of N7G may play in chromosome breakage (clastogenicity) resulting from attempted replication past a transient strand break itself resulting from processing of such an abasic site.

O^6-methylguanine DNA methyltransferase (MGMT) also plays an important role in the correction of alkylated DNA, and is primarily responsible for the removal of O^6-alkylG in a single-step reaction, where the alkyl group from the adducted base is transferred to an internal cysteine residue within the active centre of the enzyme.[26,31] This is a suicide process that results in irreversible inactivation of MGMT, so one repair molecule will only remove one O^6G adduct, and hence the cell will only have a finite capacity for this type of repair. As MGMT expression is induced in response to DNA damage, a cell's capacity to repair O^6G lesions is dependent upon the rate at which it can synthesize MGMT.[32] As with MPG, MGMT is also most efficient at removing methyl adducts, but it is able to remove larger adducts (e.g. ethyl, propyl, butyl adducts), albeit at a lower efficiency.[31] As O^6G is a highly mutagenic lesion, it is suspected to be mainly involved with point mutation induction, although chromosome breakage events can also be induced by this lesion.[33] However, the mammalian MGMT enzyme, unlike its bacterial counterpart, is inefficient at repairing O^4-alkylT or O^2-alkylT, which is reflected by the persistence of these lesions *in vivo*, where their half-lives are 30× longer than O^6-alkylG.[31,34,35]

These repair pathways are therefore very important in governing DNA protection against alkylating agents, and it is only when they fail to remove lesions that the opportunity arises for the damage to become fixed as permanent point mutations or chromosomal aberrations. For example, it has been shown that in MGMT-deficient human cells, eightfold more GC mutations are observed following exposure to the alkylating agent ENU due to increased persistence of O^6-ethylG.[36]

With regards to the alkyl methanesulfonates, at low doses, BER may be responsible for removing the N7-alkylG lesions induced by MMS and EMS, while the MGMT enzyme may cope with the low levels of O^6-alkylG adducts, thus resulting in their NOELs for the induction of chromosomal damage and point mutations, respectively. In support of this theory, previous genotoxic studies *in vitro* have highlighted a potential role for MGMT in altering the shape of dose responses. In both bacterial and mammalian cells, MGMT knockouts result in more linear-shaped mutational dose responses in contrast to the sublinear shapes in the wild-type cells.[37–39] Recently, MGMT gene expression has been shown to be substantially upregulated by MMS at doses below the threshold for MMS-induced point mutations (1.25 µg/mL; Fig. 7.5). Thus, this boost in MGMT expression at low doses may be responsible for repairing O^6-methylG lesions before they are fixed as permanent base substitutions.[24] However, this was not the case with regards to chromosomal damage, as this LOEL for MMS is lower than for point mutations at 0.85 µg/mL. The evidence therefore indicates that O^6-alkylG is unlikely to be primarily responsible for the clastogenicity observed at these lower doses, because despite the MGMT upregulation observed at 1 µg/mL, at this concentration, significant chromosomal damage can already be detected. Hence, removal of O^6-alkylG by MGMT appears to have limited influence on the chromosomal damage threshold for MMS, suggesting that O^6-alkylG is not a key clastogenic adduct. Consequently, it seems that at low doses, O^6-methylG lesions are responsible for MMS mutagenicity, while N7-methylG may be the predominant cause of MMS clastogenicity.

Unexpectedly, at concentrations higher than the LOEL, MGMT expression returned to base level (Fig. 7.5[24]) The reason for this is unknown; p53 activation might be involved, as it modulates both basal- and genotoxic stress-induced MGMT expression.[40–43] However, it may also be possible that MGMT is the more dominant

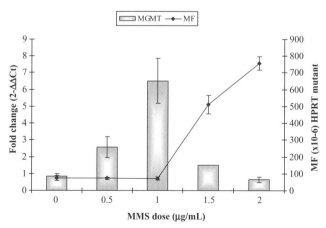

Figure 7.5   Relative fold change in MGMT mRNA expression compared with the point mutation frequency dose-response curve that results after exposure to increasing concentrations of the direct acting alkylating agent MMS. *MF*, mutation frequency (the number of 6-thioguanine resistant clones/106 clone-forming cells; Doak et al.[13,24]).

means of adduct removal at low doses, while at higher exposure levels, alternative DNA repair pathways are triggered in the cell by the genotoxic responses. Indeed, this has been observed in resistance to the chemotherapeutic agent BCNU.[44] Furthermore, N7-alkylG and O[6]-alkylG are also substrates for mismatch repair (MMR) and nucleotide excision repair (NER), respectively, particularly when MGMT is overloaded,[26,27,45–47] but further analysis is required to substantiate this theory with regards to monofunctional alkylating agents.

It therefore appears that the threshold dose responses that have been shown experimentally for direct-acting genotoxins MMS and EMS are probably due to efficient repair of the lesions induced at low doses. Although data to support this theory is now emerging, further evidence is required to clearly demonstrate the interplay between DNA damage profiles and repair pathways in governing thresholded dose responses. A full understanding of the biological mechanisms of action imposing genotoxic thresholds is fundamental to accepting the plausibility of these thresholds.

7.2.1   Statistical Assessment of Dose Response Datasets

In order to assess the dose response of genotoxins, it is imperative that the most sensitive tests available are employed to achieve sufficient power to calculate the NOEL, LOEL, and the inflection point. For the purposes of this chapter, a threshold is defined as the point below which there was no dose response. A threshold can only be described statistically by detailed analysis of the dose response data, and has a characteristic called the inflection point that is the point where the change in gradient is at its maximum. When these methods of analysis have been carried out, the dose response can be categorized as either being linear or as having a threshold. A fundamental requirement for such data analysis is starting with high-quality dose response data. Poor quality data is not amenable to such statistical modeling. In order to accurately assess the dose response of a genotoxin, sensitive tests must be used, and adequate replicates are needed to ensure that spurious effects are avoided. Closely spaced doses are also necessary to better define any changes in the shape of the dose response. The more closely spaced the doses, the better the resolution of any threshold effects. Logarithmic graphs can complicate the dose response and can artificially suggest nonlinearity, hence these should be avoided and the data plotted on linear–linear graphs.

Thresholded responses can be calculated by using the hockey stick model incorporated in the statistical analysis package described by Lutz and Lutz.[48] If fitting of the more complex hockey stick model explains a greater proportion of the variation than the linear model, then it is a threshold dose response with a defined inflection point. Figure 7.6 describes some of the potential dose responses that can be fitted to genotoxicity data in this way. Detailed knowledge of the dose response relationship of a given compound is paramount in the area of genetic toxicology.

The hockey stick package provided by Lutz and Lutz[48] attempts to fit two straight line segments to the data. A line with zero slope at low dose is forced and then joined to a line with positive slope at higher dose. The junction between these two line segments is a point of inflection at which increasing dose begins to cause

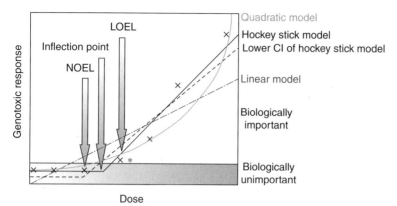

Figure 7.6   Lutz and Lutz hockey stick model showing linear v quadratic v hockey stick responses. Also showing the main outputs of the analysis (NOEL/LOEL, confidence intervals and point of inflection). Taken from Johnson et al.[14]

a measurable response. The change in gradient is at its maximum at this point of inflection. Confidence intervals are also calculated, and the lower confidence interval for the inflection point is presented graphically as a dotted line in the output, and this can be used as the worst-case scenario. Further parameters are also calculated, including the gradient of the line above the inflection point, the Y-intercept, and the probability value for fitting the linear model to a greater degree than the hockey stick.

As an alternative, the fitting of linear and quadratic models can be carried out using SPSS v. 13.0 (IBM) or similar software. A straight line (with two parameters, intercept and slope) is first fitted to the data. This is generally significant, but not necessarily a good visual fit to the data. Then a quadratic (with additional parameter) is fitted. In both cases, the variation in response explained statistically by dose, is determined by the coefficient of determination ($R2$). If the $R2$ value on fitting the quadratic is significant, then the quadratic is deemed a significantly better fit to the data than the linear model. The inflection point of the quadratic can then be regarded as a threshold.

Once the dose response has been defined, then further statistical analyses can be used to determine the LOEL. One approach is the Dunnett's test. This is a widely used and well regarded analysis method for dose response data. Dunnett's test is a multiple comparison post hoc method, performed after a one-way analysis of variance (ANOVA) by comparing all treatment data versus the control.

Another suitable approach uses the ANOVA+ t-test method designed and kindly provided to us by the BioStatistics Department at Covance Laboratories UK in 2008, for the analysis of linear versus threshold dose responses. It takes the response below the inflection point into consideration, and, unlike the Dunnett's, it is not affected when there is increased error at high concentrations. This method is carried out as follows.

1. The controls (group 0) are compared with the lowest concentration (group 1) using a one-sided two-sample t-test.

2. Groups 0 and 1 pooled are compared with the next highest concentration (group 2) using a one-sided two-sample t-test.

3. The process from this point forward is to compare each concentration against the previous three pooled, after first testing for homogeneity of the means.

For example, groups 0, 1, and 2 are compared for homogeneity of the means using one-way ANOVA. Group 3 is then compared with groups 0, 1, and 2 combined together, using a one-sided two-sample t-test. The testing continues to higher doses, each time testing the high dose with the three preceding lower doses, when these do not show heterogeneity of means. If statistically significant differences ($p < 0.05$) are found in Step 1 or 2, or in the homogeneity of means test, these differences are taken into account when later steps are interpreted. The process, however, moves onto the next step regardless of the statistical significance. A potential threshold value is defined as a concentration that produces a statistically significant difference from the preceding three concentrations, with all subsequent concentrations having the same or higher response. When such a potential threshold concentration is identified, the process of t-testing stops.

In general, to refute the linear dose response, more complex models (as discussed above) are fitted to the data to attempt to describe any nonlinearity and any thresholded effects. The threshold dose can only be described statistically and is highly dependent upon the quality of the data available.

7.2.2 Extrapolation from One Thresholded Chemical to Another

Currently, genotoxic thresholds need to be identified on a chemical by chemical basis. As the number of identified thresholds is still very low, it is currently not possible to extrapolate from known threshold effects for one chemical to other chemicals within a similar chemical class. As yet, the best proof of genotoxic thresholds is available only for EMS, as both *in vitro* and *in vivo* evidence supports this. Its sister chemical, MMS, is clearly thresholded *in vitro*, and it would be fair to assume that MMS would also display a threshold *in vivo*; however, there is currently little proof to confirm this. At present, it is not appropriate to assume that dose responses can be predicted due to chemical class, DNA adduct profile, or mechanism of action. However, in the future, with more data available on thresholds induced by many more chemicals, it may be possible to predict with some degree of certainty a dose response for a chemical, based purely on existing data from similar chemicals, or from chemicals with similar mechanisms of action.

7.2.3 Extrapolation of Thresholds to Populations?

Given that DNA repair appears to be centrally involved in the existence of genotoxic thresholds, and also given that there is population level variation in DNA repair genes, it can be assumed that this genetic variation may alter susceptibility to

TABLE 7.4   **Polymorphisms in DNA Repair Genes Reported to Modulate Risk of Cancer**

Gene	Polymorphism	Cancer type affected	Reference
XRCC1	−71 T/C	Lung cancer link	Vineis et al.[53]
MGMT	I143V	Oesophageal adenocarcinoma	Doecke et al.[54]
MGMT	K178R	Lung cancer	Crosbie et al.[55]
MGMT	56 C/T	Colorectal cancer	Ogino et al.[56]
MGMT	K178R	Lung cancer	Povey et al.[57]
APEX	I64V	Lung cancer	Zienolddiny et al.[58]
MPG	8603 C/T, 12235 G/A	Lung cancer	Rusin et al.[59]

genotoxins in the low-dose region. Indeed, it has previously been suggested that defining a genotoxic threshold for a population might be impossible, due to genetic variation among individuals.[49] There is certainly the possibility that individuals will exist in a population who are more sensitive to a genotoxin due to possession of a DNA repair variant protein with lower than average efficiency. Table 7.4 summarizes some of the polymorphisms known to be present in several DNA repair genes pertinent to alkylating agent induced DNA damage. As can be see from Table 7.4, possession of some of these variant alleles is linked to increased risk to several cancer types, presumably due to lower DNA repair capacity. It is, however, fair to say, that conflicting evidence is present in the literature that requires some resolution.

Unpicking the haplotypes (combinations) of DNA repair gene polymorphisms, which influence susceptibility to mutation and cancer, is likely to be a complex process. This is discussed in more detail elsewhere.[50] Theoretically, if mismatch repair (MMR) were found to be the main mediator of a threshold response to a genotoxin, and safe exposures levels in humans were calculated based on a threshold dose in proficient models, then patients with hereditary nonpolyposis colorectal cancer (HNPCC; a deficiency in MMR) would be more susceptible to mutation and perhaps cancer, while the general population would be tolerant of exposure. In short, the threshold dose calculated in this example would not necessarily apply for these HNPCC individuals. Of course, the fact that mismatch repair (MMR) (and indeed other repair processes) can unwittingly facilitate chromosome damage induction[33] complicates this view, as efficient MMR can drive chromosome damage, and may represent a double edged sword in mutagenesis. Moreover, due to the overlapping specificity of the different DNA repair processes, other functional counterpart pathways may well compensate the reduced efficiency of one pathway. Therefore, failure of more than one pathway may be necessary to radically alter any population level threshold dose. Repair haplotypes may better define susceptible individuals, allowing a better understanding of risk assessment in terms of exposure to genotoxic carcinogens. Furthermore, while it is accepted that MGMT and BER are centrally involved in the repair of alkylating agent-induced DNA damage, nucleotide excision repair (NER) can also contribute to this repair effort as shown by increased alkylation sensitivity in NER deficient cells.[46] This is particularly true for larger alkyl groups (ethyl, isopropyl) compared with methyl groups.[51]

Certainly, safety factors used in risk assessment need to take account of genetic variation in DNA repair genes (currently included for inter-individual variation in general), particularly when risk assessing a genotoxin with a thresholded dose response. Mechanistic studies to better understand the biological basis for genotoxic thresholds are essential, as they highlight the key protective factors (like DNA repair) underlying the thresholds. In fact, before suggesting safe exposure limits to known genotoxins (thresholded or not), adequate characterization of any protective mechanisms should be undertaken in order to inform the risk assessments necessary. The identification of these protective processes and the genes involved can then lead to the search for susceptible groups before setting safe exposure levels. This may require confirmatory genotoxicity testing in appropriate model systems (e.g. DNA repair deficient) to examine the likely risks to populations with deficiencies in key DNA repair pathways.

7.3   CONCLUSIONS

Genotoxic thresholds exist and have now been well described for a small number of chemicals. The biological basis for these thresholds can involve multiple cellular and extracellular mechanisms (e.g. functional redundancy, DNA repair). Understanding the biological mechanism behind specific thresholded dose responses is fundamental to accepting that these responses are genuine and also can be useful in highlighting susceptible subpopulations.

However, at this point in time, there are insufficient data to apply this on a wider basis to genotoxic carcinogens in general. Thus, individual investigations are required. It is, however, hoped that by the conduct of further studies across a range of different chemical classes, that a more thorough understanding of the existence of thresholds will be gained, and that this will ultimately be used to refine current methodologies, resulting in an approach that better reflects the actual level of risk.

ACKNOWLEDGMENTS

We are indebted to Hoffman LaRoche and the European Chemical Industry Council/Long-Range Research Initiative for funding ongoing and previous research at Swansea University into genotoxic thresholds. Research in this area at Swansea University is also currently funded by Unilever plc.

REFERENCES

1. Williams GA, Iatropoulos J, Jeffrey AM. 2000. Mechanistic basis for nonlinearities and thresholds in rat liver carcinogenesis by the DNA-reactive carcinogens 2-acetylaminofluorene and diethylnitrosamine. *Toxicol. Pathol.* 28:388–395.
2. Bailey GS, Reddy AP, Pereira CB, et al. 2009. Nonlinear cancer response at ultra-low dose: A 40800-animal ED001 tumor and biomarker study. *Chem. Res. Toxicol.* 22:1264–1276.

3. Henderson L, Alberini S, Aardema M. 2000. Thresholds in genotoxicity responses. *Mutat. Res.* 464:123–128.

4. Elhajouji A, Tibaldi F, Kirsch-Volders M. 1997. Indication for thresholds of chromosome non-disjunction versus chromosome lagging induced by spindle inhibitors in vitro in human lymphocytes. *Mutagenesis* 12:133–140.

5. Lynch A, Harvey J, Aylott M, et al. 2003. Investigations into the concept of a threshold for topoisomerase inhibitor-induced clastogenicity. *Mutagenesis* 18:345–353.

6. Committee on Mutagenicity (COM). 2001. *Statement on Risk Assessment of In-Vivo Mutagens (and Genotoxic Carcinogens)*. COM/01/S3. Available at http://www.iacom.org.uk/statements/COM01S3.htm (accessed March 2010).

7. Perera FP. 1988. The significance of DNA and protein adducts in human bio-monitoring studies. *Mutat. Res.* 205:255–269.

8. Zito R. 2001. Low doses and thresholds in genotoxicity: From theories to experiments. *J. Exp. Clin. Cancer Res.* 20:315–325.

9. Swenberg JA, Fryar-Tita E, Jeong YC, et al. 2008. Biomarkers in toxicology and risk assessment: Informing critical dose-response relationships. *Chem. Res. Toxicol.* 21:253–265.

10. Hanawalt PC. 1994. Transcription-coupled repair and human disease. *Science* 23:1957–1958.

11. Elhajouji A, Van Hummelen P, Kirsch-Volders M. 1995. Indications for a threshold of chemically-induced aneuploidy in vitro in human lymphocytes. *Environ. Mol. Mutagen.* 26:292–304.

12. Smart DJ, Halicka HD, Schmuck G, et al. 2008. Assessment of DNA double-strand breaks and gamma H2AX induced by the topoisomerase II poisons etoposide and mitoxantrone. *Mutat. Res.* 641:43–47.

13. Doak SH, Johnson G, Quick E, et al. 2007. Mechanistic influences for mutation induction curves after exposure to DNA-reactive carcinogens. *Cancer Res.* 67:3904–3911.

14. Johnson GE, Doak SH, Griffiths SM, et al. 2009. Non-linear dose-response of DNA-reactive genotoxins: Recommendations for data analysis. *Mutat. Res.* 678:95–100.

15. Johnson GE, Parry EM. 2008. Mechanistic investigations of low dose exposures to the genotoxic compounds bisphenol-A and rotenone. *Mutat. Res.* 651:56–63.

16. Chequer FMD, Angeli JPR, Ferraz ERA, et al. 2009. The azo dyes Disperse Red 1 and Disperse Orange 1 increase the micronuclei frequencies in human lymphocytes and in HepG2 cells. *Mutat. Res.* 676:83–86.

17. Platel A, Nesslany F, Gervais V, et al. 2009. Study of oxidative DNA damage in TK6 human lymphoblastoid cells by use of the in vitro micronucleus test: Determination of no-observable-effect levels. *Mutat. Res.* 678:30–37.

18. Cosentino L, Heddle JA. 1999. A comparison of the effects of diverse mutagens at the LacZ transgene and the dld locus in vivo. *Mutagenesis* 14:113–119.

19. Jansen JG, Vrieling H, van Teijlingen CM, et al. 1995. Marked differences in the role of O6-alkylguanine in hprt mutagenesis in T-lymphocytes of rats exposed in vivo to ethylmethane sulphonate N (2-hydroxyethyl) –N-nitrosourea, or N-ethyl-N-nitrosourea. *Cancer Res.* 55:1875–1882.

20. Gocke E, Ballantyne M, Whitwell J, et al. 2009. MNT and Mutamouse studies to define the in vivo dose response relations of the genotoxicity of EMS and ENU. *Toxicol. Lett.* 190:286–297.

21. Calabrese EJ, Baldwin LA. 2003. Toxicology rethinks its central belief. *Nature* 421:691–692.

22. Crebelli R. 2000. Threshold-mediated mechanisms in mutagenesis: Implications in the classification and regulation of chemical mutagens. *Mutat. Res.* 464:129–135.

23. Kirsch-Volders M, Vanhauwaert A, Eichenlaub-Ritter U, et al. 2003. Indirect mechanisms of genotoxicity. *Toxicol. Lett.* 140–141:63–74.

24. Doak SH, Brusehafer K, E Dudley E, et al. 2008. No-observed effect levels are associated with up-regulation of MGMT following MMS Exposure. *Mutat. Res.* 648:9–14.

25. Guttenplan JB. 1990. Mutagenesis by N-nitroso compounds: Relationships to DNA adducts, DNA repair and mutational efficiencies. *Mutat. Res.* 233:177–187.

26. Drablos F, Feyzi E, Aas PA, et al. 2004. Alkylation damage in DNA and RNA—Repair mechanisms and medical significance. *DNA Repair* 3:1389–1407.

27. Wyatt MD, Pittman DL. 2006. Methylating agents and DNA repair responses: Methylated bases and sources of strand breaks. *Chem. Res. Toxicol.* 19:1580–1594.

28. Krokan HE, Standal R, Slupphaug G. 1997. DNA glycosylases in the base excision repair of DNA. *Biochem J.* 325:1–16.
29. Kunkel TA, Alexander PS. 1986. The base substitution fidelity of eucaryotic DNA polymerases. Mispairing frequencies, site preferences, insertion preferences, and base substitution by dislocation. *J. Biol. Chem.* 261:160–166.
30. Boysen G, Pachkowski BF, Nakamura J, et al. 2009. The formation and biological significance of N7-guanine adducts. *Mutat. Res.* 678:76–94.
31. Pegg AE. 2000. Repair of O-6-alkylguanine by alkyltransferases. *Mutat. Res.* 462:83–100.
32. Grombacher T, Eichhorn U, Kaina B. 1998. p53 involved in regulation of the DNA methyltransferase (MGMT) by DNA damaging agents. *Oncogene* 17:845–851.
33. Armstrong MJ, Galloway SM. 1997. Mismatch repair provokes chromosome aberrations in hamsters cells treated with methylating agents or 6-thioguanine, but not with ethylating agents. *Mutat. Res.* 373:167–178.
34. Yarosh DB. 1985. The role of O6-methylguanine-DNA transferase in cell survival, mutagenesis and carcinogenesis. *Mutat. Res.* 145:1–16.
35. den Engelse L, Menkveld GJ, de Brij RJ, et al. 1986. Formation and stability of alkylated pyrimidines and purines (including imidiazole ring opened 7-alkylguanine) and alkylphosphotriesters in liver DNA of adult rats treated with ethylnitrosourea or dimethylnitrosamine. *Carcinogenesis* 7:393–403.
36. Bronstein SM, Cochrane JE, Craft TR, et al. 1991. Toxicity, mutagenicity and mutational spectra of N-ethyl-N-nitrosourea in human cell lines with different repair phenotypes. *Cancer Res.* 51:5188–5197.
37. Rebeck GW, Samson L. 1991. Increased spontaneous mutation and alkylating sensitivity of Escherichia coli strains lacking the ogt O6 methylguanine DNA repair methyltransferase. *J. Bacteriol.* 173:2068–2076.
38. Kaina B, Fritz G, Ochs K, et al. 1998. Transgenic systems in studies on genotoxicity of alkylating agents: Critical lessons, thresholds and defense mechanisms. *Mutat. Res.* 405:179–191.
39. Sofuni T, Hayashi M, Nohmi T, et al. 2000. Semi-quantitative evaluation of genotoxic activity of chemical substances and evidence for a biological threshold of genotoxic activity. *Mutat. Res.* 464:97–104.
40. Nutt CL, Loktionova NA, Pegg AE, et al. 1999. O6- methylguanine-DNA methyltransferase activity, p53 gene status and BCNU resistance in mouse astrocytes. *Carcinogenesis* 20:2361–2365.
41. Rafferty JA, Clarke AR, Sellappan D, et al. 1996. Induction of murine O-6-alkylguanine-DNA-alkyltransferase in response to ionising radiation is p53 gene dose dependent. *Oncogene* 12:693–697.
42. Hengstler JG, Tanner B, Moller L, et al. 1999. Activity of O6-methylguanine-DNA methyltransferase in relation to p53 status and therapeutic response in ovarian cancer. *Int. J. Cancer* 84:388–395.
43. Srivenugopal KS, Shou J, Mullapudi SRS Jr, et al. 2001. Enforced expression of wild-type p53 curtails the transcription of the O6-methylguanine-DNA methyltransferase gene in human tumor cells and enhances their sensitivity to alkylating agents. *Clin. Cancer Res.* 7:1398–1409.
44. Bobola MS, Berger MS, Silber JR. 1995. Contribution of O^6-methylguanine-DNA methyltransferase to resistance to 1,3-(2-chloroethyl)-1-nitrosourea in human brain tumor-derived cell lines. *Mol. Carcinog.* 13:81–88.
45. Glaab WE, Tindall KR, Skopek TR. 1999. Specificity of mutations induced by methyl methanesulfonate in mismatch repair-deficient human cancer cell lines. *Mutat. Res.* 427:67–78.
46. Op het Veld CW, van Hees Stuivenberg S, Van Zeeland AA, et al. 1997. Effect of nucleotide excision repair on HPRT mutations in rodent cells exposed to DNA ethylating agents. *Mutagenesis* 12: 417–424.
47. Plosky B, Samson LD, Engelward BP, et al. 2002. Base excision repair and nucleotide excision repair contribute to the removal of N-methylpurines from active genes. *DNA Repair* 1:683–696.
48. Lutz RW, Lutz WK. 2009. Statistical model to estimate a threshold dose and its confidence limits for the analysis of sub-linear dose-response relationships, exemplified for mutagenicity data. *Mutat. Res.* 678:118–122.
49. Lutz WK. 2000. A true dose in chemical carcinogenesis, cannot be defined for a population, irrespective of the mode of action. *Hum. Exp. Toxicol.* 19:566–568.

50. Jenkins GJS, Johnson G, Zair Z, et al. 2010. Genotoxic thresholds, mechanisms, DNA repair, and susceptibility in human populations. *Toxicology* (in press).
51. Kaina B, Christmann M, Naumann S, et al. 2007. MGMT: Key node in the battle against genotoxicity, carcinogenicity and apoptosis induced by alkylating agents. *DNA Repair* 6:1079–1099.
52. Beranek DT. 1990. Distribution of methyl and ethyl adducts following alkylation with monofunctional alkylating agents. *Mutat. Res.* 231:11–30.
53. Vineis P, Manguerra M, Kavvoura FK, et al. 2009. A field synopsis on low penetrance variants in DNA repair genes and cancer susceptibility. *J. Natl. Cancer Inst.* 101:24–36.
54. Doecke J, Zhao ZZ, Pandeya N, et al. 2008. Polymorphisms in MGMT and DNA repair genes and the risk of oesophageal adenocarcinoma. *Int. J. Cancer* 123:174–180.
55. Crosbie PAJ, McGowan G, Thorncroft MR, et al. 2008. Association between lung cancer risk and single nucleotide polymorphisms in the first intron and codon 178 of the DNA repair gene, O-6-alkylguanine-DNA-alkyltransferase. *Int. J. Cancer* 122:791–795.
56. Ogino S, Hazra A, Tranah GJ, et al. 2007. MGMT germline polymorphism is associated with somatic MGMT promoter methylation and gene silencing in colorectal cancer. *Carcinogenesis* 28:1985–1990.
57. Povey AC, Margison GP, Santibanez-Koref MF. 2007. Lung cancer risk and variation in MGMT activity and sequence. *DNA Repair* 6:1134–1144.
58. Zienolddiny S, Campa D, Lind H, et al. 2006. Polymorphisms of DNA repair genes and risk of non-small cell lung cancer. *Carcinogenesis* 27:560–567.
59. Rusin M, Samojedny A, Harris CC. 1999. Novel genetic polymorphisms in DNA repair genes: O(6) methylguanin-DNA-methyltransferase (MGMT) and N-methylpurine-DNA glycosylase (MPG) in lung cancer patients from Poland. *Hum. Mutat.* 14:269–270.

CHAPTER 8

GENOTOXIC IMPURITIES: A RISK IN PERSPECTIVE

Dave Elder
Jim Harvey

8.1 INTRODUCTION

The primary objective of the following chapter is to put into context the risk posed to humans from low levels of genotoxic impurities (GIs) present in medicinal products. To do this, this chapter will explore the significance of the typical exposure to GIs experienced by humans arising from natural sources, both endogenous and exogenous, and compare and contrast the relative levels of these with those permitted in pharmaceuticals.

That exposure to genotoxic substances arising from sources other than low-level contaminants in pharmaceuticals is already partially acknowledged within the CHMP (Committee for Medicinal Products for Human Use) guidelines[1,2]. It states that a "TTC (threshold of toxicological concern) higher than 1.5 μg/day may be acceptable under certain conditions, for example for short-term exposure, when life expectancy is much shorter than 5 years, or where the impurity is a known substance and human exposure will be much greater from other sources, for example food. This of course only addresses the rare occasion where an identical GI arising via the synthesis, also occurs naturally, for example formaldehyde. It does not address the huge gulf in terms of relative levels of exposure (the fundamental "dose issue"), which is explored in depth in the forthcoming chapter. However, this is not a new debate. For nearly two decades, the issue of the safety implications of exposure to toxic synthetic chemicals, in the context of parallel exposure to higher levels of naturally occurring toxins (mainly from the diet), has been actively discussed.[3,4]

This chapter will summarize those factors impacting on DNA damage, look at the body's intrinsic defense mechanisms, and evaluate the role of diet and pretreatment of food and drink as risk factors. It will also explore in depth the significant exogenous exposure to volatile aldehydes, epoxides, and nitroso/*N*-nitroso compounds and other potential mutagens. Finally, it will examine herbal products and the clear disconnect that exists in terms of level of controls between such products and pharmaceuticals.

Genotoxic Impurities: Strategies for Identification and Control, Edited by Andrew Teasdale
Copyright © 2010 by John Wiley & Sons, Inc.

8.2 FACTORS IMPACTING ON DNA DAMAGE

Historically, it has been always assumed that there are no safe levels for *in vivo* genotoxins as they have "the ability to damage DNA at any level of exposure and that such damage may lead/contribute to tumor development." [2] However, the existence of *in vivo* mechanisms leading to meaningful thresholded levels is increasingly acknowledged even for genotoxic compounds, for example alkylating agents, such as EMS and ENU.[5] Even for those direct-acting DNA genotoxins, the CHMP guideline[2] contains the following comment that "extrapolation from high to low concentrations may not be justified due to the presence of several protecting mechanisms which operate effectively at low doses," that is implying that direct acting genotoxins may well have NOELs (no observable effect levels).

Damage to DNA plays a significant role in a number of processes, including ageing, as well as carcinogenicity and mutagenicity. This damage is caused by exposure to either exogenous and/or endogenous genotoxins/carcinogens, leading to formation of either DNA adducts, or hydrolysis and/or oxidation of DNA. In particular, damage has been linked with exposure to reactive oxygen species (ROS) and other activated metabolites.[6]

It is recognized that the environment is a major contributor to the development of cancer; the environment constitutes a multitude of variables such as diet, smoking/smoke, radiation, sunlight, occupation, drugs, and those socioeconomic factors that affect exposures in addition to substances in air, water, and soil.[7] However, inconsistencies in the definition of what constitutes "environmental exposure" makes accurate estimates of the size of its contribution to human cancer virtually impossible, with estimates ranging from 1%–3% to 19% for involuntary exposures, such as those linked to air, water, soil, or food pollutants,[8] including occupational exposures,[9] to 10%–70% being attributable to diet, with the most likely figure being about 35%.[10,11]

Most of the body's DNA defense mechanisms have evolved to limit levels of ROS, from both exogenous and endogenous sources ultimately to limit the resulting damage they can cause.[12] The endogenous production of ROS occurs during mitochondrial respiration and the levels formed are considerable. Up to 5% of oxygen is converted to the superoxide anion free radical; this is then converted to hydrogen peroxide via the enzyme superoxide dismutase, which in the presence of transition metals forms the highly reactive hydroxyl free radical.

Another common endogenous DNA oxidizing agent is the peroxynitrite species. This is formed via the reaction of nitric oxide (a vaso-relaxant and neurotransmitter) and superoxide, and is a potent oxidant both directly and indirectly via hydroxyl free radicals.[13] In addition, endogenously produced *N*-nitroso compounds, which are potent genotoxins, can be formed from nitrite species in the buccal cavity, stomach, lungs, and from bacteria and macrophages in inflamed tissues,[14] as well as from tobacco smoke and cooked food.

DNA can also be damaged by the endogenous formation of reactive substances, including oxidants, for example hydroperoxide and peroxide radicals and reactive carbonyls via the oxidation of lipids. The aldehydic by-products of lipid oxidation are all genotoxic in nature (e.g. formaldehyde, acetaldehyde, crotonaldehyde, acrolein, glyoxal, 4-hydroxynonenal [HNE], and malondialdehyde [MDA]), and they damage DNA via the formation of exocyclic base adducts. MDA is the most mutagenic volatile aldehyde that is formed; whereas HNE is the most toxic.[15] Glyoxal can also be formed endogenously via auto oxidation of sugars and oxidative degradation of deoxyribose.[16] Methylglyoxal is another reactive carbonyl endogenously formed via glucose metabolism, but also seen in many foodstuffs and beverages.[17]

Guanine adducts (7-[2-hydroxyethyl]-guanine) can also be formed by exposure to endogenously produced ethylene oxide, a known mutagen and carcinogen. This is metabolically formed from ethane, which is another by-product of lipid oxidation, as well as intestinal gut flora metabolism.[18]

The body also synthesizes endogenous alkylating agents that are important mediators of cell metabolism. The most important of these are *S*-andenosylmethionine (SAM) used in the enzymatic methylation of DNA, which helps regulate gene expression.[19] However, SAM can also nonenzymatically methylate DNA.[20] Other endogenously produced alkylating agents are betaine, choline, as well as simple alkylating agents, for example *N*-nitroso compounds. Although these alkylating agents may be formed from cellular precursors, they also arise exogenously from environmental sources, for example tobacco smoke and diet. Exposure from all sources appears to be inevitable, and it is difficult to accurately apportion the exogenous and endogenous contributions.[21]

The glycoside bond linking the base pairs to deoxyribose in DNA can be cleaved by heating, akylation of the bases, or enzymatically. This leads to abasic sites, which are produced spontaneously, but also mediated by ROS.[22] These abasic sites are very common and occur very frequently, that is 10,000 modifications/cell/day,[23] but are considered mutagenic due to the preferred incorporation of adenine opposite abasic sites by DNA polymerases during the replication process.[24]

8.3   NATURAL DEFENSE MECHANISMS

The numbers of naturally occurring toxic chemicals is significant, it is estimated that between 5000 and 10,000 different natural pesticides and their breakdown products are toxic to humans/animals.[25] Animals have, of necessity, developed broad-based defense mechanisms. First, a continuous shedding of external cells exposed to exogenous and endogenous toxins. The surface layers of mouth, esophagus, and the remainder of the gastrointestinal (GI) tract, as well as the skin are shed every few days.[4]

Second, the mobilization of the so-called electrophile response attack. This involves the induction of phase II enzymes; such as glutathione-*S*-transferases (GST), NAD(P)H-quinone acceptor oxidoreductases (QRs), UDP glucosonyltransferase (UGT), and epoxide hydrolase (EH), as well as elevation of intracellular levels of reduced glutathione in peripheral tissues, in response to a variety of electrophiles and antioxidants.[26]

Third, the active efflux via P-glycoprotein mediated mechanisms, or similar, of planar hydrophobic molecules, both natural and synthetic, out of the GI tract and liver cells. Fourth, the body's effective and inducible DNA repair mechanisms against electrophile-induced DNA-adduct formation, hydrolysis, and oxidation via

ROS. Finally, the body's effective olfactory and gustatory senses that have the ability to discern bitter, pungent, astringent, or acidic chemicals, often at low concentrations, and the ability to consciously or unconsciously (the latter via vomiting and/or diarrhea) remove these offending foodstuffs and beverages from the body.[4]

8.4 ELECTROPHILES AND OXIDANTS IN FOOD

Plants produce toxins to prevent infection and/or predation by fungi, insects, and animals. There are estimated to be about 10,000 natural pesticides and antioxidants and their structurally related breakdown products, which are biosynthesized by plants, and which are present in foods. Less than 1% have been adequately tested in animals, and about half of these are mutagenic or carcinogenic.[3,4] Ames et al.[3] estimated that the American diet contained about 1.5 g of these natural pesticides/day, and this figure would undoubtedly be higher in vegetarians. Average exposure in common foods is high and covers all different types of foodstuffs, including those promoted as being essential for health and well-being, for example fruits and vegetables. The principal known genotoxic and/or carcinogenic components of food are summarized in Table 8.1.

TABLE 8.1 Estimated Daily Exposure from Natural Mutagens/Carcinogens Derived From Foods, Spices and Beverages (Abstracted from Berkeley Carcinogenic Potency Database[27])

Food source	Natural mutagen/ carcinogen	Alerting structural motif	Estimated daily exposure (µg/day)	Ames test result
Mustard, horseradish	Allyl isothiocyanate	Isothiocyanate	28	+
Common mushrooms	Agaritine	Hydrazine	224	+
Lettuce, tomatoes, apples, coffee	Caffeic acid	Michael Receptor	40,580	−
Coffee	Catechol	Phenolic	1160	−
Cinnamon	Coumarin	Michael Receptor	65	+
Various spices	Estragole	Phenolic	54	−
Various foods, e.g. bread, coffee	Furfural	Volatile Aldehyde	3640	+
Common mushrooms	Hydrazinobenzoic acid	Hydrazine	59	+
Various spices, coffee	Methyl eugenol	Phenolic	424	−
Celery, parsnip, parsley	8-Methoxy oxypsoralen	Furan	11	+
Various spices	Safrole	Phenolic	1200	−

Source: Berkeley Carcinogenic Potency Database: Carcinogenic in rodents, http://potency.berkeley.edu/pdfs/herp.pdf[27] (accessed September 22, 2010).

NR, Not reported.

These naturally toxic compounds will be discussed in more detail in the ensuing text. Ames et al.[3] reported that allyl isothocyanate was among the most toxic compounds investigated,[28] and is a mutagen at very low concentrations.[29] Allyl isothiocyanate was reported to be clastogenic at concentrations of about 0.5 ppb.[3]

The fava or broad bean is a common Mediterranean vegetable, but contains the toxins vicine and convicine at levels of about 2% of its dry weight. Reduced levels of glucose-6-phosphate dehydrogenase in southern European populations' results in low glutathione levels. This results in a marked increase in sensitivity to these fava bean toxins, often leading to a severe hemolytic anemia.[3,4]

Certain furocoumarins, for example psoralen and its derivatives are potent photo-induced carcinogens and mutagens. They are widespread in plants of the *Umbelliferae* family, for example celery, parsnips, and the *Moraceae* family, for example figs. The levels in celery (800 ppb–1 ppm dried weight) can increase markedly (100-fold) if the plant is damaged or diseased. Agricultural workers exposed to celery commonly develop skin rashes on their hands and arms. The introduction of a new "insect-resistant" celery in the mid-1980s led to a plethora of photo-induced rashes/burns in consumers. Levels of psoralens were about sixfold higher, that is *ca.* 6 ppm.[30] Oil of bergamot contains very high levels of psoralen, and was used as an ingredient in a leading sun tan lotion in France, as psoralens, when photo-activated, induced tanning more rapidly. However, following epidemiological studies that linked the use of psoralen containing sunscreens to melanoma, these products were subsequently withdrawn from use.

Edible mushrooms contain many toxins (mainly carcinogenic hydrazines), including the rodent carcinogen glutamyl-4-hydrazinobenzoate. One of the most popular edible mushroom, *false morel* (*Gyromitra esculenta*), contains 11 hydrazines, at least three of which are rodent carcinogens. One of these volatile hydrazines, N-methyl-N-formyl hydrazine, is present at a concentration of 500 µg/g of dried mushroom, and induces tumors in mice via the oral route at low doses <50 µg/day (based on a TD50 in mice of 2.37 mg/kg/day).[3,4]

The most common commercial mushroom, *Agaricus bisporus*, contains about 300 mg of agaritine (on a dried basis), as well as smaller amounts of other related carcinogens. Unfortunately, agaritine is not affected by cooking and is metabolized to the corresponding diazonium compound (4-[hydroxymethyl] benzenediazonium ion), which is a very potent carcinogen; for instance, a single dose of 400 µg/g of agaritine gives 30% occurrence of stomach tumors in mice. In addition, agaritine can decompose to produce N'-acetyl-4-hydroxymethylphenylhydrazine, 4-hydroxymethylphenylhydrazine, as well as the corresponding diazonium compound.[3,4]

The catecholic phenols, for example tannin, caffeic acid, and their esters, that is chlorogenic and neochlorogenic acid, are widely distributed in the plant kingdom. They are reported to have beneficial antioxidant and antimicrobial effects via ROS mechanisms. However, although neither chlorogenic nor neochlorogenic acids have been tested for carcinogenicity, they are metabolized to caffeic acid and catechol, which are both carcinogens. Chlorogenic acid is clastogenic at 150 ppm, a similar concentration to the levels found in apples and other fruits, but over 100 times less than the concentrations found in coffee.[3,4] Both chlorogenic and caffeic acids are mutagenic. Interestingly, as with many chemicals shown to be carcinogenic at high doses,[31] caffeic acid is reported to be anticarcinogenic at lower doses.[32]

Flavonoids are a widely distributed group of secondary plant metabolites, which are commonly found in foodstuffs and beverages.[33] Additional enzymatic modifications yield related compounds: flavanols (for example, quercetin, rhamnazin), flavones (for example, luteolin, apigenin), dihydroflavonols (for example, taxifolin, dihydroxyquercertin, and dihydroxykaempferol), and anthocyanins (for example, cyanidin, malvidin).[34]

The therapeutically beneficial effects of fruit, vegetables, tea, and, more contentiously, red wine have been attributed to flavonoid compounds rather than to known vitamins or nutrients. Flavonoids can be found in many dietary sources. All citrus fruits, berries, onions, parsley, pulses, tea, red wine, dark chocolate, and many herbal preparations, for example *Ginko biloba*, *Sorbus aucuparia*, contain flavonoids.[35,36]

Like most food-derived antioxidants, flavonoids have anticancer effects *in vitro* and *in vivo* animal models, as well as clinically for the treatment of certain cancers.[37,38] Conversely, those same molecules are often shown to have toxic, genotoxic, or carcinogenic effects at higher levels.[39,40]

Their efficacy and toxicology effects may be both related to their inhibition of DNA topoisomerase activity. On the beneficial front, inhibition of topoisomerase activity has been suggested as being an important factor in chemotherapy,[41] and many topoisomerase poisons are commonly used in chemotherapy, for example topotecan and etoposide.[42] Ironically, their toxic effects are probably also linked with their role as topoisomerase poisons.[43–45] Flavonoids may interfere with topoisomerase activity by binding to the DNA template primer, or competitively inhibiting the enzyme. The former inhibition could be by an intercalative mechanism due to the planar aromatic structures of the flavonoids. Other intercalalator agents, such as acridines and anthracyclines, are toxic via inhibition of topoisomerase activity.[46]

High doses of specific flavonoids, for example myricetin, derived from dietary supplements, could cause topoisomerase-mediated genotoxicity and resulting carcinogenic effects; but in contrast, dietary intake of foods rich in fruit and vegetables, which will contain natural levels of flavonoids, are considered safe and have been associated with a reduced cancer risk.[47]

Curcumin is the principal curcuminoid of the spice tumeric, which is itself obtained from the ground root of *Curcuma longa*. The curcuminoids are polyphenols linked by two α,β unsaturated carbonyl groups, which can act as Michael acceptors, undergoing nucleophilic addition reactions. Curcumin acts as a free radical scavenger and antioxidant, which inhibits lipid peroxidation and resultant oxidative DNA damage.[48]

In addition to its use as a food preservative, food colorant and flavoring agent, it has been used as a traditional herbal medicine for centuries for the treatment of many disorders, including certain cancers. Indeed, accumulating epidemiological, clinical and preclinical evidence suggests that curcumin does have anticancer properties.[49] Experimental evidence is also available to suggest that curcumin enhances the therapeutic efficacy of both chemotherapy and radiotherapy of certain agents.[50]

However, despite evidence of beneficial clinical efficacy, there is also evidence suggesting that curcumin may be a topoisomerase inhibitor capable of inducing DNA complex formation. It is established that curcumin can induce DNA strand breaks.[51] In fact, curcumin can induce 8-oxoguanisine formation in both cell systems and isolated DNA,[51,52] and it is known that 8-oxoguanisine induces the formation of topoisomerase I-DNA complexes. Curcumin has been shown to induce topoisomerase II-DNA complexes *in vitro*.[53] López-Lázaro et al.[54] demonstrated that curcumin induced topoisomerase I and II-DNA complex formation in leukemia cells, and that the levels of those DNA complexes formed were higher than those induced by several topoisomerase I (e.g. camptothecin) and topoisomerase II poisons (e.g. etoposide, idarubicin, amsacrine, and mitoxantrone) at equi-toxic doses. Interestingly, unlike standard topoisomerase I and II poisons, ROS may mediate the formation of these DNA complexes as the presence of the antioxidant *N*-acetylcysteine, inhibits complex formation.

In a recent study, Cao et al.[55] showed that at higher concentrations (8 and 16 µg/mL) curcumin displayed a small but significant increase in the frequency of micro-nucleated cells linked with ROS and resulting DNA damage. In contrast, at lower concentrations (2 µg/mL) curcumin significantly reduced micro-nucleated cell formation induced by the cytotoxic chemotherapeutic agent, cyclophosphamide. Thus demonstrating that curcumin shows both genotoxicity and antigenotoxicity dependant on the concentration. This is again a telling point, and equally germane to the discussion of the potential impact on human health of low levels of GIs (<TTC) in medicinal products.

Safrole (1-allyl-3,4-methylenedioxybenzene), estragole (1-allyl-4-methoxybenzene), and methyleugenol (1-allyl-3,4-dimethoxybenzene) are found in many edible plants, yet are rodent carcinogens. Oil of sassafras contains about 75% safrole. In contrast, black pepper contains small amounts of safrole and large amounts of the analogue, piperine (*ca.* 10% by weight). Safrole used to be used as a food additive, but was subsequently banned following studies that demonstrated the material was carcinogenic in rodents. Similarly, its use in soaps and perfumes has been banned. The estimated average intake of safrole, estragole, and methyleugenol equates to between 0.3 and 0.5 mg/day, 4.3–8.7 mg/day 13–36 mg/day, respectively.[56–58] Safrole is clastogenic at concentrations of about 100 ppm, roughly similar to the concentration in black pepper and about 30 times less than the concentration in nutmeg.

Extracts of black pepper cause tumors in mice at a variety of sites at a dose of extract equivalent to 4 mg of dried pepper/day over 3-month period. Capsaicin, the active ingredient in hot peppers, is a mutagen, and there is some evidence for its being a carcinogen.[3]

Mutagenic aflatoxins, which are found in moldy corn and peanuts, have been linked to human liver cancer. Epidemiological studies using biomarkers indicative of aflatoxins in Africa and China, where there are high rates of liver cancer, show high levels of aflatoxin exposure.[59] Eleven mould toxins are reported to be carcinogenic,[3] whereas 19 mould toxins have been demonstrated to be clastogenic.[28] Interestingly, it is the metabolic activation of aflatoxin B_1 to the corresponding 8,9-epoxide that is responsible for its toxicity.

Foods that are consumed in accordance with a standardized "*European diet*,"[60] and where low levels of aflatoxin contamination would be anticipated

(<20 µg/kg, i.e. <20 ppb), are expected to yield a mean estimated intake of 19 ng/ person/day of aflatoxin.[61] This equates to about 0.3 ng/kg body weight/day, which is in good accord with national data from a Swiss study of 0.25 ng/kg body weight/ day of aflatoxin.[62] However, if food intake is aligned to a standardized "*Far Eastern diet*,"[60] where higher levels of exposure would be anticipated, but where contamination is again limited to <20 µg/kg, the mean estimated intake of aflatoxin is over 10-fold higher than in Europe (125 ng/person/day). This equates to about 2.0 ng/kg body weight/day. Contamination of the four common aflatoxins (B_1, B_2, G_1, and G_1) in the diet have been limited to <4 ppb in the United Kingdom, <10 ppb in Japan, and <20 ppb in United States.[63] In contrast, aflatoxins are excluded from the pharmaceutical TTC on the basis that their extreme toxicity precludes a safe level.

Meaningful quantitative data on genotoxic components of food is fairly sketchy and shows patterns of extensive variability. A good example of this is the toxic glycoalkaloids α-chaconine and α-solanine found in potatoes, which are referred to generically as solanine. These glycoalkaloids are strong cholinesterase inhibitors and possible teratogens and are present in amounts of about 75 µg/g (75 ppm) in dried potato. This is less than a 10-fold safety margin compared with the toxic dose in man.[64] Additionally, both glycoalkaloids because of their lipophilicity are concentrated in the tissues of humans.[65]

The levels are impacted by growing conditions, storage and handling, tuber size and age, and are highest in the potato skin and "eyes," and the levels are inversely proportional to tuber size. It was shown that solanine levels in potatoes grown in Germany in 1922 (which was a very poor growing year), when compared with 1923 (which was significantly improved) ,were statistically different[64] (see Table 8.2). They found that sunshine and rainfall were the biggest determinants of solanine concentrations, and that in poorer years, the exposure was just under one-fifth of the acceptable total daily intake. This safety margin would be eroded further for those individuals with greater consumption, and it becomes clearer why there are occasional incidences of solanine poisoning.[66]

Occasionally, other drivers will impact on the acceptable safety margins. In the 1970s, the U.S. Department of Agriculture developed the *Lenape* variety of potato, which had resistance to late blight, coupled with unusually high solids content, giving it excellent processability characteristics. Unfortunately, the solanine

TABLE 8.2 Solanine Concentrations in Potatoes Grown in Germany during the Period 1922–1923 (Abstracted from[64])

Crop year	No. of separate analyses	Average levels of solanine (µg/g)	Range (µg/g)	Percentage of LAEL (200 mg in man)
1922	5	35.8	2.4–58.3	17.9
1923	5	2.7	2.0–3.4	1.4

LAEL, lowest adverse effect level.

concentrations were several times higher than normal (>20 μg/g of dried potato), and the variety was withdrawn by the U.S. Food and Drug Administration (FDA).[67]

The pyrrolizidine alkaloids are known to be carcinogenic, mutagenic, and teratogenic, and are present in many different plant species, often at levels greater than 1% by weight. Some of these plants are ingested by humans, particularly as herbs and herbal teas, for example comfrey, and sometimes in honey. Petasitenine and senkirkine have been linked with the carcinogenicity of two types of coltsfoot, used in traditional herbal remedies in Japan, *Petasites japonicus* and *Tussilago farfara*.[68] The edible comfrey, *Symphytum officinale*, contains symphytine, a potent rodent carcinogen.

Pyrrolizidine alkaloid poisonings in man causes both lung and liver lesions. The phorbol esters present in the herb *Euphorbiaceae* are used as folk remedies and in herbal teas. These are mitogens, and have been linked to nasopharyngeal cancer in China[69] and esophageal cancer in Curacao.[70]

A diet low in fats and high in antioxidants derived from plants appears to reduce the risk of cancer, and this has prompted growth in the use of vitamins that have antioxidant properties (E and C) and phenolic phytochemicals. Interestingly, several studies have shown that these supplements show no clear observable benefit and in contrast may cause DNA damage. This suggests that balanced diets are more important than individual antioxidants in cancer prevention.[71]

Bruce Ames and Lois Gold[3] categorically stated that no human diet could be free of those naturally occurring chemicals that have been shown to be rodent carcinogens.

In addition, of those chemicals that are naturally ingested as part of our diet, 99.99% are natural, and less than one hundredth of 1% are synthetic. Sugimura[63] concurred, and indicated that "It is likely that people believe that naturally occurring substances to be safe, but industrially derived materials to be dangerous." The illogicality of trying to avoid the hypothetical risk of small numbers of synthetic genotoxins and neglecting or ignoring these natural genotoxins/carcinogens in food was exemplified by Kava and Flynn,[72] who recently prepared an ACSH (American Council on Science and Health) Holiday dinner menu. This is reproduced with permission from the authors in Table 8.3.

The Committee on Comparative Toxicity of Naturally Occurring Carcinogens, National Research Council,[73] concluded that based on available exposure data, the great majority of these naturally occurring (and in a few cases synthetic) chemicals seen in the diet are present at levels below which adverse biological effects are likely and at levels unlikely to pose an appreciable cancer risk. The committee also indicated that they had greater concerns regarding the natural carcinogens rather than the synthetic components, but this concern needed additional studies to confirm the proposition. Finally, they decided that the health benefits of the many antigenotoxic compounds present in food outweighed the risk, emphasizing that a diet rich in vegetables and fruits is associated with a reduced incidence of certain human cancers. Epidemiological data also shows that there are reduced risks of cancer associated with diets rich in antioxidants.[74] However, the real conundrum is that these antioxidants, while having genuine antimutagenic activity at low concentrations, are often themselves mutagenic at high concentrations.

TABLE 8.3   ACSH Holiday Dinner Menu (Reproduced with Kind Permission from the Authors: Kava and Flynn[72])

Course	Menu option	Naturally occurring mutagens/carcinogens
Appetizers	Cream of mushroom soup	Hydrazines
Fresh relish tray	Carrots	Aniline, caffeic acid
	Cherry tomatoes	Benzaldehyde, caffeic acid, hydrogen peroxide, quercetin glycosides
	Celery	Caffeic acid, furan derivatives, psoralens
Assorted nut dishes	Mixed roast nuts	Aflatoxins, furfural
Green salad	Tossed lettuce and arugula with basil-mustard vinaigrette	Allyl isothiocyanate, caffeic acid, estragole, methyl eugenol
Entrees	Roast Turkey	Heterocyclic amines
	Bread stuffing (with onions, celery, black pepper and mushrooms)	Acrylamide, ethyl alcohol, benzo(a) pyrene, ethyl carbamate, furan derivatives, furfural, dihydrazines, d-limonene, psoralens, quercetin glycosides, safrole
	Cranberry sauce	Furan derivatives
	Roast beef with parsley sauce	Benzene, heterocyclic amines, psoralens
Vegetables	Broccoli	Allyl isothiocyanate
	Baked potato	Ethyl alcohol, caffeic acid
	Sweet potato	Ethyl alcohol, furfural
Side dish	Bread roll and butter	Actetaldehyde, benzene, ethyl alcohol, benzo(a)pyrene, ethyl carbamate, furan derivatives, furfural
Desserts	Pumpkin pie	Benzo(a)pyrene, coumarin, methyl eugenol, safrole
	Apple pie	Acetaldehyde, caffeic acid, coumarin, estragole, ethyl alcohol, methyl eugenol, quercetin glycosides, safrole
Fruits	Apples, pears, mangos, grapes, pineapple	Acetaldehyde, benzaldehyde, caffeic acid, d-limonene, coumarin, estragole, ethyl acrylate, quercetin glycosides
Beverages	Red wine/White wine	Ethyl alcohol, ethyl carbamate
	Coffee	Benzo(a)pyrene, benzene, benzofuran, caffeic acid, catechol, 1,2,5,6-dibenz(a)anthracene, ethyl benzene, furan, furfural, hydrogen peroxide, hydroquinone, d-limonene, 4-methylcatechol
	Tea	Benzo(a)pyrene, quercetin glycosides
	Jasmine tea	Benzyl acetate

8.5 FOOD AND BEVERAGE TREATMENT

Historically, it is well established that pretreatment of foods (particularly during cooking) and of beverages (for example, fermentation), produces chemical by-products that are a concern in terms of their carcinogenic potential.[27]

Cooking food is acknowledged as a contributor to the overall risk of cancer. A wide variety of mutagenic and carcinogenic chemicals are formed during cooking, particularly at elevated temperatures, for example barbequing. These include furans (in particular furfural), nitrosamines, polycyclic hydrocarbons, and heterocyclic amines (HCAs) (see Table 8.4).

Furfural, a by-product of thermolysis of sugars, is a widespread component of most food flavors, and it is reported to be Ames positive. The average coffee drinker in the U.S. imbibes 2.1 mg/day of furfural.[75] Brusick[76] wryly commented that the daily mutagenic exposure from this one source alone was three orders of magnitude greater than the permitted daily intake of a genotoxic impurity in an API taken over a 12-month period.

TABLE 8.4 Estimated Daily Exposure from Natural Mutagens/Carcinogens Derived From Cooked Foods, Spices and Processed Beverages (Abstracted from Berkeley Carcinogenic Potency Database[27])

Food source	Natural mutagen/ carcinogen	Alerting structural motif	Estimated daily exposure (μg/day)	Ames test result
Bacon	N-Diethylnitrosamine	Nitrosamine	0.019	+
Bacon	N-Dimethylnitrosamine	Nitrosamine	0.057	+
Bacon	N-Nitrosopyrrolidine	Nitrosamine	0.324	+
Beer	N-Dimethylnitrosamine, N-Nitrosopyrrolidine, N-Nitrosopiperidine	Nitrosamine	0.016	+
Carbohydrate (pan fried), biscuits, bread, coffee beans	Acrylamide	Michael acceptor	40	+
Hamburger (pan fried)	PhIP (2-amino-1-methyl-6-phenylimidazol [4,5-b]pyridine)	Heterocyclic amines	0.176	+
Hamburger (pan fried)	MeIQ (2-amino-3,4-dimethylimidazol [4,5-f]quinoline)	Heterocyclic amines	0.038	+
Hamburger (pan fried)	IQ (2-amino-3-methylimidazol[4,5-f] quinoline)	Heterocyclic amines	0.006	+
Toasted bread, beer	Ethyl carbamate (urethane)	Ethyl carbamate	1	+

Acrylamide is formed when both proteins (5–50 ppb) and carbohydrates (150 ppb–4 ppm) are heated, and the highest levels are found in potato crisps and "french fries."[77] Conversely, acrylamide could not be detected in unheated food or food that was simply boiled. In Norway, the mean exposure to acrylamide was between 410 and 420 ng/kg body weight/day.[78] An American survey showed very similar mean levels (430 ng/kg body weight/day) of acrylamide.[79] This survey also indicated a higher exposure in paediatric populations. Acrylamide is genotoxic, neurotoxic, and carcinogenic in laboratory animals.[80]

It has been known for over half-century that polycyclic aromatic hydrocarbons (PAHs), for example benzo[a]pyrene can be formed when food is charred.[81] Similarly, coffee roasting induces the formation of PAHs and volatile aldehydes, for example methylglyoxal and glyoxal.[82]

Several genotoxic and carcinogenic heterocyclic aromatic amines (HCAs) are produced by excessive cooking, particularly barbequing and charring, of meat, poultry, and fish. These HCAs, for example 2-amino-1-methyl-6- phenylimidazo [4,5-b]pyridine (PhIP), 2-amino-3,4-dimethylimidazo [4,5-f]quinoline (MeIQ) and 2-amino-3,8-dimethylimidazo[4,5-f]quinoxaline (MEIQx), are trans species, multiple organ carcinogens, and are clearly mutagenic providing a plausible mechanism for the carcinogenic mechanism of action. Under normal cooking conditions, levels of HCAs are in the low ppb range; but levels in the general diet from all sources are at least as high and probably higher than reported in Table 8.4.[83] Exposure data for PhIP is scarce, with exposure estimates of 1–17[7] and 4.8–7.6 ng/kg[61] body weight/ day being reported.

Alcoholic beverages cause buccal, esophageal, and liver cancers and epidemiological studies indicate that increase consumption increases the risk.[27] Alcohol itself is deemed to be the single most important teratogen in humans. Given that the average consumption of alcohol in the United States is greater than 1 unit/person/ day and that 5 units/person/day poses a carcinogenic risk to humans, society appears to be markedly unconcerned with the abuse potential of this common beverage.

Human exposure to ethyl carbamate (urethane) is also typically linked with excessive consumption of alcoholic beverages. Exposure from foods and beverages, including wine (300 mL), was estimated to be 70 ng/kg body weight/day. This increased markedly when brandy (60 mL) was included in the assessments (2000 ng/ kg body weight/day). For comparison purposes, the exposure levels from food alone were 20 ng/kg body weight/day.[84]

Uthurry et al.[85] looked at the mechanism of formation of ethyl carbamate in red wine. Based on principal component analysis (PCA), they correlated elevated levels of ethyl carbamate with ethyl lactate and acidity, suggesting that urea was the one of the precursors, and carbamyl fermentation by-products was the other main precursor, reacting with ethanol to form the ethyl carbamate. The authors reported that in all cases the wines studied had ethyl carbamate levels below limits established by Canadian authorities (30 ppb), but some were outside U.S. FDA limits (15 ppb). Levels were reported in the range 3–25 μg/L (3–25 ppb).[86]

The U.K. Foods Standard Agency[87] (FSA) surveyed the levels of ethyl carbamate in over 200 whisky samples. The majority (83%), contained levels of ethyl carbamate in the range 10–40 μg/L (10–40 ppb), with a mean level of 29 μg/L (29 ppb), which was significantly lower than earlier surveys in 1990 and 1992, where the mean values were in the range 45–54 µg/L (45–54 ppb). This reduction has arisen through scientific understanding of the issue and the Brewing Industry's subsequent awareness that the utilization of the right barley varieties, with naturally low level occurrence of the precursors of ethyl carbamate, was critical. In parallel, a greater understanding of the distillation process is apparent. Copper catalyses the formation of ethyl carbamate. Ironically, if ethyl carbamate levels can be maximized early in the distillation process, then the nonvolatile impurity is not carried over into the product. Hence, distillation is typically performed in the presence of sacrificial copper, and an additional, third distillation has been included to minimize levels.

The FSA report[87] indicated that ethyl carbamate was rapidly metabolized to carbon dioxide, water, and ammonia. It concluded that "The levels and intake of ethyl carbamate in the U.K. diet are generally low, any risks to health resulting from these intakes are small, and are likely to be much less than the known risks of consuming alcoholic beverages."

In parallel, the U.S. FDA[88] reported that the U.S. wine industry has embarked on a similar program. They are encouraging the minimization of fertilization for vines that do not require a high level of nitrogen in the soil, as this increases arginine levels, leading to higher urea and alkyl carbamate levels. They are also introducing a different type of yeast (*prise de mousse*), which forms lower indigenous levels of urea. Finally, they have also modified their distillation processes, introducing sacrificial copper, and recommending enhanced cleaning to remove alkyl carbamate or its precursors.

FDA[88] reported that levels of alkyl carbamate were reduced significantly over a 4-year period (1987 to 1991) across all alcoholic beverages. Foreign importers had made some strides, but residual levels were still higher than the corresponding domestic produce. The data are summarized in Table 8.5.

TABLE 8.5   Ethyl Carbamate Levels (µg/L or ppb) in U.S. and Foreign Alcoholic Beverages (1987–1991)[88]

Alcoholic beverage	1987 Ethyl carbamate levels (ppb)	1991 Ethyl carbamate levels (ppb)	1991 Ethyl carbamate levels (ppb)
Origin	U.S. domestic	U.S. domestic	Foreign
Wine	13	10	13
Fortified wine			
Sherry	130	10	40
Port	60	23	26
Spirits			
Sake	300	55	60
Rum	20	2	5
Grape brandy	40	10	45
Fruit brandy	1200	5	255
Bourbon	150	70	55
Whisky	5	—	55

It is perhaps interesting to reflect on the extensive measures taken to reduce levels of ethyl carbamate, and to consider how they appear analogous with the stringent controls taken in respect to GIs in pharmaceuticals. In both cases, it is a matter of debate/conjecture as to whether they have in any appreciable way impacted on/reduced the overall risk relating to the total exposure to genotoxins. Certainly the value of concerted effort focused on isolated examples seems a relatively ineffective way of tackling the overall risk. This is especially so for ethyl carbamate, when the risk posed by the ethanol itself would appear to far outweigh any concerns arising from a minor by-product (ethyl carbamate) present in the beverage.

However, if the potential risk due to exposure to such compounds from alcoholic beverages gives the consumer cause for concern, then there can be no solace by turning to coffee. Roasted coffee contains at least 826 volatile compounds,[89] at least 21 of these have been tested chronically, and 16 are rodent carcinogens. In addition, there are some nonvolatile carcinogens, for example caffeic acid. It has been estimated that a typical cup of coffee contains as much as 10 mg (or 40 ppm) of carcinogens, including caffeic acid, hydroquinone, hydrogen peroxide, catechol, and furfural.[3]

A significant proportion of this overall exposure was attributed to hydrogen peroxide. Percolated coffee can generate hydrogen peroxide on standing in the presence of atmospheric oxygen.[90] Instant coffee is reported to produce *ca*. 200 ppm of hydrogen peroxide after dissolving the powder in hot water.[90]

8.6 REACTIVE ALDEHYDES

Volatile aldehydes are the major by-products of lipid oxidative degradation. They are also extremely biologically reactive, and are positive in various genotoxicity tests, forming adducts with DNA, proteins, and phospholipids. Lipid oxidation is strongly linked with many diseases, including cancer, mutagenesis, arthritis, and inflammation.[91]

The major by-product of lipid oxidation is formaldehyde, which has been clearly shown to be a rodent carcinogen via the inhalation route.[92,93] Likewise, acetaldehyde has been shown to be a rodent carcinogen via the inhalation route.[27] In contrast, formaldehyde, malonaldehyde, acrolein, and glyoxal are not considered to be carcinogenic via the oral route,[94-96] and, likewise, a risk assessment of acetaldehyde indicated it is also unlikely to be carcinogenic via the oral route.[97]

Formaldehyde is ubiquitous and is present in the environment from multiple sources. It is present in the atmosphere, particularly from automobile exhaust fumes, in the home, in occupational settings, and finally as a naturally occurring component of meats, fish, vegetables, and fruit. The daily formaldehyde exposure alone from dietary sources is estimated at between 1.5 to 14.0 mg/day.[98]

All biological organisms are equipped with enzyme systems capable of metabolizing formaldehyde and other related volatile aldehydes. This is almost certainly as a result of formaldehyde's endogenous formation. Formaldehyde undergoes rapid oxidation to formic acid, catalyzed by glutathione and formaldehyde dehydrogenase.[98]

The body's endogenous exposure to formaldehyde is truly staggering. The formaldehyde content within the body has been estimated at between 1.75 and 2.6 mg/kg, equating to 122.5–182 mg for a 70 kg adult. Based on the lower estimate (122.5 mg) and a half-life of 1.5 min this equates to a metabolic rate of 41 mg/minute. These calculations would suggest that the daily endogenous turnover of formaldehyde is 31–59 g.[98]

In contrast, the body's exogenous exposure is two orders of magnitude less. Therefore, it seems to be clear that while formaldehyde is a well-documented local irritant of the skin, lungs, nose, and GI tract,[99,100] the body's metabolic clearance mechanism, linked to the short half-life, makes it unlikely that exogenous oral exposure is a serious issue.

In addition, some pro-drugs are known to release formaldehyde as a result of bioconversion to the active drug. Dhareshwar and Stella[98] reviewed the metabolic fate of formaldehyde that can be generated from such pro-drugs as: cerebyx, aquavan, spectracef, fosphenytoin, hespera, etc. They concluded that in comparison to the daily endogenous exposure from metabolism, as well as the exogenous exposure from food and the environment, the total exposure from pro-drugs is minute and not likely to cause any significant systemic toxicity in humans. The same arguments will hold equally true for the presence of formaldehyde in medicinal products from other sources, for example as impurities in API or from auto-oxidizable excipients.

8.7   EPOXIDES

Like volatile aldehydes, epoxides are ubiquitous and are present in the environment from multiple sources; in the air, water, soil, microorganisms, food, and, in particular, lipids.[101] They are present in some biochemical pathways, as key metabolites of certain compounds, for example polyaromatic hydrocarbons and medicinal products, for example carbamazepine, menatetrenone. Although exposure is almost certainly guaranteed via these different sources, their intrinsic high reactivity results in rapid degradation *in vivo*, and they do not tend to reach target organs, even when given in high concentrations.[102] Several authors have studied the acid-catalyzed hydrolysis of primary and secondary aliphatic epoxides. Most epoxides are rapidly hydrolyzed in acid and/or gastric media. Stella et al.[103] reported that the half life of the cytotoxic compound, rhizoxin (NSC-332598), a macrocyclic lactone with epoxides at the 1,2- and 11,12-positions, was 10.3 min in HCl at pH 2.0.

Most biological organisms are equipped with enzyme systems capable of metabolizing epoxides, for example epoxide hydralases, epoxide reductases, glutathione-*S*-transferases, etc. This suggests that cells are highly evolved to cope with some exposure to these reactive compounds, even if this is only to their own internal metabolic pathways, for example mixed function oxidases.[102]

Ethylene oxide is an interesting example of an endogenously and exogenously derived epoxide that paradoxically appears to exhibit different toxicity dependant on its target organ. Ethylene oxide is endogenously produced via metabolism of ethylene,[18] and it has been linked with the hydroxyethylation of the DNA base pair guanine and alkylation of hemoglobin. Levels of DNA adducts are very similar across species and across tissues within the same species.[104]

This class of compounds perhaps exemplifies better than any other the disconnect between the extremely tight controls relating to GIs as mandated through the EMEA and FDA regulatory guidance, with the reality of rapid *in vivo* and *in vitro* hydrolysis and exposure from other sources, including, food, flavoring agents, and many common herbal remedies.

8.8 NITROSO/*N*-NITROSO

Another group of specific concern are nitroso and the related *N*-nitrosamines; these are formed in foods via the reaction between nitrites (present either as food additives, for example sodium nitrite, or naturally occurring, derived from nitric oxide) and amines (meat and fish).

Dialkylnitrosamines, for example dimethylnitrosamine, can be produced from the corresponding amine, for example dimethylamine and nitrite under acidic conditions, and formation will occur in the stomach. Sodium nitrite levels are now strictly controlled in food; for example levels of 50 and 200 ppm in ham and sausages are enforced in Japan and the United States, respectively.[63]

Interestingly, all of the necessary ingredients for *in situ* nitroso formation are also readily available through natural dietary exposure. Amines are prevalent in fish, cereal, tobacco, and organic dyes; nitrates are available from certain foods, for example spinach; nitrites are used as food additives and are contained in human saliva, and nitrogen dioxides are abundant in the atmosphere as a consequence of pollution. *N*-Nitrosamines are also side products of normal metabolic processes, but they are mutagenic, and with metabolic activation, they have been shown to be carcinogenic. Dimethylamine in seafood is the most prevalent of these nitroso precursors,[105] and dosing of nitrite and secondary amines or amides together potentially results in carcinogenicity.[106]

Interestingly, endogenous nitrates derived from the diet also contribute to an entero-salivary circulation system. The ingested nitrate is absorbed from the GI tract, and plasma nitrate is actively transferred to and concentrated in the salivary ducts, where it is enzymatically converted to nitrite by microorganisms, for example *S. sciuri* and *S. intermedius*, which are located on the dorsal surface of the tongue. As a consequence, human saliva containing high levels of nitrite ions will form nitrous acid in the highly acidic gastric environment, which in turn can nitrate amine and phenolic compounds, such as tyrosine (4-hydroxyphenylacetic acid), which is present in both saliva and ingested proteins.

Therefore, ironically, the current healthy eating advice of "5-a-day" consumption of fruits and vegetables could well lead to increases in endogenous nitrate and nitroso formation. In addition to the formation of 3-nitrotyrosine, other commonly occurring amino acids, such as cysteine or nucleotide bases, for example guanine, can also be nitrated to form *S*-nitrocysteine or 8-nitroguanine, respectively.

Another important nitroso precursor is tyramine, produced by the fermentation of soybeans, which reacts with nitrite ions to yield the corresponding nitroso and

TABLE 8.6   Levels of MTCA derived from Different Locations and Percentage Mutagenicity Attributable to MTCA. Derived from Wakabayashi et al.[109]

Soy sauce designation	State	Country	MTCA (ppm)	Percentage mutagenicity attributable to MTCA
1	Chiba	Japan	668	44
2	Chiba	Japan	678	61
3	Chiba	Japan	378	26
4	Mie	Japan	95	16
5	Chiba	Japan	604	45
6	Chiba	Japan	521	34
7	Aichi	Japan	82	50
8	Mie	Japan	275	26
9	Hawaii	US	55	22
10	Hawaii	US	<4	
11	Hawaii	US	34	24
12	Ohio	US	<4	
13	Wisconsin	US	711	44

diazo compounds.[107] 3-Diazotyramine has been found to be carcinogenic.[108] Another nitroso precursor found at elevated levels in soy sauce is the isomeric MTCA (1-methyl-1,2,3,4-tetrahydro-β-carboline-3-carboxylic acid). After activation with nitrite, MTCA was found to be mutagenic in the Ames assay (without S9 activation). Quantitative assessment of soy sauces from different geographical locations showed pronounced differences.[109] Japanese-sourced soy sauce showed elevated levels of MCTA (82–678 ppm), whereas in contrast, levels of MCTA from soy sauces sourced from the United States showed significantly reduced levels (see Table 8.6).

Tobacco (both smoking and chewing) is another major source of exposure to N-nitrosamines, specifically N'-nitrosonornicotine and 4-(methylnitrosoamino)-1–3-pyridyl)-1-butanone.[3,4] Most nitrosamines are potent carcinogens and typical human exposure is estimated to be 0.3–1 μg/day, primarily from N-nitrosodimethylamine (DMN), N-nitrosopyrrolidine (NPYR) and N-nitrosopiperideine. The highest human exposure was to DMN in beer, which led the brewing industry to modify its processes and introduce indirect firing of malt in 1979, which led to a 30-fold reduction in levels (Glória et al., 1997). Several nitrosamines are also found in cured bacon (N-diethylnitrosamine, N-dimethylnitrosamine and NPYR).

Wakabayashi et al.[109] estimated that the MTCA consumption per person per year in Japan was 2–18 mg. Tyramine is also found in many other foods, and can react with acetaldehyde to yield MTCA. Herraiz[110] reported on the occurrence of MTCA and the related THCA (1,2,3,4-tetrahydro-β-carboline-3-carboxylic acid) in fruit juices, purees, and jams. Levels in commercial fruit juices were in the range of

10 ppb–1.45 ppm for THCA and 1 ppb–12 ppm for total MCTA (both isomers). Levels were higher in citrus juices than in other juices, for example grape, apple, pear, etc. Levels in infant preparations (purees) were 14 ppb and 68 ppb, respectively, for THCA and total MCTA. Jams and marmalades showed intermediate levels, that is 23 ppb and 101 ppb, for THCA and total MCTA, respectively.

Similar indole-related precursors that can be nitrite activated can be found in fava beans (4-chloro-6-methoxyindole), which forms the α-hydroxy-nitroso derivative after activation, Chinese cabbage (indole-3-acetonitrile, 4-methoxyindole-3-acetonitrile and 4-methoxyindole-3-acetaldehyde),[111] and cigarette smoke (1-methoxyindole) also form corresponding mutagenic nitroso compounds.[112]

The key question, as to why the body deliberately produces high nitrite concentrations in the stomach remains unclear. Nitric oxide is endogenously produced from L-arginine via NO synthetase (NOS) in mammals, and plays a key role in stimulating gastric blood flow; mucous production and nitrous acid can effectively kill many ingested bacterial pathogens.

However, interestingly, NO can also be formed by gut flora reducing endogenous nitrate to nitrite, which spontaneously decomposes to form NO under the acidic conditions prevalent in the stomach.[113] Sobko et al.[114] demonstrated that isolated strains of *Lactobacilli* generated NO *in vitro* when nitrite ions where added to the growth medium and locally generated NO could synergistically mediate some of the beneficial effects of probiotic bacteria.

The endogenous formation of nitrite via the NOS pathway is believed to be approximately similar to the sum of exogenous nitrite intake and the bacterial production of nitrite from nitrate.[115]

In addition to its key role as a potent bacteriocide, it could be that nitrated substrates, for example 3-nitrotyrosine, acts as carriers for rapid distribution of nitric oxide, which is an extremely potent biological mediator that is effective in the nanomolar range. In addition, nitrite is a potent vasodilator and cyto-protective agent in the heart and circulatory system. In contrast, nitroso/N-nitroso compounds are excluded from the pharmaceutical TTC on the basis that their extreme toxicity precludes a safe level.

8.9 HERBAL PRODUCTS

Despite the growing popularity of traditional herbal medicines, there is little clear evidence for their intrinsic safety. Indeed, unless manufacturers make specific, drug-like claims, then these medicinal products are exempted from good manufacturing practice (GMP), and they do not require premarketing approval by the FDA. Safety is primarily achieved by self-regulation of suppliers.[116] With the huge number of constituents of traditional Chinese medicines,[117,118] it is often difficult to judge what are "active" constituents and what are impurities; indeed, this differentiation is blurred further as most (if not all) constituents will have pharmacological activity because of their biological origin.

Guo and co-workers[117,118] reported on the volatile constituents of a traditional Chinese medicine (*Artemisis capillaris herba*) using gas chromatography-mass spectroscopy (GC-MS). They reported on the identity of 42 out of 75 of the resolved constituents, which accounted for nearly 90% of the total. Two of the volatile impurities accounting for nearly 5% of the total of 42 identified peaks were potentially genotoxic epoxide impurities (*cis* and *trans*-Z-α-bisabolene epoxide), obviously at levels far in excess of what are allowable in medicinal products.

Another fairly common observation is the variability of levels of both active constituents and impurities in traditional Chinese medicines, often predicated by the source of the herbal extract. The inter-sample variability of individual constituents is often marked. In the traditional Chinese medicine, ChanSun, the levels of the epoxide components have been found to vary considerably from that observed in the reference pharmacopoeial standard.

Levels of the epoxide impurity (Z-6,7-epoxyligustilide) are fairly consistent in the Danggui samples sourced from China (2.06–3.24%), but were either absent or present at two-threefold higher levels (6.83%) in alternative Danggui samples[119] sourced from either Japan or Korea (see Table 8.7). The authors indicated that the clinical efficacy of these different Danggui medicines had not been ascertained.

Herbal products that contain aristolocholic acid (*Radix aristolochiae or Aristolochia spp.*), a family of structurally related nitrophenanthrene carboxylic acids, have received several FDA warning letters in recent years.[120] Aristolocholic acid has been classed a human carcinogen by the World Health Organization.[121] IARC[122] reported an outbreak of Chinese herb nephropathy in Belgium involving mostly middle-aged woman taking weight loss products, including traditional Chinese herbal products of the *Aristocholia* species incorrectly labeled *Stephania tetrandra*. While there was significant batch-to-batch variability in the chemical

TABLE 8.7 **Percentage of Major Components of Danggui from Different Sources and Levels of Epoxide Impurity in Same Samples. Adapted from Lao et al.[119]**

Phthalides (% of total extracted)	Sample 1[a,1]	Sample 2[a,1]	Sample 3[a,1]	Sample 4[a,2]	Sample 5[b,3]	Sample 6[b,4]	Sample 7[c,5]
Z-ligustide	50.93	53.19	53.09	37.68	17.57	27.37	19.22
E-ligustide	11.02	10.04	8.02	7.84	7.72	9.12	7.78
Z-6,7-epoxyligustide	2.06	2.30	2.19	3.24	6.83	ND	ND
Total extracted (%)	6.17	5.83	5.90	3.80	1.79	1.62	1.75

[a] *Angelica sinensis.*

[b] *Angelica acutiloba.*

[c] *Angelica gigas.*

[1] Sourced from Gansu.

[2] Sourced from Yunnan.

[3] Sourced from Hokkaido.

[4] Sourced from Toyama.

[5] Sourced from Korea.

ND, not detected.

composition of the herbal products implicated in the outbreak, aristolochic acid-DNA adducts were found in urothelial tissues from all of the urothelial cancer patients affected, providing compelling evidence of the involvement of *Aristolochia* herbal products.

It is interesting that the regulatory authorities seem to view the perceived risk of GIs from medicinal and herbal products from very different perspectives. The EMEA's Herbal Medicinal Products Committee (HPMC) has issued a draft guideline[123] on the assessment of genotoxic constituents of herbal medicines. However, in contrast to the CHMP guidance for medicinal products, HPMC have highlighted that the growth in use of herbal medicines for self-treatment is unlikely to be impacted by this guidance, and cautioned that regulatory authorities should not be overzealous in banning such products based on "extrapolated suspicions." HPMC stressed the need to develop robust risk–benefit assessments for herbal products. They conceded that the complex and variable (e.g. season to season, geographical origin, or mode of preparation) nature of herbal products presents additional challenges compared with standard medicinal products. The HPMC indicated that "the complete composition is very difficult to unravel, so one can argue that there are always many unknown constituents and thus there may be hidden dangers."

The committee cautioned that even for well-established genotoxins with known safety profiles, the complexity of the herbal medicine may make it difficult, if not impossible, to establish a TTC. In addition, they conceded that the herbal product could also contain variable levels of radical scavengers (antioxidants) and even anticarcinogens, making the assessment even more complicated. The arguments used in connection with herbal products[123] that because control is difficult, with respect to genotoxic constituents, it therefore may not be necessary, seems incompatible with the arguments used within the guidelines addressing pharmaceuticals,[1,2] which are based on the principle of the maximal level of control achievable, that is ALARP (as low as reasonably achievable). This is especially troubling when in many cases, there may be no proven clinical efficacy associated with many herbal medicines, and, furthermore, the levels of potential GIs in such products dwarfs the levels in licensed pharmaceuticals as controlled by the TTC.

8.10   CONCLUSION

In conclusion, it can be clearly seen that genotoxic exposure from other sources, both endogenous and exogenous, is much higher, indeed probably several orders of magnitude higher, than any contribution from GIs present in pharmaceutical products.

Ames and Gold[75] have concluded that the cancer hazard from natural carcinogens is higher than from their synthetic cousins based on the HERP Index (Human Exposure/Rodent Potency). These findings were corroborated by the U.K. National Research Council,[73] who indicated that they had greater concerns regarding natural, rather than synthetic carcinogens. However, several researcher's commented on the logic disconnect that the lay public appears to believe that naturally occurring substances to be safe, but industrially derived materials to be dangerous.[63]

As in all cases, moderation is the key, and we need to remember that the basic tenant of toxicology, as outlined by Paracelsus. is that all compounds (natural or synthetic) are toxic, if given at high enough doses. Ames et al.[3,4] have suggested that if we eat a balanced diet and avoid overexposure to food that presents other more relevant epidemiological risks, for example fatty fried food, then in addition to lowering the risks associated with high cholesterol, we also address many, but not all of the risks of genotoxins in food, for example ethyl carbamate, acrylamides, HAs (PhIP, MeIQ, IQ), etc. A constant finding of much research is that the danger of overeating is translated into a greater exposure to natural and synthetic carcinogens, which in turn translates into a greater incidence of cancer, when viewed over a life time basis.

A diet low in fats and high in antioxidants derived from plants appears to reduce the risk of cancer, and this has prompted growth in the use of vitamins that have antioxidant properties (E and C) and phenolic phytochemicals. Interestingly, several studies have shown that these supplements are not beneficial and in contrast may cause DNA damage. This suggests that balanced diets are more important than individual antioxidants in cancer prevention.[71] However, the real conundrum is that these antioxidants found in food, while having genuine antimutagenic activity at low concentrations, are often themselves mutagenic at higher concentrations.

The body's daily exposure to natural genotoxins is staggering, based on the quantity (5000–10,000 different natural genotoxins and their breakdown products,[3,4,25] diversity (from simple volatile aldehydes, for example formaldehyde to complex phytochemicals), and absolute exposure (about 1.5 g/day of naturally occurring genotoxins[3]). However, the body is well adapted to cope with this onslaught, and has a well-developed protection mechanism that includes inducible metabolic responses (the so called Electrophile Response Attack[26]). Based on this precedent, it perhaps seems illogical to believe that exposure to low levels (<TTC) of GIs should in anyway constitute a substantive threat to public safety.

In addition, the generally accepted adage that individuals can chose their lifestyle, for example eating, drinking, smoking etc., but cannot chose the quality of their therapeutic medicines and therefore that these need to regulated (or over-regulated) to control intrinsic levels of genotoxins, appears to be fatally flawed especially in light of the huge endogenous exposure to naturally produced genotoxins and carcinogens, for example formaldehyde. It is acknowledged by toxicologists that the TTC level is conservative, and as such lends itself to regulatory interpretation, rather than necessarily absolute adherence and conformation. At present, though, there seems to be little deviation away from rigid application of the TTC concept.

In contrast, the less rigid standards applied to the control of GIs in herbal medicines is difficult to understand against the background of stringent controls for pharmaceuticals. This is especially troubling, when in many cases, there is no proven efficacy associated with many herbal medicines, and furthermore, the levels of potential GIs in such products dwarfs the levels in licensed pharmaceuticals.

That controls over the level of residues of genotoxic reagents in pharmaceuticals are required is beyond doubt; however, what is questionable is the limit defined by the TTC and its rigid application. This is especially so given the overall burden that as a person one is exposed to naturally, simply as a consequence of daily living, for example through the diet.

ACKNOWLEDGMENTS

Drs. Kava and Flynn from the American Council on Science and Health for permission to reproduce the ACHS Holiday Dinner Menu. Dr. Robert Rees (GSK) for reviewing the manuscript.

REFERENCES

1. Food and Drug Administration, Center for Drug Evaluation and Research (CDER). December 2008. *Genotoxic and Carcinogenic Impurities in Drug Substances and Products: Recommended Approaches*. Draft guidance. Available at http://www.fda.gov/cder/guidance/7834dft.pdf (accessed January 10, 2008).
2. Committee for Medicinal Products for Human Use (CHMP). *Guidelines on the limits of genotoxic impurities*. London, June 26, 2006. CPMP/SWP/5199/02, EMEA/CHMP/QWP/251344/2006.
3. Ames BN, Profet M, Gold LS. 1990. Dietary pesticides (99.99% all natural). *Proc. Natl. Acad. Sci. USA* 87:7777–7781.
4. Ames BN, Profet M, Gold LS. 1990. Nature's chemicals and synthetic chemicals: Comparative toxicology. *Proc. Natl. Acad. Sci. USA* 87:7782–7786.
5. Lutz WK. 2009. The Viracept (nelfinavir)—Ethyl methansulfonate case: A threshold risk assessment for human exposure to a genotoxic drug contaminant? *Toxicol. Lett.* 190:239–242.
6. De Bont R, van Larebeke N. 2004. Endogenous DNA damage in humans: A review of quantitative data. *Mutagenesis* 19:169–185.
7. Jameson CW. 2009. U.S. Department of Health and Human Services, Public Health Service, National Toxicology Program. *Report on Carcinogens*, Eleventh Edition. Available at www.ntp.niehs.nih.gov/ntp/roc/toc11.html (accessed September 22, 2010).
8. Boffetta P, McLaughlin JK, Vecchia C, et al. 2007. 'Environment' in cancer causation and etiological fraction: Limitations and ambiguities. *Carcinogenesis* 28:913–915.
9. Prüss-Üstun A, Corvalán C. 2006. *Preventing Disease through Healthy Environments. Towards An Estimate of the Environmental Burden of Disease*. WHO, Geneva.
10. Doll R, Peto R. 1981. The causes of cancer: Quantitative estimates of avoidable risks of cancer in the United States today. *J. Natl. Cancer Inst.* 66:1191–1308.
11. Doll R. 1998. Epidemiological evidence of the effects of behaviour and the environment on the risk of human cancer. *Rec. Res. Cancer Res.* 154:3–21.
12. Slupphaug G, Kavli B, Krokan HE. 2003. The interacting pathways for prevention and repair of oxidative DNA damage. *Mutat. Res.* 531:231–251.
13. Richeson CE, Mulder P, Bowry VW, et al. 1998. The complex chemistry of peroxynitrite decomposition: New insights. *J. Am. Chem. Soc.* 120:7211–7219.
14. Tricher AR. 1997. *N*-nitroso compounds and man: Sources of exposure, endogenous formation and occurrence in body fluids. *Eur. J. Cancer Prev.* 6:226–268.
15. Esterbauer H, Eckl P, Ortner A. 1990. Possible mutagens derived from lipids and lipid precursors. *Mutat. Res. Rev. Genet. Toxicol.* 238:223–233.
16. Abordo EA, Minhas HS, Thornalley PJ. 1999. Accumulation of α-oxaloaldehydes during oxidative stress: A role in cytotoxicity. *Biochem. Pharmacol.* 58:641–648.
17. Roberts MJ, Wondrak GT, Laurean DC, et al. 2003. DNA damage by carbonyl stress in human skin cells. *Mutat. Res.* 522:45–56.
18. Törnqvist M, Gustaffson B, Kautiainen A, et al. 1989. Unsaturated lipids and intestinal bacteria as sources of endogenous production of ethene and ethylene oxide. *Carcinogenesis* 10:39–41.

19. Holliday R, Ho T. 1998. Gene silencing and endogenous DNA methylation in mammalian cells. *Mutat. Res.* 400:361–368.

20. Rydberg B, Lindhal T. 1982. Nonenzymatic methylation of DNA by the intracellular methyl group donor S-adenosyl-L-methionine is a potentially mutagenic reaction. *EMBO J.* 1:211–216.

21. Zhao C, Tyndyk M, Eide I, et al. 1999. Endogenous and background DNA adducts by methylating and 2-hydroxyethylating agents. *Mutat. Res.* 424:117–125.

22. Nakamura J, La DK, Swenburg JA. 2000. 5′-Nicked apurinic/apyrimidinic sites are resistant to β-elimination by β-polymerase and are persistent in human cultured cells after oxidative stress. *J. Biol. Chem.* 275:5323–5328.

23. Lindahl T. 1993. Instability and decay of the primary structure of DNA. *Nature* 362:709–715.

24. Jackson AL, Loeb LA. 2001. The contribution of endogenous sources of DNA damage to the multiple mutations in cancer. *Mutat. Res.* 477:7–21.

25. Maarse H, Visscher CA, eds. 1989. *Volatile Compounds in Foods.* CIVO-TNO, Zeist, The Netherlands.

26. Prestera T, Zhang Y, Spencer SR, et al. 1993. The electrophile counterattack response: Protection against neoplasia and toxicity. *Adv. Enzyme Regul.* 33:281–296.

27. Gold LS. *Berkeley Carcinogenic Potency Database.* Available at http://potency.berkel.edu/pdfs/herp.pdf (accessed September 22, 2010).

28. Isihidate M, Harnois MC, Sofuni T. 1988. A comparative analysis of data on the clastogenicity of 951 chemical substances tested in mammalian cell cultures. *Mutat. Res.* 195:151.

29. McGregor DB, Brown A, Cattanach P, et al. 1998. Responses of the l5178y tk⁺/tk⁻ mouse lymphoma cell forward mutation assay: III. 72 Coded chemicals. *Environ. Mol. Mutagen.* 12:85–154.

30. Beier RC. 1990. Natural pesticides and bioactive components in foods. *Rev. Environ. Contam. Toxicol.* 113:47–137.

31. Lutz U, Lugli S, Bitsch A, et al. 1997. Dose response for the simulation of cell division by caffeic acid in forestomach and kidney of the male F344 rat. *Fund. Appl. Toxicol.* 39:131–137.

32. Park H-Y, Nam M-H, Lee H-S, et al. 2009. Isolation of caffeic acid from Perilla Frutescens and its role in enhancing γ-glutamylcysteine and synthetase activity and glutathione levels. *Food Chem.* 119:724–730.

33. López-Lázaro M, Willmore E, Austin CA. 2007. Cells lacking DNA topoisomerase II beta are resistant to genistein. *J. Nat. Prod.* 70:763–767.

34. Anon. 2009. Wikipedia. Available at http://en.wikipedia.org/wiki/Flavonoid.

35. Justestan U, Knuthsen P. 2001. Composition of flavonoids in fresh herbs and calculation of flavonoid intake by use of herbs in traditional Danish dishes. *Food Chem.* 73:245–250.

36. Ewald C, Fjelkner-Modig S, Johansson K, et al. 1999. Effect of processing on major flavonoids in processed onions, green beans, and peas. *Food Chem.* 64:231–235.

37. López-Lázaro M. 2002. Flavonoids as anticancer agents: Structure- activity relationship study. *Curr. Med. Chem. Anticancer Agents* 2:691–714.

38. Ren W, Qiao Z, Wang H, et al. 2003. Flavonoids: Promising anticancer agents. *Med. Res. Rev.* 23:519–534.

39. Strick R, Strissel PL, Birgers S, et al. 2000. Dietary bioflavonoids induce cleavage in the *MLL* gene and may contribute to infant leukaemia. *Proc Natl. Acad. Sci. USA* 97:4790–4795.

40. Galati G, Brien PJO. 2004. Potential toxicity of flavonoids and other dietary phenolics: Significance for their chemopreventive and anticancer properties. *Free Radic. Biol. Med.* 37:287–303.

41. Cho KH, Pezzuto JM, Bolton JL, et al. 2000. Selection of cancer chemopreventive agents based on inhibition of topoisomerase II activity. *Eur. J. Cancer* 36:2146–2156.

42. Mittra B, Saha A, Chowdhury AR, et al. 2002. Luteolin, an emerging anti-cancer flavonoid, poisons eukaryotic DNA topoisomerase I. *Biochem. J.* 366:653–661.

43. Felix CA. 1998. Secondary leukaemias induced by topoisomerase-targeted drugs. *Biochem. Biophys. Acta* 1400:233–255.

44. Felix CA. 2001. Leukemias related to treatment with DNA topoisomerase II inhibitors. *Med. Pediatr. Oncol.* 36:525–535.

45. Mistry AR, Felix CA, Whitmarsh RJ, et al. 2005. DNA topoisomerase II in therapy-related acute promyelocytic leukemia. *N. Eng. J. Med.* 352:1529–1538.

46. Liu LF. 1989. DNA topoisomerase poisons as antitumor drugs. *Ann. Rev. Biochem.* 58:351–375.

47. Spector LG, Xie Y, Robinson LL, et al. 2005. Maternal diet and infant leukaemia: The DNA topoi-somerase II inhibitor hypothesis: A report from the children's oncology group. *Cancer Epidem. Biomarkers Prev.* 14:651–655.

48. Shukla PK, Khanna VK, Khan MY, et al. 2003. Protective effect of curcumin against lead neuro-toxicity in rat. *Hum. Exp. Toxicol.* 22:653–658.

49. Sharma RA, Gescher AJ, Steward WP. 2005. Curcumin: The story so far. *Eur. J. Cancer* 41:1955–1968.

50. Li M, Zhang Z, Hill DL, et al. 2007. Curcumin, a dietary component. *Cancer Res.* 67:1988–1996.

51. Scott DW, Loo G. 2004. Curcumin-induced GADD153 gene up-regulation in human colon cancer cells. *Carcinogenesis* 25:2155–2164.

52. Sakano K, Kawanishi S. 2002. Metal-mediated DNA damage induced by curcumin in the presence of human cytochrome P450 isozymes. *Arch. Biochem. Biophys.* 405:223–230.

53. Martin-Cardero C, López-Lázaro M, Galvez M, et al. 2003. Curcumin as a DNA topoisomerase II poison. *J. Enzyme Inhib. Med. Chem.* 18:505–509.

54. López-Lázaro M, Willmore E, Johnson A, et al. 2007. Curcumin induces high levels of topoisom-erase I– and II–DNA complexes in K562 leukaemia cells. *J. Nat. Prod.* 70:1884–1888.

55. Cao J, Li-Ping J, Liu Y, et al. 2007. Curcumin-induced genotoxicity and antigenotoxicity in HepG2 cells. *Toxicon* 49:1219–1222.

56. European Commission, Health and Consumer Protection Directorate General. 2002. *Opinion of the Scientific Committee on Food on the safety of the presence of safrole (1-allyl-3,4-methylene dioxy benzene) in flavourings and other food ingredients with flavouring properties.* SCF/CS/FLAV// Flavour/6 ADD3 Final, 9 January.

57. European Commission, Health and Consumer Protection Directorate General. 2001. *Opinion of the Scientific Committee on food on estragole (1-allyl-4-methoxy benzene).* SCF/CS/FLAV//Flavour/6 ADD2 Final, 26 September.

58. European Commission, Health and Consumer Protection Directorate General. 2001. *Opinion of the Scientific Committee on food on methyleugenol (4-allyl-1,2-dimethoxy benzene).* SCF/CS/FLAV// Flavour/4 ADD1 Final, 9 September.

59. Groopman JD, Zhu JQ, Donahue PR, et al. 1992. High-affinity monoclonal antibodies for aflatoxins and their application to solid-phase immunoassays. *Cancer Res.* 52:45–52.

60. WHO. 1998. *Global Environment Monitoring System—Food Contamination Monitoring and Assessment Programme (GEMS/Food).* Available at http://www.who.int/foodsafety/chem/gems/en/index.html.

61. O'Brien J, Renwick. AG, Constable A, et al. 2006. Approaches to the risk assessment of genotoxic carcinogens in food: A critical appraisal. *Food Chem. Toxicol.* 44:1613–1635.

62. Lutz WK, Schlatter J. 1992. Chemical carcinogens and overnutrition in diet-related cancer. *Carcinogenesis* 13:2211–2216.

63. Sugimura T. 2000. Nutrition and dietary carcinogens. *Carcinogenesis* 21:387–395.

64. Jadhav SJ, Scharma RP, Salunkhe DK. 1981. Naturally occurring toxic alkaloids in foods. *Crit. Rev. Toxicol.* 9:21–104.

65. Harvey MH, Morris BA, Mcmillan M, Marks V. 1985. Measurement of potato steroidal alkaloids in human serum and saliva by radioimmunoassay. *Hum. Toxicol.* 4:503–512.

66. McMilland M, Thompson JC. 1979. An outbreak of suspected solanine poisoning in schoolboys: Examination of criteria of solanine poisoning. *Q. J. Med.* 48:227–243.

67. Barceloux DG. 2008. *Medical Toxicology of Natural Substances: Foods, Fungi, Medicinal Herbs, Toxic Plants, and Venomous Animals.* John Wiley & Sons, Hoboken, NJ, pp. 77–83.

68. Hirono I, Mori H, Yamada K, Hirata Y, Haga M. 1977. Carcinogenic activity of petasitenine, a new pyrrolizidine alkaloid isolated from *Petasites japonicus* Maxim. *J. Natl. Cancer Inst.* 58:1155–1157.

69. Hirayama T, Ito Y. 1981. A new view of the etiology of nasopharyngeal carcinoma. *Prev. Med.* 10:614–622.

70. Hecker E. 1981. Cocarcinogenesis and tumor promoters of the diterpene ester type as possible carcinogenic risk factors. *J. Cancer Res. Clin. Oncol.* 99:103–124.

71. Lee KW, Lee HJ, Lee CY. 2004. Vitamins, phytochemicals, diets, and their implementation in cancer chemoprevention. *Crit. Rev. Food Sci. Nut.* 44:437–452.

72. Kava R, Flynn L. *ACSH Holiday Dinner Menu.* Available at http://www.acsh.org/publications/pubID.103_detail.asp.

73. Estabrooke R. 1996. Carcinogens and anticarcinogens in the human diet. A comparison of naturally occurring and synthetic substances. Available at www.nap.edu/books/0309053919/html/index.html (accessed September 22, 2010).

74. Loft S, Poulson HE. 1996. Cancer risk and oxidative DNA damage in man. *J. Mol. Med.* 74:297–312.

75. Gold LS, Ames BN. 2001. Natural and synthetic chemicals in the diet: A critical analysis of potential cancer Hazards. In: *Food Safety and Food Quality*, edited by RE Hester, RM Harrison. Royal Society of Chemistry, Cambridge, UK, pp. 95–128.

76. Brusick DJ. 2009. A perspective on testing of existing pharmaceutical excipients for genotoxic impurities. *Reg. Toxicol. Pharmacol.* 55:200–204.

77. Tareke E, Rydberg P, Karlsson P, et al. 2002. Analysis of acrylamide, a carcinogen formed in heated foodstuffs. *J. Agric. Food Chem.* 50:4998–5006.

78. Dybing E, Sanner T. 2003. Risk assessment of acrylamide in foods. *Toxicol. Sci.* 75:7–15.

79. Dybing E, O'Brien JO, Renwick AG, Sanner T. 2008. Risk assessment of dietary exposures to compounds that are genotoxic and carcinogenic—An overview. *Toxicol. Lett.* 180:110–117.

80. Schlatter J, Knaap A (chairs). Summary Report, EFSA Scientific Colloquim No. 11. Acrylamide carcinogenicity. New evidence in relation to dietary exposure. May 22–23, 2008, Tabiano (PR), Italy. Available at www.efsa.europa.eu/en/events/event/colloque080522.htm (accessed on September 22, 2010).

81. Kuratsune M. 1956. Benzo[*a*]pyrene content of certain pyro- genicmaterials. *J. Natl. Cancer Inst.* 16:1485–1496.

82. Kuratsune M, Hueper WC. 1960. Polycyclic aromatic hydrocarbons in roasted coffee. *J. Natl. Cancer Inst.* 24:463–469.

83. Keating GA, Bogen KT. 2001. Methods for estimating heterocyclic amine concentrations in cooked meats in the US diet. *Food Chem. Toxicol.* 39:29–43.

84. Zimmerli B, Schlatter J. 1991. Ethyl carbamate: Analyticalmethodology, occurrence, formation, biological activity and risk assessment. *Mutat. Res.* 259:325–350.

85. Uthurry CA, Varela F, Colomo B, et al. 2004. Ethyl carbamate concentrations of typical Spanish red wines. *Food Chem.* 88:329–336.

86. Foulke JE. 1993. *FDA Consumer: Urethane in alcoholic beverages under investigation.* U.S. Food and Drug Administration, Jan–Feb.

87. Johns S. May 2000. Foods Standard Agency UK. Survey of ethyl carbamate in whisky, Report No. 02–00. Available at www.food.gov.uk/science/surveillance/fsis2000/2whisky (accessed September 22, 2010).

88. Butzke CE, Bisson LF. Ethyl carbamate or urethane. *Information on Ethyl Carbamate (Urethane) in Foods and Beverages.* Ethyl Carbamate Preventative Action Manual. Available at www.fda.gov/Food/FoodSafety/FoodContaminantsAdulteration/.../EthylCarbamateUrethane/ucm078521.htm (accessed September 22, 2010).

89. Stofberg J, Grundschober F. 1987. The consumption ratio and food predominance of flavoring materials. *Perfum. Flavor.* 12:27–56.

90. Fujita Y, Wakabayashi K, Nagao M, et al. 1985. Implication of hydrogen peroxide in the mutagenicity of coffee. *Mutat. Res.* 144:227–230.

91. Shibamoto T. 2006. Analytical methods for trace levels of reactive carbonyl compounds formed in lipid peroxidation systems. *J. Pharm. Biomed. Anal.* 41:12–25.

92. Axelson O, Berglund B, Calamari D. 1989. IPCS Environmental health criteria no. 89, Formaldehyde. Available at http://www.inchem.org/documents/ehc/ehc/ehc89.htm (accessed September 22, 2010).

93. Gerim M (chair). 2006. *IARC monographs on the evaluation of carcinogenic risks to humans: Formaldehyde, 2-butoxyethanol and 1-tert-butoxypropan-2-ol,* Vol. 88.

94. Federal Register. Docket no. 97F-0440, 1998, Vol. 63, No. 124.

95. Aito O, Axelson O, Blair A, et al. 1999. *Re-evaluation of some organic chemicals, hydrazine and hydrogen peroxide.* IARC Monographs on the Evaluation of Carcinogenic Risks to Humans, Vol. 71.

96. Parent RA, Caravello HE, Long JE. 1991. Oncogenicity study of acrolein in mice. *J. Am. Coll. Toxicol.* 10:647–659.

97. Morris JB, Robinson DE, Vollmuth TA, et al. 1996. A parallelogram approach for the safety evaluation of ingested acetaldehyde. *Regul. Toxicol. Pharmacol.* 24:251–263.

98. Dhareshwar SS, Stella VJ. 2008. Your pro-drug releases formaldehyde: Should you be concerned? No! *J. Pharm. Sci.* 97:4184–4193.

99. Collins JJ, Acquavella JF, Esmen NA. 1997. An updated meta-analysis of formaldehyde exposure and upper respiratory tract cancers. *J. Occup. Environ. Med.* 39:639–651.
100. Arts JHE, Rennen MAJ, de Heer C. 2006. Inhaled formaldehyde: Evaluation of sensory irritation in relation to carcinogenicity. *Regul. Toxicol. Pharmacol.* 44:144–160.
101. Fer M, Goulitiquer S, Dreano Y, et al. 2006. Determination of polyunsaturated fatty acid mono-epoxides by high performance liquid chromatography-mass spectrometry. *J. Chromatographr. A* 1115:1–7.
102. Manson MM. 1980. Epoxides—Is there a human health problem? *Br. J. Ind. Med.* 37:317–336.
103. Stella VJ, Umprayn K, Waugh WN. 1998. Development of parenteral formulations of experimental cytotoxic agents. I. Rhizoxin (NSC-332598). *Int. J. Pharm.* 43:191–199.
104. Bolt HM. 1996. Quantification of endogenous carcinogens: The ethylene oxide paradox. *Biochem. Pharmacol.* 52:1–5.
105. Ishidate M, Tanimura A, Ito Y, et al. 1972. Secondary amines, nitrites and nirosamines in Japanese foods. In: *Topics in Chemical Carcinogenesis*, edited by W Nakahara, S Takayama, T Sugimura, et al. University of Tokyo Press, Tokyo, Japan, pp. 313–321.
106. Sander J, Burkle G, Schweinsberg F. 1972. Induction of tumours by nitrite and secondary amines or amides. In: *Topics in Chemical Carcinogenesis*, edited by W Nakahara, S Takayama, T Sugimura, et al. University of Tokyo Press, Tokyo, Japan, pp. 313–321.
107. Ochiai M, Wakabayashi K, Nagao M, et al. 1984. Tyramine is a major mutagen precursor in soy sauce, being convertible to a mutagen by nitrite. *Gann* 75:1–3.
108. Fujita Y, Wakabayashi K, Takayama S, et al. 1987. Induction of oral cavity cancer by 3-diazotyramine, a nitrosated product of tyramine present in foods. *Carcinogenesis* 8:527–529.
109. Wakabayashi K, Ochiai M, Saito H, et al. 1983. Presence of 1-methyl-1,2,3,4-tetrahydro-beta-carboline-3-carboxylic acid, a precursor of a mutagenic nitroso compound, in soy sauce. *Proc. Natl. Acad. Sci. USA* 80:2912–2916.
110. Herraiz T. 1998. Tetrahydro-β-carboline alkaloids occur in fruits and fruit juices. Activity as anti-oxidants and radical scavengers. *J. Agric. Food Chem.* 46:3484–3490.
111. Wakabayashi K, Nagao M, Ochiai M, et al. 1985. A mutagen precursor in Chinese cabbage, indole-3-acetonitrile, which becomes mutagenic on nitrite treatment. *Mutat. Res.* 143:17–21.
112. Ochiai M, Wakabayashi K, Sugimura T, et al. 1986. Mutagenicity of indole and 30 derivatives after nitrite treatment. *Mutat. Res.* 172:189–197.
113. Benjamin N, O'Driscoll F, Dougall H, et al. 1994. Stomach NO synthesis. *Nature* 368:502.
114. Sobko T, Reinders CL, Jansson E, et al. 2005. Gastric intestinal bacteria generate nitric oxide from nitrate and nitrite. *Nitric Oxide* 13:272–278.
115. Tannerbaum SR. 1979. Endogenous formation of nitrite and *N*-nitroso compounds. In: *Naturally Occurring Carcinogens-Mutagens and Modulators of Carcinogenesis*, edited by EC Miller, JA Miller, I Hirono, et al. Jap.Sci.Soc.Press, Tokyo/University Park Press, Baltimore, pp. 211–220.
116. van Breemen RB, Fong. HHS, Farnswort NR. 2007. The role of quality assurance and standardization in the safety of botanical dietary supplements. *Chem. Res. Toxicol.* 20(4):577–582.
117. Guo F-Q, Liang Y-Z, Xu C-J, et al. 2003. Determination of the volatile chemical constituents of *Notoptergium incium* by gas-chromatography-mass spectrometry and iterative or non-iterative chemometrics resolution methods. *J. Chromatographr. A.* 1016:99–110.
118. Guo F-Q, Liang Y-Z, Xu C-J, et al. 2004. Analyzing of the volatile chemical constituents in *Artemisia capillaris herba* by GC–MS and correlative chemometric resolution methods. *J. Pharm. Biomed. Anal.* 35:469–478.
119. Lao SC, Li SP, Kan KKW, et al. 2004. Identification and quantification of 13 components in *Angelica sinensis* (Danggui) by gas chromatography–mass spectrometry coupled with pressurized liquid extraction. *Anal. Chim. Acta* 526:131–137.
120. Schwetz BA. 2001. Safety of Aristolochic acid. *JAMA* 285:2705.
121. WHO Pharmaceuticals Newsletter, No. 1 (2002).
122. IARC. International Agency for Research on Cancer. 2002. *Aristolochia Species and Aristolochic Acids*, Vol. 82. IARC, Lyon, France.
123. Committee for Medicinal Products (CHMP), European Medicines Agency. 2006. *Concept paper on the development of a guideline on the assessment of genotoxic constituents in herbal substances/preparations* (EMEA/HPMC/413271/2006). London, October 25, 2006.

PART 4

ASSESSMENT OF GENOTOXIC RISK: QUALITY PERSPECTIVE

CHAPTER *9*

STRATEGIES FOR THE EVALUATION OF GENOTOXIC IMPURITY RISK

Andrew Teasdale
Dave Elder
Simon Fenner

9.1 INTRODUCTION

Since the publication of the European Medicines Evaluation Agency (EMEA) position paper in 2002 on limits for genotoxic impurities, it has been necessary for pharmaceutical companies to consider the potential risk posed by genotoxic impurities within their products. This has therefore driven the need to develop an effective strategy that both identifies and assesses the risk posed by any genotoxic impurity within the process used to manufacture the active pharmaceutical ingredient (API), and any subsequent change to the synthesis.

In order to synthesize APIs efficiently, it is necessary to build up the molecular structure through the combination of simple structural motifs. This typically involves the formation of carbon–carbon, carbon–nitrogen, and carbon–oxygen bonds. The current status of synthetic methodology is such that this is impractical to achieve without the use of electrophilic species that fall into the broad class of alkylating agents, and are hence potentially genotoxic.

Thus, many intrinsically reactive starting materials, intermediates, and reagents used in the synthesis of APIs are potentially genotoxic, and furthermore may present as residual impurities within the API. Although avoidance is generally considered to be the preferable option from a regulator's perspective, there is tacit acceptance of the fact that this is generally impractical, and hence rather than avoidance, the issue becomes one of control.[1]

Several organizations have published details of their approach,[2-4] and these are discussed below; all are based on the same general principal.

- First, materials present in the synthesis are screened for potential genotoxicity, typically through the application of an appropriate structure activity relationship (SAR) process, using commercial systems such as DEREK® (Lhasa Limited,

Genotoxic Impurities: Strategies for Identification and Control, Edited by Andrew Teasdale

Leeds, UK) and/or MCase® (Multicase Inc., Beachwood, OH) to predict for mutagenicity.

- Then, for materials flagging as potentially (PGI) or actually genotoxic (GI), this is followed by an evaluation of the likelihood of the material in question to carry through to the API, taking into consideration the properties of the compound in question, and the downstream process conditions.

This chapter describes this evaluation process in detail. A structured approach is defined based on the principals of quality by design (ICH Q8[5]) and risk assessment (ICH Q9[6]), providing an effective, robust process that identifies and addresses the risk posed by genotoxic impurities. This also examines the scope of such activities and the critical factors to consider when assessing risk. The relationship between analytical and safety testing, as well as the relative timing of such activities, is also considered.

The practical application of this process is then demonstrated in several case studies.

9.2 SCOPE

9.2.1 General

Both the adopted EMEA guideline,[7] and the draft FDA guideline,[8] are stated to be only applicable to new products and those currently in clinical development. However, the principles of the assessment process are also equally applicable to the assessment of a marketed product, in circumstances where these guidelines are deemed to be retrospectively applicable.

9.2.2 Impurities: API and Formulated Product

While it is likely that the scope of the assessment is focused on starting materials, raw materials, reagents, and intermediates within the synthetic process, the EMEA guideline also stipulates the need to take "probable" impurities and degradants into consideration. The guideline specifically defines the scope as probable impurities, and thus any evaluation of impurities should be framed in this context. It is impractical and unnecessary to attempt to evaluate every conceivable product derived from increasingly improbable side reactions. Further definition of "probable" is pertinent and will be explored in more detail in Section 9.3.1.

It is important to note that the guidelines also stipulate the need for consideration of any additional impurities that are observed in the formulated product.

9.2.3 Degradants

Although the threat posed by genotoxic impurities originates principally from the synthetic process used for the manufacture of the API, genotoxic impurities can also be formed as a result of degradation in either the API and/or the drug product. It is thus important that the genotoxic impurity risk assessment takes into consideration information related to degradants gained during stability and/or degradation studies. This is examined in detail in Chapter 15.

9.2.4   Excipients

Established excipients are generally considered to be outside of the scope of the EMEA guideline.[7] The principles behind this exclusion are similar to those that exclude existing marketing products, being based on safety data established through use within existing products. Furthermore, many excipients are also used in other applications, particularly food, and some are also listed on the FDA GRAS (generally regarded as safe) list.[9] This area has been thoroughly reviewed by Brusick.[10]

However, the guideline is considered applicable when considering novel excipients, and in such cases, the same assessment principles described in this document may also be applied.

It is recommended that compatibility is taken into consideration should there be any potential for reaction between an API and an excipient (see Chapter 15). In most instances where such incompatibilities arise, it is likely to lead to replacement of that particular excipient, or where unavoidable, a specific grade or form designed to minimize the interaction should be selected. This mirrors the approach employed during API development, in which a thorough understanding of the science is combined with a strategy to reduce or control the formation of the PGI material of concern. For example, an inerting atmosphere might be selected for the processing of liquid or semi-solid formulations, and/or addition of antioxidants made to prevent or limit oxidatively-mediated degradation processes. Similarly, the use of low moisture excipients, low moisture processing (e.g. direct compression or dry granulation), and highly protective container closures (e.g. cold-form aluminium blisters) would be recommended to preclude moisture-mediated hydrolysis processes. As with API synthetic routes, the rejection of the formulation in question and the development of an alternative one is typically the least favored option.

9.2.5   Metabolites

Neither the EMEA guideline nor the draft FDA guideline makes specific reference to potentially genotoxic metabolites of APIs. Separate guidance is available covering the approach to take for significant metabolites.[11]

However, there may be occasions where a process intermediate, impurity, or degradant may also be a human metabolite. In such cases, the overall risk assessment should take into account total exposure, that is, to both the process related material and metabolite. The evaluation of genotoxic risk associated with metabolites is discussed in detail in Chapter 6.

9.2.6   Quality Risk Management Process

The need for quality risk management of pharmaceutical processes and procedures has been fully discussed within ICH Q9.[6] Risk management is based on an evaluation of two key factors:

- the probability or likelihood of occurrence; and
- the severity or impact of the resulting outcome.

It is a systematic process that evaluates:

- what can go wrong;
- what is the likelihood of it going wrong;
- what are the consequences; and
- what can be done to either eliminate or control the risk.

A further factor in risk evaluation is the level of effort taken to evaluate the risk. This should be directly related to the level of the risk, as should the efforts taken to eliminate or reduce it.

In the context of an assessment of risk posed by genotoxic impurities, the threshold of toxicological concern (TTC) effectively establishes a limit in terms of defining "acceptable risk." The requirement is therefore to assess the likelihood of a genotoxic impurity exceeding this threshold in API/DP, and where a significant likelihood is identified, to provide adequate assurance of its effective control. Such a process is described below.

A key aspect of the process is its multidisplinary nature. For such a process to be efficient, it must necessarily draw on the collective skills of personnel from disciplines, such as chemistry, toxicology, formulation, and analytical.

9.3 GI RISK ASSESSMENT PROCESS

The process begins with the evaluation of the synthetic route for postulated and/or known impurities. This is followed by structural assessment of agreed "probable" impurities, along with other route materials and reagents where appropriate, hazard classification, quantification and/or safety testing, risk assessment and finally establishment of control measures where required.

The evaluation process is represented schematically in Figure 9.1.

The process should be flexible; each API/DP synthesis has its own distinctive features, and, where appropriate, the ordering of the steps described may be changed; however, the overall process should generally remain the same.

There is a clear link between the assessment of risk and the permitted level for a genotoxic impurity. Any such evaluation should therefore take into account the phase of development, the intended dose and likely clinical trial study duration. Permissible limits are based on the "staged TTC" principle. Limits cited in the EMEA Q&A Supplement[12] to the main guideline are given in Table 9.1.

The EMEA guideline also states that values higher than the TTC may be acceptable under certain conditions, including short-term exposure, for treatment of a life-threatening condition, when life expectancy is less than 5 years or when there is greater exposure from other sources such as food.

It is recommended that a permitted limit, for example staged TTC, is established in advance of instigating the formal evaluation, with the caveat that this limit will change dependant on both time (duration of clinical phase) and dose (absolute level of exposure).

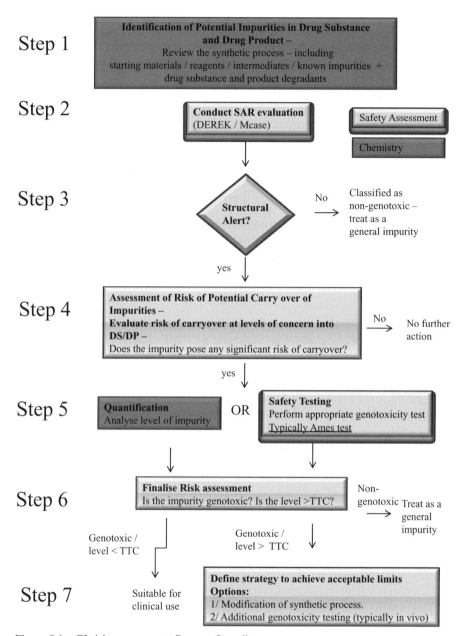

Figure 9.1   GI risk assessment—Process flow diagram.

TABLE 9.1   Adopted Allowable Daily Intakes (μg/day) for GIs during Clinical Development, a Staged TTC Approach Depending on Duration of Exposure

	1 day	2 days to 1 month	>1–3 months	>3–6 months	>6–12 months	>12 months
ADI * (μg/day) for different duration of exposure (as normally used in clinical development)	120[a] Or 0.5%[c] Whichever is lower	60[a] Or 0.5%[c] Whichever is lower	20[a] Or 0.5%[c] Whichever is lower	10[a] Or 0.5%[c] Whichever is lower	5[a,c]	1.5[b]

[a] Probability of not exceeding a 10^{-6} risk is 93%.

[b] Probability of not exceeding a 10^{-5} risk is 93%, which considers a 70-year exposure.

[c] Other limits (higher or lower) may be appropriate and the approaches used to identify, qualify and control ordinary impurities during developed should be applied.

ADI, allowable daily intake.

9.3.1   Step 1: Evaluation of Drug Substance and Drug Product Processes for Sources of Potentially Genotoxic Impurities

The responsibility for this step is likely to fall to the chemists and analysts responsible for the design and development of the API synthetic process, with additional input from pharmaceutical development groups who can comment on issues arising from stability and degradation studies, as well as excipient compatibility.

An evaluation of the synthetic route, focused on starting materials, intermediates, reagents, catalysts and solvents is carried out to identify materials which could possibly survive the process and present in the API as impurities. It should also include consideration of other potential impurities that may arise from the synthetic route, particularly in the final stages. These could include related substances of the API or intermediates, through to materials derived from interactions between reagents and solvents. However, care should be exercised when considering the scope of impurities to be included in the assessment. The EMEA guideline contains the following advice:

> As stated in the Q3A guideline, actual and potential impurities most likely to arise during the synthesis, purification and storage of the new drug substance should be identified, based on sound scientific appraisal of the chemical reactions involved in synthesis, impurities associated with raw materials that could contribute to the impurity profile of the new drug substance, and possible degradation products. This discussion can be limited to those impurities that might reasonably be expected based on scientific knowledge of the chemical reactions and conditions involved.

Such impurities could include, for example, a regioisomer of an alerting intermediate that does not react as per the main component in a cyclization reaction, leaving the regioisomer to potentially pass unreacted into the API. Other examples include side reactions between sulfonic acids and alcohols to yield sulfonate esters (although such reactions can be very effectively controlled—see Chapter 14).

Potentially genotoxic impurities that might be present in API generally fall into the following categories:

- Unreacted contributory materials or intermediates with alerting substructures that have survived processing (e.g. unreacted nitroaromatic in a nitrogen heterocycle API, due to incomplete hydrogenation or a positional isomer unable to cyclize).

- Substances closely related to contributory materials, intermediates, or the API itself that contain an alerting structural motif (e.g. a chloroalkyl analogue of a hydroxyalkyl containing API following treatment with hydrochloric acid during processing).

- Unrelated substances formed by combinations of solvents and reagents with each other or with contributory materials or intermediates (e.g. isopropyl tosylate formed as a result of isopropanol damp hydroxylated intermediate being used in a reaction with tosyl chloride).

This is fully aligned with the tenets of ICH Q9,[7] which focuses on the probability of an event occurring, combined with an evaluation of the impact of the event occurring, leading to a consideration of the risk posed. The magnitude of the risk is therefore related to the probability of the PGI being present. Hence, the greatest risk is posed by those agents used in the late stages of the API synthesis that possess well-established alerting structural motifs, and these should be the main focus of the evaluation.

At an appropriate point in the development of an API, the risk assessment should also include consideration of materials arising from degradation during manufacture or on long term storage of the API or its formulated product. This review may be based on a combination of factors, including scientific knowledge and *in silico* predictions of the typical degradation pathways of the API and formulated product based on the chemical structure and literature precedent. The conduct of such assessments is described in detail in Chapter 15.

Another factor for consideration when defining the scope of the evaluation is the level of an impurity and the extent of characterization. It was confirmed through the EMEA Q&A[12] supplement to the main guideline that no action is required for any unidentified impurity below the ICH identification threshold. Hence, there is no requirement to identify and assess every impurity observed within the API and the resulting formulated product, the threshold for identification being defined by ICH Q3A/B.[13,14]

Having agreed a list of materials, which might comprise structurally contributing raw materials, intermediates, known process impurities, other probable process impurities, as well as significant degradation products, these should then be subjected to a formal structural assessment for genotoxicity.

9.3.2 Step 2: Structural Assessment

Both EMEA and FDA draft guidelines recognize the use of structural assessment as a valid means by which an assessment of genotoxic potential can be made. The use of *in silico* systems is generally recommended; the most commonly applied are the

Structural Alerts for Mutagenicity

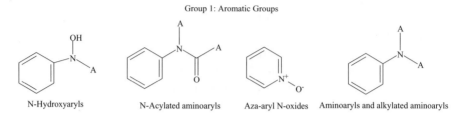

Group 1: Aromatic Groups

N-Hydroxyaryls · N-Acylated aminoaryls · Aza-aryl N-oxides · Aminoaryls and alkylated aminoaryls

Purines or Pyrimidines, Intercalators, PNAs or PNAHs

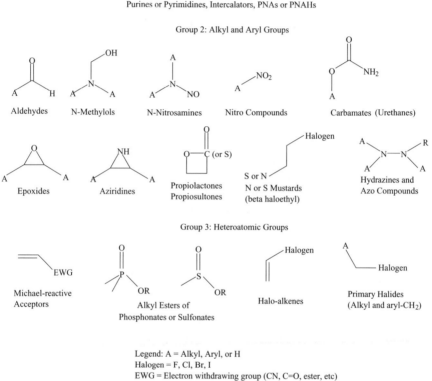

Group 2: Alkyl and Aryl Groups

Aldehydes · N-Methylols · N-Nitrosamines · Nitro Compounds · Carbamates (Urethanes)

Epoxides · Aziridines · Propiolactones Propiosultones · S or N N or S Mustards (beta haloethyl) · Hydrazines and Azo Compounds

Group 3: Heteroatomic Groups

Michael-reactive Acceptors · Alkyl Esters of Phosphonates or Sulfonates · Halo-alkenes · Primary Halides (Alkyl and aryl-CH$_2$)

Legend: A = Alkyl, Aryl, or H
Halogen = F, Cl, Br, I
EWG = Electron withdrawing group (CN, C=O, ester, etc)

Figure 9.2 Structural alerts.

commercial packages DEREK® and MCase®; often used in tandem, these are described in more detail in Chapter 4. Evaluations are primarily focused on mutagenicity (Ames positive) due to this being recognized as the most appropriate indicator for direct interaction with DNA.

Smaller organizations may find these systems to be prohibitively expensive, in which case a simple system based on Ashby and Tennant alerts[15] (see Fig. 9.2) is available.

In addition to using commercial databases, some organizations have developed their own *in silico* systems utilizing in-house data that allow for further refinement of predictions.

9.3.3   Step 3: Classification

Once a structural assessment has been completed, each impurity should be categorized according to its genotoxic hazard. The five-class classification scheme, defined by Mueller et al.,[16] has been widely adopted for this purpose, and this is shown in Table 9.2.

It is important to be aware that the SAR evaluation procedures can only be as good as the databases and rule sets that underpin the systems. It is known that there are deficiencies in the models for some compound classes, for example those relating to anilines and heteroaromatic amines. It may be advisable to treat these cases individually, with the option to consider safety testing (Ames test) where this is deemed necessary.

Although *in silico* systems are comprehensive in terms of the compound classes covered, there are nevertheless examples of classes that are not covered and for which there is no closely related data in the underlying database. This point was made by Dobo et al.[2] in respect of heteroaromatic nitro compounds. Hence, it is important for the recipients of the SAR output to scrutinize the findings. If an impurity has no flags for genotoxicity, but is used in the process as an electrophile, then it would be prudent to seek expert judgment with respect to the strength of the underlying dataset.

Evaluation of genotoxic risk can also be augmented by data derived from within the public domain. Included within these is TOXNET, a searchable database provided by the U.S. Library of Medicine. This provides access to a series of databases through a common portal:

- HSDB: Hazardous Substances Databank;
- CCRIS: Chemical Carcinogenesis Research Information System; and
- IRIS: Integrated Risk Information System)

that provide an excellent source of safety data for many common chemicals. Another related system is the Berkeley database.[17] Indeed, as described in Chapter 5, it is often

TABLE 9.2   Impurity Classification

Classification	Definition
Class 1	Known genotoxic carcinogens, based on evidence of carcinogenicity derived from animal/human carcinogenicity studies
Class 2	Impurities known to be genotoxic (mutagenic) with unknown carcinogenic potential. Genotoxic potential typically identified by a positive response in an Ames test.
Class 3	Impurities judged to be alerting for genotoxicity by SAR analysis, but for which no data on genotoxic potential exist.
Class 4	Impurities judged to be alerting for genotoxicity by SAR analysis, but for which the alert in question is common to one also present in the parent API. Provided that the API has been adequately assessed for mutagenicity and shown to negative, such impurities can be considered qualified and controlled as a normal impurity
Class 5	Impurities for which there is no identified structural alerts and no additional data to suggest the existence of any mutagenic potential. Such impurities are controlled as normal impurities

possible with common reagents to locate sufficient safety data to allow genotoxic risk to be assessed on a compound specific basis rather than simply applying the TTC. This is defined as an allowable approach within the recent FDA guideline.[8]

9.3.4 Step 4: Assessment of Risk of Potential Carry over of Impurities

Once impurities with a potential genotoxic safety concern have been identified by the SAR evaluation process, the next step is to consider the likelihood of a particular impurity being present in the isolated API, often referred to as impurity fate mapping.

The impurities under consideration are by nature often highly reactive, hence their removal during downstream processing is facilitated by this intrinsic activity. Acidic and/or basic work-up conditions frequently encountered in manufacturing processes may lead to decomposition and/or removal of the material of concern. Similarly, other reagents used in downstream processing may react with the material, rendering it less reactive and thereby "safe." Factors that contribute to removal of such impurities are reviewed in depth in the following section.

Such impurity fate assessments have largely been based on the theoretical knowledge and experience of the evaluating chemist. Unfortunately, however compelling the arguments developed, they have often been viewed as nonquantitative from a regulatory perspective. Thus, in many cases, there is a need to provide further analytical data to substantiate the impurity fate assessment. Hence, a quality by testing (QbT) approach is adopted rather than a quality by design (QbD) approach.

There would be considerable value from an industry and regulatory perspective in defining a standardized approach to such assessments. It should be possible to assess fate at least semi-quantitatively based on factors linked to the impurity's physicochemical properties (and taking in to account those of the API and intermediates), and the process conditions employed in the route of manufacture to the API. Pierson et al.[3] have suggested that an assumption could be made of a 10-fold reduction per synthetic stage. In many cases, this would suffice and indeed may even be a cautious estimate of the risk. However, in certain circumstances, for example an unreactive genotoxic reagent or intermediate used in a "telescoped" process (no isolations between stages), this may be too simplistic. For this reason, a more quantitative approach, based on actual process conditions and the physicochemical properties of the genotoxic impurity in question, has been sought, and is outlined below.

A number of contributory factors have been defined that should be taken into account for such an assessment; these are described below.

9.3.4.1 Reactivity
As already described, many of the PGIs/GIs that are likely to be of concern are intrinsically reactive. For example, acyl halides are compounds that are so reactive that there would be little practical value in monitoring their presence in the outcome of the reaction. Moreover, should there be any residual analyte; this would be effectively eliminated through procedures such as an aqueous quench or even a simple water wash of the resulting product.

Even in processes where there is a likelihood that some residue may remain in an intermediate, for many such compounds, there is a high probability of reaction

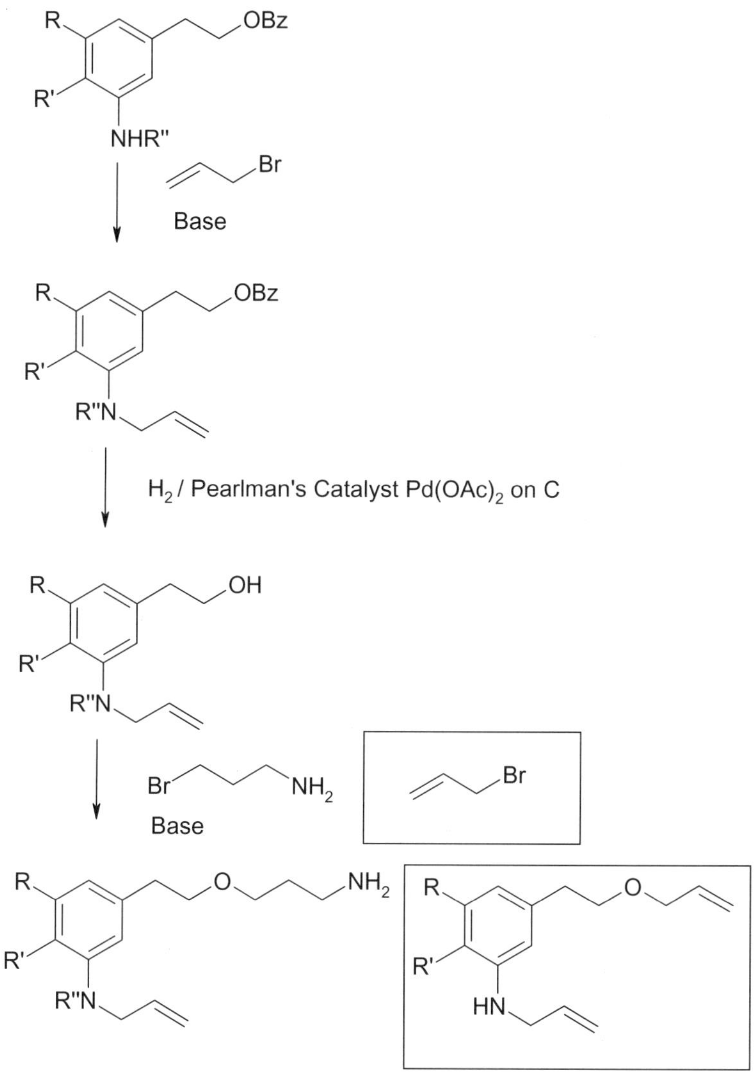

Figure 9.3 Example reaction scheme illustrating a process involving two alkylation steps and the likely fate of any residual allyl bromide used in Step 1.

in a subsequent process stage. Consider, for example, an alkyl halide used early in a synthesis; should a further alkylating agent be used downstream in the process, any residual quantities of the initial alkyl halide are highly likely to be consumed in the latter stage (see Fig. 9.3). In this process, any residual allyl bromide remaining after stage 1 may carry through into stage 3 where, if still present, it would be expected to react to produce the allyl analogue of the desired product.

On the basis of *chemical* reactivity, it is proposed that genotoxic compounds could be placed into one of three categories (see Table 9.3).

TABLE 9.3 Genotoxic Compounds classified based on Reactivity

Reactivity class	Genotoxic groups
Highly reactive[a]	Epoxides/aldehydes/sulfonate esters/acyl halides/aziridines/hydrazines
Moderate reactivity	N or S mustards/Michael reactive acceptors/halo-alkenes, primary halides
Low reactivity	Amino aryls, nitro compounds, purines or pyrimidines, carbamates

[a] Susceptible to attack by a wide range of potential nucleophiles.

NB: This table is intended to be used simply as a guideline. Chemical reactivity should be evaluated on a case-by-case basis for each process.

9.3.4.2 *Solubility—Isolated Stages*

Many of the reagents/intermediates that are highly electrophilic (and hence often genotoxic) are introduced into the synthetic process at those stages specifically designed to optimize the yield and product quality. A critical factor in most processes is that reactants are physically able to react with one another; in practical terms, this is best achieved by the reactants being in solution. By inference, this means that the genotoxic reactant in question is likely to be highly soluble in the reaction solution selected for the process. Thus, should the process concerned result in the isolation of the product as a solid, then the genotoxic reactant should remain in the reaction mother liquors and thus be removed, provided the deliquoring process is efficient. This can be augmented further by washing the cake with a solvent in which the genotoxic reagent is freely soluble and the product is not. Often isolation may involve some form of solvent replacement; where this is the case, the solubility of the genotoxic reagent should be evaluated in the replacement solvent in order to define the appropriate purge factor.

9.3.4.3 *Volatility*

A number of the genotoxic materials likely to be encountered within a typical synthetic process are volatile, including low molecular weight alkyl halides, aldehydes, and nitrogen or sulphur haloethyl "mustards." Distillation is frequently used to lower or completely remove the volume of reaction solvent present, and this can be effective in reducing or eliminating any residual genotoxic material, dependant on the volatility of the genotoxin relative to the boiling point of the solvent.

9.3.4.4 *Ionizability*

Aromatic amines are perhaps the most obvious example of potentially genotoxic materials that contain an ionizable group. The majority of APIs and some intermediates will be potentially ionizable. Where this is the case, and there is a suitable difference in the ionisability of the genotoxin of concern and the matrix in which it is potentially present, it should be possible to reduce the level of the former by manipulation of the pH of the aqueous phase and extraction into an organic solvent.

Reduction of a nitro compound to an amine is an example where such a process would be very effective. Although they generally possess a common genotoxic metabolic intermediate (a nitrenium ion), the nitro compound in question may be found to genotoxic, whereas its amine analogue may not. In such circumstances, the removal of the nitro precursor is desired, particularly if the nitro compound concerned is unreactive in the downstream process, and there is the potential for it to carry through the process in its original form.

Where there is a need to remove excess nitro compound, this can be achieved very effectively through a liquid/liquid extraction by employing a two-phase system with an acidic aqueous layer. Any nonionizable nitro compound will reside in the organic layer, whereas the ionized amine will reside in the aqueous layer. The organic layer would then be discarded, and amine then simply back extracted in a new organic solvent layer following basification.

In the synthesis of the common painkiller paracetamol, the penultimate stage involves the reduction of 4-nitrophenol to the corresponding amine.[18] The reaction mixtures are extracted with toluene, basified, and the amine is extracted.

In addition to classical liquid/liquid extractions, solid-phase extraction (SPE) can also be employed. By exploiting both the physical properties (ionisability) and chemical properties (polarity), this technique may confer an advantage over liquid/liquid extraction. The variety of stationary phases available, which can separate analytes according to different chemical properties, is another favorable characteristic of SPE. Most stationary phases are based on silica, and increasingly, this has been modified by attachment of a specific functional group. Modifying functional groups include:

- hydrocarbon chains of varying length (for reversed phase SPE);
- quaternary ammonium or amino groups (for anion exchange); and
- sulfonic acid or carboxyl groups (for cation exchange).

The main drawback of solid phase extraction has been its practicality at a manufacturing scale.

9.3.4.5 Chromatography
The technique of chromatography offers a range of options to remove or reduce a potential genotoxic impurity from API or an intermediate. Techniques range from simple "filtration" through a silica bed to preparative liquid chromatography.

Preparative chromatography is typically performed in normal phase mode, that is the use of a polar (typically silica) stationary phase and a nonpolar mobile phase (organic solvent system). The reason for the use of normal phase mode (most analytical chromatography is now performed in reverse phase mode) is due to the practical need to isolate the compound in question—normal phase using volatile solvents that are easily removed. Reverse phase can be used, but the difficulty in removing aqueous-based solvent systems limits the applicability, although it is possible to employ freeze drying as a means of removal. Another potential alternative is Super-critical fluid chromatography (SFC); this has the advantage of a readily removable eluent (CO_2).

Preparative HPLC is a now a standard technique within the pharmaceutical industry for the reduction or removal of impurities, with multi-kilo capability present in the larger companies, as well as a range of contract manufacturers. Improvements in the quality and range of stationary phases, as well as the supporting hardware, have greatly increased the scope of this technique, and there are few separations that cannot be achieved in this fashion.

The removal of a GI can be considered a subset of the standard chromatographic challenge of impurity removal, and typically will be approached in the same way. Additional considerations for GIs may exist, for example, "what is the stability of the PGI?" or "is there any risk of producing additional PGIs?" from the systems being considered. Indeed, with respect to the first consideration, Welch et al.[19] (Merck USA) have published work on the removal of an unwanted oxime via its high reactivity to a packing material; the resin/packing material can simply be stirred with the reaction solution, or cycled though a preparative column.

Bandichhor et al.[20] reported the purification of rizatriptan, a serotonin 5-HT receptor agonist. A genotoxic dimer impurity generated in the synthesis could not be removed to an acceptable limit of mass fraction 0.01% by conventional processes, such as fractional crystallization and recrystallization. A reverse phase method was developed using careful pH and ionic strength modification to increase the selectivity between the rizatriptan and the genotoxic dimer. The genotoxic dimer was strongly retained on the column, and the loadability optimized to give maximum productivity without any appreciable breakthrough of the genotoxic dimer into the product. Here, the retention of the rizatriptan was kept to a minimum, and the genotoxic dimer washed off between injections. The authors reported a decrease in the level of the genotoxic dimer from ca. 40,000 ppm to 40–80 ppm (yield >95%). Full details of the method are available in the paper.

9.3.4.6 Recrystallization Perhaps one of the most effective ways in which to remove impurities from API or intermediates, including those that are potentially genotoxic, is recrystallization. This involves selecting a solvent in which the API or intermediate is highly soluble when hot and virtually insoluble when cold. The impure API or intermediate is dissolved in the smallest practical volume of the solvent at an elevated temperature. The hot solution is then typically filtered to remove any impurities insoluble in the hot solvent for clinically destined API as a GMP against extraneous solid contamination. The filtered solution is then allowed to cool under carefully controlled conditions until the product crystallizes out of the cooling solvent. Impurities that are more soluble in the cold solvent remain in solution. The product is then isolated by filtration, leaving impurities in the filtrate (mother liquors).

The process can be further refined through the introduction of seed crystals (previously isolated product material); although typically used to determine or modify a specific property, for example morphic form, it can help to improve the selectivity of the recrystallization.

9.3.4.7 Other Techniques As well as the techniques described above, there are a variety of other "niche" techniques that can be applied. Two examples are activated charcoal and resins.

Activated Charcoal Activated charcoal is used in a variety of industries, including the water industry and alcoholic beverage (e.g. vodka, rum) industry to remove a range of impurities. Activated charcoal is, however, a complex material in terms of its physicochemical properties, and the effect of charcoal is very difficult to predict. In some circumstances, and often in combination with a recrystallization process, it can prove to be very effective in removing certain species, particularly colored impurities.

Scavenger Resins   Polymer scavengers are functionalized polymers that are designed to react with and bind reagents and by-products. The concept is analogous to that of other extraction and partitioning techniques, the genotoxic impurity of interest binds to the resin and can thus be removed by filtration as the desired product remains in solution. Such resins have found widespread applicability in the combinatorial chemistry arena.

Some of the types of resin available and their potential applicability are described in Table 9.4.

TABLE 9.4   Example Scavenger Resins

Scavenger (functional group)	Structure	Application
Benzaldehyde		Scavenges nucleophiles including primary amines, hydrazines
Isocyanate		Scavenges nucleophiles including amines
Amine		Scavenges acid chlorides, sulfonyl chlorides and miscellaneous electrophiles
Thiophenol		Scavenges alkylating agents e.g. alkyl halides
Trisamine		Scavenges acid chlorides, sulfonyl chlorides and miscellaneous electrophiles
Hydrazide		Scavenges Aldehydes

A recent publication examined the potential use of such resins to remove sulfonate esters.[21] The successful removal of methyl sulfonate esters was reported; however, related ethyl and isopropyl esters were only partially removed. Nevertheless, the authors concluded that the used of such resins showed some potential, and suggested that this could be extended to other classes of genotoxins, for example alkyl halides.

A drawback to date of such polymer-based resins has been their stability in aggressive organic solvents such as tetrohydrofuran (THF). Leaching of the monomer has been observed, hence a procedure to remove potentially genotoxic impurities may lead to the potential contamination of the product with another material. Depending on the nature of the monomer in question, this could introduce a bigger problem, and this factor has largely precluded the use of such resins in large-scale synthetic processes.

9.3.4.8   *Overall Quantification of Risk*   In order to make a quantitative assessment of the level of carryover of a particular material into an API or downstream intermediate, a number of mitigating criteria have been selected and are defined in Table 9.5. For each mitigating criteria, a purge factor can then be selected according to the characteristics of the material under consideration. The numerical scale has been developed to link individual process steps to the physicochemical properties of the individual impurity in question. Each factor is scored (high–low) in terms of its ability to purge the impurity, thus the higher the score, the greater the likelihood that the impurity would be purged from the process.

Hence, if a material is identified three steps from API, given the characteristics of the material concerned, and the nature of the three downstream processing stages, an overall purge factor can be assigned by multiplying the purge factors arising from

TABLE 9.5   Definitions of Mitigating Criteria and Purge Factors

Nature of Process	Purge factor
Reactivity—compound class	Highly reactive = 100
	Moderate reactivity = 10
	Low reactivity = 1
Solubility	Freely soluble = 10
	Moderately soluble = 3
	Sparingly soluble/insoluble = 1
Volatility	Boiling point >20°C below that of solvent = 10
	Boiling point +/– 10°C of solvent = 3
	Boiling point >20°C of solvent or in-volatile = 1
Ionisability	Ionization potential of GI significantly different to API/matrix = 10
Chromatography	Chromatography—GI elutes prior to API = 100
	Chromatography—GI elutes after API = 10
	Others—evaluated on a individual basis
Recrystallization	Factor = 10
Others, e.g. resins	Evaluated on a individual basis

each separate stage. Based on this value, a decision can be made as to what if any further action may be required.

Where a purge factor of greater than 10,000 is assigned, the likelihood of the genotoxic impurity in question being present in API at ppm levels is very low. Unless the daily API dose were 1 gram per day or greater, this theoretical evaluation alone should provide sufficient justification to take no further action, with no specific controls considered necessary.

For purge factors between 100 and 10,000, additional verification of the purge capabilities of the process should be considered. This would typically take the form of spiking studies.

If a purge factor less than 100 is assigned, formal process controls should be considered in addition to spiking studies. This will typically reflect the scenario where the genotoxic impurity in question is introduced or formed in the final or penultimate bond forming step.

The use of a semi-quantitative assessment process such as that described would shift the focus of effort to those genotoxic impurities with a high likelihood of being present in API, and hence could pose a significant risk to patient safety.

A number of case studies that examine the utility of such an approach are outlined below in Section 9.6.

9.3.5 Step 5: Further Evaluation

Having compiled an initial list of potential impurities, retained those that are known or suspected genotoxins, and evaluated which of these is likely to be present in API based on the material characteristics, origin in the process, and ability to survive the process intact, a shortlist of remaining materials is produced.

There are now two ways by which the risk of such potential genotoxic impurities may be mitigated.

1. *Safety testing:* Demonstrating that a material is nongenotoxic will allow it to be addressed under ICH Q3A/B.

2. *Analytical testing:* Demonstrating that a material is below the permitted TTC or staged TTC limit.

Which approach to take will depend on the unique nature of the project and the impurity concerned, and may be influenced by factors such as the availability of pure samples of the material of concern, and/or availability of appropriate analytical methodology with which to determine levels.

9.3.5.1 *Safety Testing*   For any impurity identified as being potentially geno-toxic (based on SAR evaluation) and assessed as having a high likelihood of carry-over into the API, the next step is often to carry out *in vitro* safety testing.

If *in vitro* testing is selected, it is recommended that the synthesized or isolated impurity is tested for mutagenicity as an individual impurity. However, where this is impractical, then spiked samples or batches of material that contain elevated levels of the impurity of concern may be tested. The latter approach is not generally encour-aged by regulatory authorities, and in such cases, an early dialogue with the relevant regulatory authority is recommended.

It is generally accepted that a single point bacterial mutation assay, such as the Ames test, has the necessary sensitivity and specificity to detect nonthresholded genotoxic chemicals.

However, some structural groups, such as carbamates, are known to be inefficiently detected in bacterial genotoxicity tests. In such situations, a mammalian cell assay (e.g. *in vitro* mouse lymphoma TK assay to detect chromosomal aberrations or chromosome damage in cultured human lymphocytes) should be considered. Such testing is examined in detail in Chapter 3.

A positive result in one or more of these tests is generally sufficient evidence to define the impurity as genotoxic, in which case it will be then necessary to adopt the appropriate TTC approach. Occasionally, a thresholded mechanism can be argued based on available safety data. If an impurity is found to be negative, it is considered nongenotoxic (qualified for genotoxicity), and can then be treated as a normal impurity under ICH Q3A/B.[13,14]

The genotoxic potential of *in vitro* positive materials may be further evaluated *in vivo* in order to establish the biological relevance of the *in vitro* findings; this is examined in detail in Chapter 3.

9.3.5.2 *Quantification of Level Present*

For potential GIs that have been assessed as having a reasonable likelihood of being present in API at levels of concern, it may be appropriate to attempt to determine the level, in parallel with, or instead of the safety testing described above. The level of concern will be set by the staged TTC for the phase of development, which is related to the maximum clinical dose and the maximum duration of the proposed trial(s). This in turn will have an effect on the choice of analytical technique.

- *Choice of technique?*: The nature of the impurity (analyte), the characteristics of the API or intermediate (matrix) and the level to be determined will influence the detection technique employed. Many organizations have developed specific strategies for refining such selections, and an example strategy is presented in Chapter 11.

- *Where in the process to test?*: Testing may be performed on upstream intermediates, API, or drug product as appropriate. It is often desirable to test as close as possible to the point of introduction of a GI/PGI into the process. This approach may permit standard techniques such as HPLC with UV detection to be used, if this is allied to spiking experiments demonstrating the removal in the downstream process. While development laboratories may be equipped with more sensitive techniques suitable for analysis at the low ppm level, manufacturing quality control laboratories are unlikely to have such facilities. In addition, there would be resistance to outsourcing these more esoteric analyses, since the goal of the modern quality control laboratory is a rapid turnaround of a minimum set of controls.

- *Quantitative assay or limit test*: Both types of methods are used in the analysis of genotoxic impurities. Quantitative tests are useful to furnish data for process development and to support further process modifications to reduce or more consistently control levels of a PGI. Having established a validated process, limit tests are likely to be favored for routine QC testing.

Limit tests are also more likely to be applied to upstream testing at an intermediate stage, where they are used in conjunction with demonstrated evidence of further reduction through processing.

Quantitative assays are usually applied at the final isolated API, as they provide a measure of true levels of the PGI/GI that would be administered in the drug product. Since the staged TTC concept for acceptable levels of PGIs/GIs is routinely applied during clinical stages of development, a quantitative test is generally desirable since acceptable levels vary as the clinical program develops. However, limit tests may be appropriate at the API or DP stage if this figure is well below the staged TTC control level.

9.3.6   Step 6: Overall Risk Assessment

Once analytical and/or safety test data are available, these are used to finalise the risk assessment.

Possible outcomes include;

- A PGI returns a negative Ames test result and thus no longer requires control as a genotoxic impurity, but defaults to ICH Q3 levels of control.[13,14]

- A PGI returns a positive Ames test result, but analytical testing demonstrates adequate process control over levels, that is level well below appropriate TTC limit.

- Analytical data demonstrates that a PGI/GI is below a current staged TTC, but above future dose duration levels. In such circumstances, this may necessitate a modification of the process to reduce or eliminate the impurity in question. If the material is potentially genotoxic rather than a known genotoxin, the expedient of safety testing, with the possibility of a negative Ames test result, would remove the need for further process development and analytical control at trace levels.

- Analytical and safety data reveal an Ames positive material above a staged TTC level for a planned clinical study.* In such a scenario, it is likely that the material in question would need to be reprocessed, unless a compelling case could be made for the benefit of the treatment over the risk posed (see ICH S9[22] for example). In most cases, the process would need to be redeveloped to bring levels of the genotoxin in question within the TTC for the envisaged marketed product dose and duration.

This is not meant to be an exhaustive list, but serves to illustrate some of the potential outcomes and likely courses of action in each case.

---

* Should it be discovered that the level of a GI is above permitted levels in material currently used in clinical trials, then this may lead to suspension of the trial and expedited reporting under 15-day rules to regulatory authorities.

It should be recognized that the evaluation of genotoxic risk is an iterative process, and needs to be updated in line with any process related changes and/or emerging information relating to impurities and/or degradants in drug substance (or drug product). Other factors such as a change in the trial duration, trial population, and/or dose may also require a review of the risk assessment.

9.3.7 Further Evaluation of Risk–Purge (Spiking) Studies

Alongside the theoretical evaluation of risk described above, there is often the need to examine this experimentally through the conduct of appropriate purging or spiking experiments. This is most likely to required where a moderate to high risk of potential carryover into the API has been defined. Spiking refers to the practice of adding in a fixed quantity, or spike, of the material to be followed in order to have a quantifiable baseline. Purging refers to the aim of defining the extent to which the material in question is purged out of the downstream material, or API.

Pierson et al. [3] reported on a generic approach to the assessment, testing strategies and analytical assessments of genotoxic impurities in API, encompassing the use of spiking experiments. Their approach was influenced by the point in the synthetic process at which the potential genotoxic impurity was introduced or identified. Introduction or identification of a source of a GI in the final stage of the API was defined as the worst-case scenario, and in most cases, such an outcome would necessitate the introduction of specifications and analysis. However, they stated that omission of routine controls could be justified if supported by purge studies where these conclusively demonstrated absence of the material of concern from the API.

If a potentially genotoxic impurity was introduced in the penultimate step, but was shown to be below the proposed TTC limit for the final API, they also proposed that there should be no further action. This was demonstrated with reference to a recent project in which an alkylating agent (substituted benzyl bromide) was formed in the penultimate step, and a limit of 20 ppm was assigned (based on the TTC, taking account of the dose). Testing of the isolated final intermediate revealed levels of only 2 ppm; hence, it was concluded that there was no need for a specification or testing of the API.

The authors also proposed that where the potential genotoxic impurity was introduced three to four stages upstream from the API, then a risk assessment based on chemistry rationale and/or spike/purge experiments would be required to evaluate the ability of the downstream process to remove or reduce the impurity to acceptable levels. If these evaluations indicated that carry through to API was likely, then controls in the API would be required.

Finally, if the potential genotoxic impurity was introduced greater than three to four stages upstream from the API, then risk assessment based on chemistry rationale alone was typically required.

The use of purge studies was further examined by Liu et al. [4] who reported on the analytical control strategy for five potential genotoxic impurities in a novel oncology product, pazopanib hydrochloride (see Fig. 9.4—GIs highlighted as boxed items). They described the approach in the terms of quality by design (QbD), with levels of genotoxic impurities being thought of as critical quality attributes (CQAs).

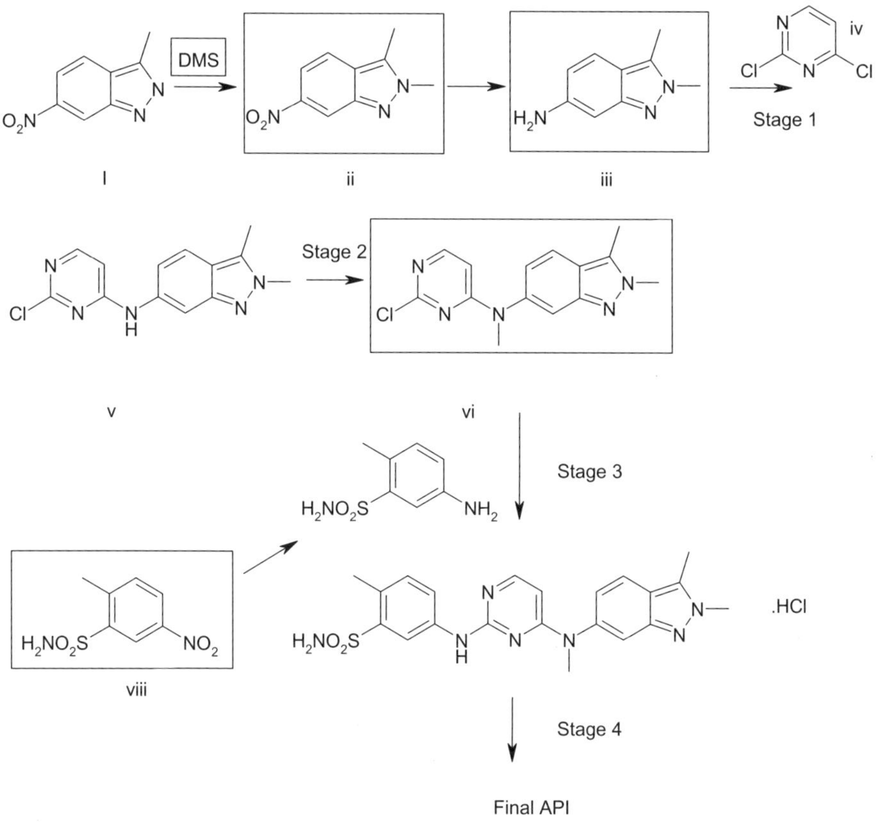

Figure 9.4   Manufacturing process of pazopanib HCl (genotoxic impurities are boxed).

Each of the impurities in question was spiked at elevated levels (as high as 5% in some cases) into the process. Impurity fate mapping was then used to demonstrate the serial reductions of levels in downstream products. For example, the stage 1 product contained 670 ppm of compound (ii), Stage 2 product 23 ppm, while Stage 3 product, intermediate grade API and final API contained less than 1.7 ppm of (ii). This enabled them to focus on upstream control in starting materials or intermediates, and avoided the need for control in the drug substance. The attractiveness of this approach is that it permits control limits to be set at higher levels, with the assurance that downstream purging will reduce the levels of materials of concern to acceptable levels. It also allows the control strategy to be based on less sophisticated and sensitive analytical methods, which are more aligned to a routine quality control environment.

9.4   CONCLUSION

The need to adequately assess the risk posed by GIs, and to limit the level present in API/DP is clearly established in the EMEA[7] and draft FDA[8] guidelines. It is the opinion of the authors of this chapter that the most effective way to achieve this is to establish control strategies based on a combination of semi-quantitative assessment, allied to analytical results and data from appropriate purging studies. Such an approach should ensure that any actual GI related risk is clearly identified and managed.

9.5 ACKNOWLEDGMENTS

The authors would like to thank Dr Stephen Smith (AstraZeneca) for the provision of advice and data relating to the chromatographic removal of GIs.

9.6 CASE STUDIES

9.6.1 Case Study 1

The following example from the synthesis of omeprazole (see Fig. 9.5) is presented to demonstrate how the fate of a genotoxic nitroaniline starting material was assessed. Using the scoring system defined in Table 9.5, the following factors were assigned:

9.6.1.1 Calculated Risk

Reactivity Based on the relative ease of the nitro reduction stage, the nitroaniline (I) was categorized as highly reactive, and therefore a factor of 100 was applied. A further factor of 10 was applied to the subsequent cyclization step, giving an overall reactivity factor of 1000.

Solubility The nitroaniline is freely soluble in the solvents employed within the process, and thus any residual amounts remaining after completion of the reaction would be expected to be removed in the mother liquors. A factor of 10 was therefore applied.
No other purge factors were deemed applicable.
Therefore, the total purge factor is $10,000 \times 10 = 10,000$.
Based on which, it would be anticipated that levels would be <100 ppm.

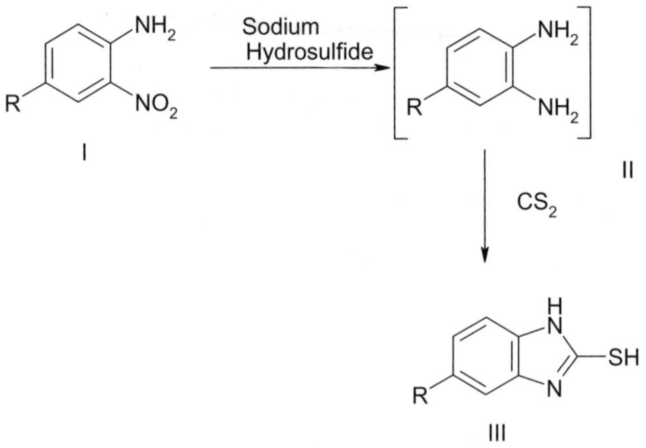

Figure 9.5 Synthesis of omeprazole intermediate III.

9.6.1.2 *Experimental Results* No nitroaniline (<5 ppm) was observed in multiple batches of the isolated cyclised product; these results show a clear and accurate correlation with the theoretical prediction.

9.6.2 Case Study 2

The second case study is presented as an example of a potentially genotoxic impurity, nitropyridine (A), within a starting material, again with reference to the synthesis of omeprazole (see Fig. 9.6). If present within the starting material, there was a concern that nitropyridine (A) might carry-over in the downstream process, hence a risk assessment was undertaken.

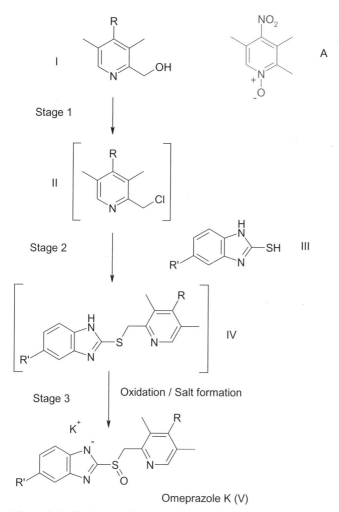

Figure 9.6 Synthesis of omeprazole potassium salt.

9.6.2.1 Calculated Risk This is a three-step reaction; however, none of the intermediates are isolated.

Reactivity The nitropyridine (A) is unreactive under the reaction conditions employed for all three steps; hence a purge factor of 1 is applied, since it is unlikely that it will be removed as a result of reaction in the downstream process.

Solubility The nitropyridine (A) is highly soluble in the solvents employed in the stages described. For a process where there are no isolations, it is therefore expected that the nitropyridine (A) would remain within the process liquors. Therefore, for stages 1 and 2, the purge factor is assigned as 1 based on solubility, meaning that no reduction in level is expected.

Volatility The nitropyridine is not volatile, hence a purge factor of 1 is again assigned, since very little will be removed as a result of any of the solvent removal or exchange processes involved.

The total purge factor to the coupled sulphide stage is calculated as $1 \times 1 \times 1 = 1$; hence no reduction in the level of nitropyridine is predicted.

Experimental Results In spiking experiments performed at a level of 3000 ppm nitropyridine (A) spiked into the starting alcohol, a level of approximately 2000 ppm was found in the stage 2 product (III). This is considered to validate the theoretical assessment that predicted no significant reduction in levels of nitropyridine in this process.

However, when the level of nitropyridine (A) was assessed in the isolated potassium salt, less than 1 ppm was detected. Due to its high solubility, the nitropyridine (A) remained in the reaction mother liquors following crystallisation of the desired product.

9.6.3 Case Study 3

In the third case study, based on the synthesis of a fluoroaryl amine, the impurities of concern were genotoxic sulfonate esters that could be potentially formed during the process, and in particular during the final crystallization stage (see Figure 9.7).

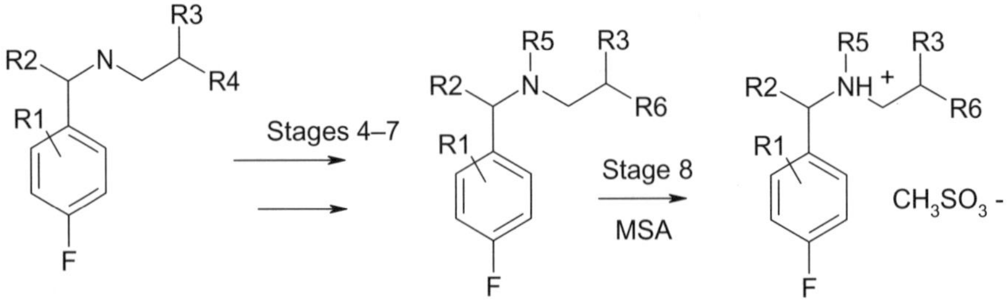

Figure 9.7 Simplified representation of the synthetic process used to manufacture the fluoroaryl amine API.

The potential carry over of these materials into the final API was a matter of concern; hence a risk assessment was performed.

9.6.3.1   Calculated Risk

Reactivity   Under the reaction conditions employed, the sulfonate esters (MMS, EMS, and IMS) are all very reactive-; therefore, a purge factor of 100 would be applied, as it is very likely that they would be removed as a result of reaction in the downstream process. Indeed, some data are available to assess relative chemical reactivity, in particular, the Swain-Scott *s* constants, which provide an assessment of the sensitivity of an electrophilic substrate to nucleophilic attack.[23] The sulfonate esters (MMS, EMS, and IMS) have different *s* values: MMS (0.83) > EMS (0.67) > IMS (0.29).[24] In this instance, because of the existence of specific data relating to reactivity, the reactivity purge factor was adjusted to allow for these differences. The individual adjusted purge factors are therefore 83 (MMS), 67 (EMS), and 23 (IMS).

Solubility   The sulfonate esters are highly soluble in the solvents employed in the final stage described. Thus, the purge factor assigned is 10.

Volatility   All of the sulfonate esters have low volatility, with boiling points (MMS [202°C], EMS [213°C], and IMS [220°C]) greater than 20°C above that of the mixed solvent used (ethyl acetate [77°C]/acetone [56°C]/iso-octane [99°C]) for the crystallization. Therefore, the assigned purge factor is 1.

No other purge factors were deemed applicable. Therefore, the total purge factors for each species were calculated as:

$$PF_{MMS} = 830$$
$$PF_{EMS} = 670$$
$$PF_{IMS} = 230$$

To examine the purge capacity of the process, Cimarosti et al.[25] crystallized the API with methane sulfonic acid (MSA) containing elevated levels (up to 5× the specification limits) of the three sulfonate esters (MMS [2500 ppm], EMS [2600 ppm], and IMS [1200 ppm]). In addition, extra quantities of the three esters (MMS [1600 ppm], EMS [2200 ppm], and IMS [2900 ppm]) were added to the mother liquors just prior to filtration.

Based on the levels spiked, the following maximum levels would be expected:

$$MMS = 4100/830 = 5 \text{ ppm}$$
$$EMS = 4800/670 = 7 \text{ ppm}$$
$$IMS = 4100/230 = 17 \text{ ppm}$$

9.6.3.2   Experimental Results   Initially, immediately after deliquoring, the residual levels of the sulfonate esters were inversely proportional to their *s* values, i.e. the most reactive ester had the lowest levels of residual ester present in the API. Thereafter, the levels of residual sulfonate ester in all cases was less than the LOD of the method (<1 ppm) (Table 9.6).

TABLE 9.6 Levels of Residual MMS, EMS, and IMS in API (Based on Cimarosti et al.[24])

	MMS	EMS	IMS
Swain–Scott Reactivity Index (s)	0.83	0.67	0.29
Relative purge factors	3.61	2.91	1.00
Wash volumes of ethyl acetate	MMS (ppm)	EMS (ppm)	IMS (ppm)
Deliquoring (0)	1	1.6	1.8
4	<1	<1	<1
8	<1	<1	<1
12	<1	<1	<1

These results again strongly support the use of the predictive tool, having successfully predicted the efficient removal of all three sulfonate esters in the process described.

REFERENCES

1. Jacobson-Cram D, McGovern T. 2007. Toxicological overview of impurities in pharmaceutical products. *Advanced Drug Delivery Reviews* 59:38–42.
2. Dobo KL, Greene N, et al. 2006. The application of structure based assessment to support safety and chemistry diligence to manage genotoxic impurities in actives pharmaceutical ingredients during drug development. *Regulatory Toxicology and Pharmacology* 44:282–293.
3. Pierson DA, Olsen BA, et al. 2009. Approaches to assessment, testing decisions and analytical determination of genotoxic impurities in drug substances. *Organic Process Research and Development* 13(2):285–291.
4. Lui DQ, Chen TK, et al. 2009. Analytical control of genotoxic impurities in the pazopanib hydrochloride manufacturing process. *Journal of Pharmaceutical and Biomedical Analysis* 50:144–150.
5. ICH. *ICH Q8 (R2)* 2005. *Pharmaceutical Development*. Available at http://www.ich.org (accessed September 2010).
6. ICH. *ICH Q9* 2005. *Quality Risk Management*. Available at http://www.ich.org (accessed September 2010).
7. EMEA. 2006. *Guideline on the limits of genotoxic impurities*. EMEA/CHMP/QWP/251344/2006.
8. FDA. 2008. *FDA draft guidance for industry genotoxic and carcinogenic impurities in drug substances and products: Recommended approaches*. Issued December 2008.
9. FDA. *GRAS List*. Available at http://www.accessdata.fda.gov/scripts/fcn/fcnNavigation.cfm?rpt=grasListing (accessed September 2010).
10. Brusick DJ. 2009. A perspective on testing of existing pharmaceutical excipients for genotoxic impurities. *Regulatory Toxicology and Pharmacology* 55(2):200–204.
11. CDER. *Guidance for Industry: Safety Testing of Drug Metabolites*. Available at http://www.fda.gov/CDER/GUIDANCE/6897ful.pdf (accessed September 2010).
12. CHMP. 2009. *Question & answers on the CHMP guideline on the limits of genotoxic impurities*. London, December 17, 2009. Doc Ref: EMEA/CHMP/SWP/431994/2007 Revision 2.
13. ICH. *ICH Q3A (R2)* 2006. *Impurities in new drug substances (revised guideline)*. CPMP/ICH/2737/99.
14. ICH. *ICH Q3B (R2)* 2006. *Impurities in new drug products (revised guideline)*. CPMP/ICH/2738/99.
15. Tennant RW, Ashby J. 1991. Classification according to chemical structure, mutagenicity to Salmonella and level of carcinogenicity of a further 39 chemicals tested for carcinogenicity by the U.S. National Toxicology Progam. *Mutation Research* 257:209–227.

16. Müller L, Mauthe RJ, Riley CM. 2006. A rationale for determining, testing and controlling specific impurities in pharmaceuticals that possess potential for genotoxicity. *Regulatory Toxicology and Pharmacology* 44:198–211.

17. *Carcinogenicity Potency Database.* Available at http://potency.berkeley.edu/ (accessed September 2010).

18. Rode CV, Vaidya MJ, et al. 1999. Synthesis of p-aminophenol by catalytic hydrogenation of nitrobenzene. *Organic Process Research and Development* 3:465–470.

19. Welch CJ, Biba M, et al. 2003. Selective removal of a pharmaceutical process impurity using a reactive resin. *Journal of Liquid Chromatography and Related Technologies* 26(12):1959–1968.

20. Bandichhor R, Reddy LA, Chakraborty S, et al. 2009. Preparative chromatography technique in the removal of isostructural genotoxic impurity in rizatriptan. *Organic Process Research and Development* 13(4):683–689.

21. Lee C, Helmy R, Strulson C. 2010. Removal of Electrophilic Potential Genotoxic Impurities Using Nucleophilic Reactive Resins. *Organic Process Research and Development* 14(4):1021–1026.

22. ICH. *ICH S9 Nonclinical evaluation for anticancer pharmaceuticals.* Step 4 (2009).

23. Swain CG, Scott CB. 1953. Quantitative correlation of relative rates. Comparison of hydroxide ion with other nucleophilic reagents toward alkyl halides, esters, epoxides and acyl halides. *Journal of the American Chemical Society* 75(1):141–147.

24. Lee GS, Blonsky KS, et al. 1992. Base alterations in yeast induced by alkylating agents with differing Swain-Scott substrate constants. *Journal of Molecular Biology* 223(33):617–626.

25. Cimarosti Z, Bravo F, Stonestreet P. 2010. Application of quality by design principles to support development of a control strategy for the control of genotoxic impurities in the manufacturing process of a drug substance. *Organic Process Research and Development* 14(4):993–998.

CHAPTER 10

ANALYSIS OF GENOTOXIC IMPURITIES: REVIEW OF APPROACHES

Dave Elder

10.1 INTRODUCTION

The issue of genotoxic impurities (GIs) in active pharmaceutical ingredients (API) has over recent years, become of considerable concern to the pharmaceutical industry. Control of GIs is addressed in the recent CHMP (Committee for Medicinal Products for Human Use) guideline[1] and draft FDA (Food and Drug Administration) guideline.[2] Both indicate that a TTC (threshold of toxicological concern) of 1.5 µg/day is appropriate for long term use, and that a staged TTC is appropriate during the clinical development phase.

As a consequence of these TTC controls at the µg/day level, there is a parallel need for stringent analytical control measures. These measures, which often necessitate control of these GI analytes at the low ppm level relative to the API, pose very significant analytical challenges. The need for specific and sensitive trace analytical methodologies, combined with the high chemical reactivity of the analytes concerned, present significant analytical challenges, especially in sample preparation. This in turn often necessitates both the application of sensitive, analytical techniques, for example gas chromatography-mass spectroscopy (GC-MS), high performance liquid chromatography-mass spectroscopy (HPLC-MS), and of sample preparation steps prior to analysis to address both selectivity and stability issues. Ironically, the same chemical reactivity issues that bedevil the analytical procedures may also ensure that many of the GIs are unlikely to survive intact the chemical synthetic clean-up procedures used in API manufacture, and even less likely to survive the aqueous-based biological environment. Such issues are addressed in detail elsewhere within this book (see Chapter 9).

This specific chapter aims to summarize the analytical approaches described in the literature that have been utilized for the assessment and control of GIs, and also aims to provide commentary on the current regulatory strategies for analysts working in this evolving field. It is linked to a series of other chapters within this

Genotoxic Impurities: Strategies for Identification and Control, Edited by Andrew Teasdale
Copyright © 2010 by John Wiley & Sons, Inc.

section of the book, and is aimed in particular at complementing the chapter specifically addressing overall analytical strategy for analysis of GIs. Information gained from the literature being a vital aspect of the overall strategy.

The chapter is subdivided into sections based on the functional groups within the analyte that are linked to genotoxicity, for example sulfonate esters, alkylating agents, etc.

In addition, this chapter will provide commentary on the related important issue of method transfer into the production environment.

10.2 SULFONATE ESTERS

Concerns surrounding sulfonate esters, a potential by-product of a reaction between sulfonic acids and alcohols, led in 2000 the European Directorate for the Quality of Medicines and Healthcare (EDQM) to issue a request for additional information on the requirement for pharmacopoeial limit tests for alkyl mesylate impurities in mesylate salts.[3] This led to significant scrutiny focused on this group of potential GIs. Subsequently, the European Pharmacopoeia (Ph. Eur.) drafted a production statement for inclusion in the monographs of all mesylate-containing APIs.[4]

These concerns were apparently vindicated in mid-2007, when the European Medicines Agency (EMEA) suspended the marketing authorization of Viracept (nelfinavir mesylate), an antiviral medicinal product, owing to concerns over the presence of elevated levels of ethyl methanesulfonate (EMS) in the drug product.[5,6] Subsequently, the CHMP assessed the corrective and preventative measures that were put in place by the Marketing Authorization Holder, these being verified by on-site inspections. CHMP were "re-assured that the contamination causes had been eliminated and that the future production of Viracept would meet the required quality standards," and recommended lifting the suspension of the marketing authorization.[7] However, following the Viracept incident, there has been much more focused regulatory attitude toward the potential formation of sulfonate esters within products utilizing sulfonic acid counterions.

Initially, attention was focused specifically on mesylates, and analysts relied on the volatility of the mesylate esters concerned and developed GC, usually with flame ionization detection (FID) and GC-MS methodologies. However, substrate interference, principally from the API, was often a restricting factor. The use of a variety of different extraction techniques, for example liquid-liquid extraction (LLE), liquid phase micro-extraction (LPME), solid-phase extraction (SPE), and solid-phase micro-extraction (SPME) were experimented with to reduce matrix interference to allow reproducible GC-MS methodologies to be developed.[8]

An alternative approach utilizes derivatization. Lee et al.[9] determined residual MMS (methyl methane sulfonate). EMS, IMS (*iso*-propyl methane sulfonate), and another potent genotoxin, dimethyl sulfate (DMS) levels utilizing alkylthiocyanate derivatives (see Fig. 10.1), which could be directly analyzed by headspace GC-MS. The limit of detection (LOD) was determined at between 0.02 ppm for the MMS and EMS esters and DMS, and 0.05 ppm for the IMS ester. The authors also assessed the LODs for the same method using FID detection, but detection levels were much

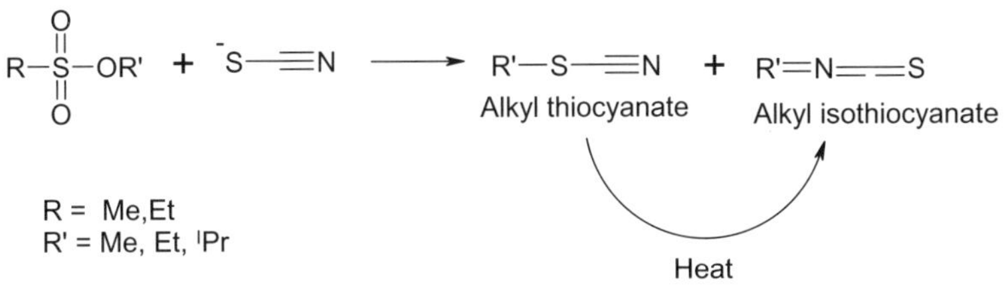
Alkyl thiocyanate
Alkyl isothiocyanate
R = Me,Et
R' = Me, Et, iPr
Heat

Figure 10.1 Derivatization of residual alkyl sulfonates esters with thiocyanate.

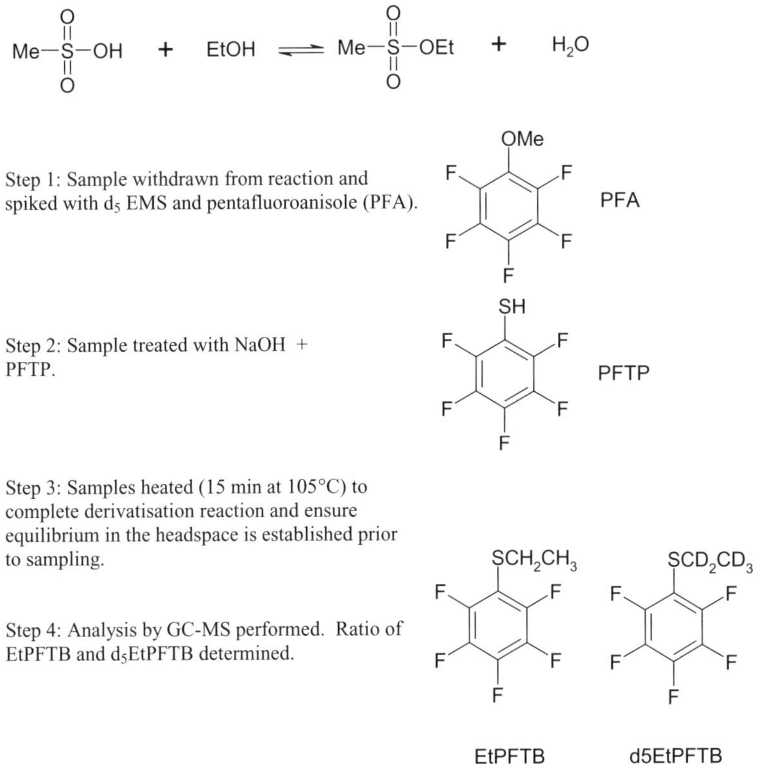
Step 1: Sample withdrawn from reaction and spiked with d5 EMS and pentafluoroanisole (PFA).
PFA
Step 2: Sample treated with NaOH + PFTP.
PFTP
Step 3: Samples heated (15 min at 105°C) to complete derivatisation reaction and ensure equilibrium in the headspace is established prior to sampling.
Step 4: Analysis by GC-MS performed. Ratio of EtPFTB and d5EtPFTB determined.
EtPFTB
d5EtPFTB

Figure 10.2 Derivatization of alkyl sulfonate ester residues with pentafluorothiophenol.

higher (5–10 ppm). An advantage of such an approach was that in derivatizing the sulfonate ester concerned; it also stabilized the analyte.

More recently, Alzaga et al.[10] also adopted a derivatization approach, using pentafluorothiophenol (PFTP) as the derivatizing agent, to form a volatile sulfide (see Fig. 10.2). A major advantage of this approach over direct analysis of the sulfonate esters is that all the derivatives are amenable to sensitive analysis using GC-MS in the single ion mode (SIM). Such an approach is not possible for the aryl sulfonate esters due to their low volatility. The authors analyzed methyl, ethyl and *iso*propyl mesylates, besylates, tosylates, and sulfates in a range of matrices with relative standard deviations (RSDs) in the range of 3%–10% at analyte concentrations of 1 µg/g (1 ppm). Matrix-dependant effects were, however, observed resulting in reduced recoveries, which necessitated the use of deuterated internal standards.

Recently, a PQRI (Pharmaceutical Quality Research Institute) subgroup published the outcomes of their investigations into the monitoring of EMS in model reaction systems).[11] They reported on the development and validation of an automated static headspace HS-GC-MS method[12] based on the previously published method of Alzaga et al.[10] The automated approach allows for unsupervised operation over extended time periods, and demonstrated excellent repeatability, linearity, and robustness. The LOD and LOQ (limit of quantitation) were <0.5 and 1 µg/mL (ppm), respectively. The method was also applicable to the determination of MMS and IMS (as well as corresponding esters of benzene sulfonic and *p*-toluene sulfonic acids).

Despite the apparent advantages given through derivatization, methods based on direct analysis of the sulfonate ester continue to be reported in the literature. Ramakrishna et al.[13] reported on the development and validation of a GC-MS method, utilizing a quadrapole MS for the simultaneous determination of MMS and EMS. The method was specific, linear over the range of 1–15 µg/mL, accurate and precise, with an LOD and LOQ of 0.3 and 1.0 µg/mL (ppm), respectively, for both analytes. The method is aligned with the limits for the individual sulfonate esters based on an upper dose of 800 mg of imatinib mesylate, and a TTC limit of <1.5 µg/day, that is 1.9 ppm.

Zheng et al.[14] also recently reported on a GC-MS method for DMS in an API intermediate. To address matrix interference, a deuterated internal standard (d_6-DMS), together with liquid/liquid extraction (LLE) using methyl-*tert*-butyl ether, was utilized. The authors used a DB-624 stationary phase with a single quadrapole MS detector in the EI (electron ionization) mode with SIM detection. The method was linear over the range of 10–60 ppm, and the LOD and LOQ were 0.3 and 1.0 ppm, respectively. The method was precise, showing RSDs of 0.1% for an 18.6 ppm DMS standard. Similarly, the accuracy was excellent, showing recoveries in the range of 102.1–108.5% for the intermediate spiked with 8.0 ppm of DMS.

As well as GC, HPLC can also be utilized for direct analysis of alkyl sulfonate esters. Direct analysis, using HPLC-MS-SIM was favored by Taylor et al.[15] They reported LODs of between 0.02 ppm and 0.05 ppm for the methyl, ethyl, and isopropyl esters of *p*-toluenesulfonic acid and methyl, ethyl, isopropyl, and *n*-butyl esters of benzenesulfonic acid in drug substances. A major issue with HPLC is the use of aqueous solvents both for chromatographic and sample preparation purposes, as the sulfonate esters are inherently unstable in aqueous environments. This means that sample solutions need to be stored prior to analysis at low temperature and analyzed within a short period of time after preparation. Such stability issues largely restrict such an approach to the more stable aryl sulfonate esters.

An elegant approach utilizing HILIC (hydrophilic interaction liquid chromatography) stationary phases was recently reported by An et al.[16] This is a generic HILIC-MS method for the determination of alkyl esters of sulfates and sulfonates in a number of different API matrices. This method uses trimethylamine as the derivatizing reagent for the methyl esters and triethylamine for the higher alkyl esters (ethyl, propyl and *iso*-propyl), see Figure 10.3. The method gave excellent precision (<4% RSD), and was linear over the analyte concentration of 0.2–20 ppm.

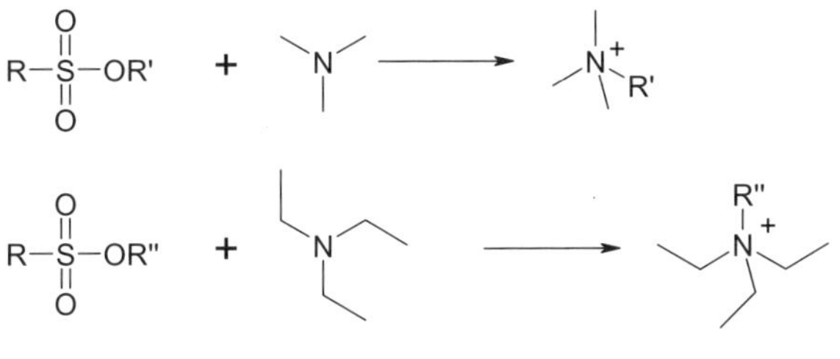

R = methyl, ethyl, aryl
R' = ethyl, propyl
R" = methyl

Figure 10.3   Derivatization of alkyl/aryl sulfonate ester residues with trimethylamine (ethyl, propyl) and triethylamine (methyl) to form quaternary ammonium derivatives.

10.3   ALKYL HALIDES AND CHLOROFORMATES

Historically, analysts have tended to rely on the volatility of alkyl halides and developed GC methodologies with FID. GC remains in many cases the preferred technique, but is now more routinely used in combination with more sensitive and selective detection techniques, such as GC-MS or electrochemical detection (ECD).

HPLC remains a key separation technique for those analytes that are insufficiently volatile and/or too thermally labile for reliable GC analysis. While many historical references employ HPLC with single wavelength ultraviolet (UV) detection, the more recent literature employs a variety of MS techniques.[17]

There are also literature references to the use of normal phase HPLC,[18] SFC,[19] ion chromatography (IC),[20] and CE techniques.[21]

Substrate interference, principally from the API, is often a restricting factor, and extraction and/or preconcentration techniques, such as headspace (HS), and, to a lesser extent LLE, are used to reduce matrix interference in GC methodologies. These approaches are routinely employed in many pharmaceutical research laboratories, as they offer the potential for generic methodologies, as demonstrated by Skett[17] and Ellison.[22]

Reverse-phase HPLC methodologies also present challenges for sample preparations due to instability of reactive analytes in the aqueous-based mobile phase preparations. The application of reduced energy mixing (vortexing vs. sonication) and reduced temperature storage of the samples has been shown to result in acceptable solution stability, thus ensuring analysis can be completed in a reasonable time frame.[23]

In a recent example, Huybrechts et al.[19] described the analytical methods used for the control of D013197, an N-chloro impurity in a novel API of undisclosed chemical structure, which was assessed as having a TTC equating to 0.67 ppm. The authors developed two complimentary and orthogonal methods—HPLC and supercritical fluid chromatography-mass spectroscopy (SFC-MS)—to determine residual levels of D013197 at sub-ppm levels.

The first method utilized HPLC-MS with SIM to monitor the designated impurity at a mass unit of m/z of 689.6. The method comprised of a 3.5 μm XBridge C18 stationary phase with a gradient mobile phase comprising of varying mixtures of 10 mM ammonium acetate with 0.25% v/v ammonium hydroxide solution and acetonitrile at 60°C. The flow rate was 1.0 mL/min, and the method gave a peak that eluted at relative retention time (RRT) 1.21. The analytical concentration of the API was 10 mg/mL.

The HPLC method was determined to be linear over the operating range of 0.2–18 ppm D013197, and had an LOD of 0.03 ppm and an LOQ of 0.1 ppm. The accuracy was acceptable, and gave recoveries in the range of 93.4–104.2% over the range of 0.2–25 ppm. Three different samples were spiked with 0.6 and 6 ppm of D013197, and the recoveries were in the range of 92.6%–111.4% at 0.6 ppm, and 83.5–126.7 ppm at 6 ppm. The repeatability of the method at the 0.5 ppm limit was assessed and found to be acceptable with a mean recovery of 0.48 ppm and RSD of 4.6%. The reproducibility of the method was determined by analysis of the same sample in a second laboratory, and found to be acceptable (RSD ≤15% and mean differences ≤30%). The analyte was found to be adequately stable in solution over a period of 48 h at room temperature.

In parallel, an orthogonal SFC-MS method combined with selective reaction monitoring (SRM) method was developed. The SFC stationary phase utilized a 2-ethylpyridine column at 35°C with a mobile phase of SFC carbon dioxide/10% methanol and 1 mM ammonium acetate. The flow rate was 2.0 mL/min, and it gave a peak that eluted at RRT of 0.71. The concentration of the API utilized was again 10 mg/mL. This also illustrates another important factor in relation to trace analysis of GIs, that because of the extremely low levels involved, it necessitates the need for high sample concentrations. This can, for many APIs and other samples (synthetic intermediates, starting materials, etc.), be a significant challenge due to limited solubility.

Both methods were claimed to be quality-control friendly at the same reporting threshold of 0.5 ppm, but no validation details were reported for the SFC procedure. The authors concluded that the analysis of GIs is neither straightforward nor trivial. The complexity is due to the large number of critical parameters, for example sample preparation, chromatography, mass spectrometry, etc.

Lee et al.,[20] when examining the application of HPLC-MS to the measurement of the relatively in-volatile alkyl halide N,N-dimethylaminoethyl chloride in diltiazem hydrochloride, demonstrated that HPLC-MS in the electrospray ionization (ESI) mode using SIM gave better responses than atmospheric pressure chemical ionization (APCI). They elected to reduce interference from the API using a reversed phase HPLC column followed by determination of the polar analyte using ion exchange chromatography. The analyte response was linear over the range of 0.2–10 ppm, with a correlation coefficient in excess of 0.999. The detection limit is in the range of 0.05–1 ppm. The repeatability of the method at the 1 ppm level was 7% RSD.

Chloroformates tend to be much more hydrolytically unstable than corresponding alkyl halides. This has prompted some authors to assess derivatization to stabilize the analyte. Liu et al.[24] reported on the determination of chloroethylchloroformate (CECF) in APIs, using 2-mercaptopyridine as the derivatizing agent

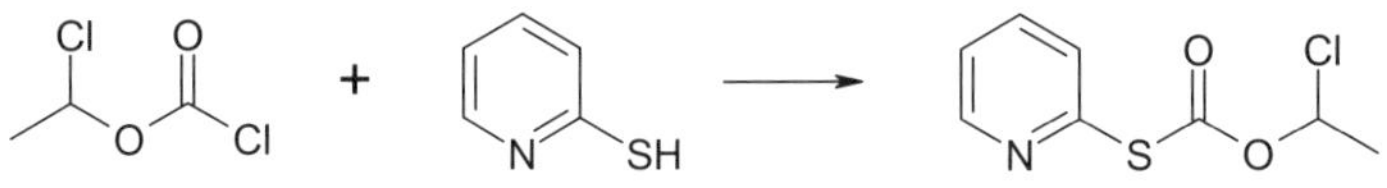

CECF

Figure 10.4   Derivatization of chloroethylchloroformate residues with 2-mercaptopyridine.

(see Fig. 10.4). The derivative is analyzed using HPLC-MS at m/z of 218, which equates to the $[M + H]^+$ ion. The authors cautioned that both glassware and solvents needed to be suitably dried in order to prevent interference from residual moisture. The LOQ was reported to be 5 ng/mL, which is equivalent to 0.1 ppm for a 50 mg/mL API concentration.

However, the presence of another chloroformate (VII) in the reaction mixture resulted in significant interference when the method was applied to the control of CECF in an intermediate. To overcome the interference, the authors utilized matrix deactivation strategies. This can be achieved by protonating the matrix or by the addition of a nucleophile scavenger. Utilizing these approaches, CECF could be analyzed in the presence of oxalyl chloride by direct injection GC-MS in methylene chloride at detection limits of 4 ng/mL, which is equivalent to 0.4 ppm in a 10 mg/mL sample.

Methodologies based on thin-layer chromatography (TLC) separations followed by visualization either by UV or via use of a variety of chemical agents would appear to be now restricted to use in pharmacopoeial monographs, and are likely to be superseded by more selective and sensitive methodologies in the future. For instance, the most recent 2009 Ph. Eur. monograph for amiodarone hydrochloride[25] still describes a TLC method for the determination of the alkylating agent 2-chloro-N,N'-diethylethanamine (Impurity H), while a HPLC-UV procedure was published in 1994.[26] Similarly, the Ph. Eur. monograph for tolnaftate[27] describes a TLC procedure for the determination of *ortho*-napthalene-2-yl chlorothioformate (Impurity C), whereas an HPLC procedure was published in 2000 by Vaidya et al.[28]

Even in cases where pharmacopoeial monographs and literature references employ the same analytical approaches, subtle differences can exist. For instance, the Ph. Eur. monograph for verapamil[29] describes the reversed phase HPLC-UV determination of 16 process impurities, including the alkylating agent, 3-chloro-N-[2-(3,4-dimethoxyphenyl)ethyl]-N-methylpropan-1-amine (Impurity D). Both Lacroix et al.[30] and Valvo et al.[31] describe similar HPLC-UV methodologies for the determination of 17 and 13 process impurities, respectively, plus the determination of the alkylating agent 2,4-dimethoxy-N-(3-chloropropyl)-N-methyl benzene ethanamine (Impurity VI). All three methods employ different stationary phases although at least they agree on the selection of 278 nm as detection wavelength.

In a few cases, differences exist in the spectrum of impurities determined. For instance, the Ph. Eur. famotidine[32] and famotidine tablet monographs[33] tabulate, respectively, seven and three related substances, while the literature[18,33,34] describes the HPLC-UV determination of four other impurities with alkylating functionality, which are not listed in the monographs. Similarly, Lambropoulis et al.[35] describes the development and validation of an HPLC-UV assay for fentanyl in fentanyl citrate injection,[36] and the determination of eight related substances, including the alkylating agent 2-bromoethylbenzene. This analyte is not included in the lists of related substances/ordinary impurities cited in the relevant Ph. Eur. monographs for both the API and drug products (fentanyl, fentanyl citrate, and fentanyl citrate injection monographs.[36–38]

In mitigation, the pharmacopoeias are legally constrained in their abilities to react and respond to changing scenarios impacting on the monographs, including newly published information. There is a well-established process for updating individual monographs that involves interactions with the relevant national licensing authorities. The latter defines the approvable levels of individual impurities, both established and new (including toxic impurities) based on clinical and preclinical data that is used to qualify each impurity. In addition, the Pharmacopoeias have to assess the robustness and general applicability of the proposed novel analytical methods, as there can be issues with these novel methods in routine use.

Following issuance of the CHMP Guideline on GIs,[1] it was not entirely clear as to how the guideline would influence the future development of pharmacopoeial monographs. However, the EDQM have recently identified the need to develop a policy for dealing with potentially GIs that can be applied during elaboration and revision of monographs.[39,40] EDQM have stated that the European Pharmacopoeia needs to derive a pragmatic approach and that for existing monographs, in the absence of new study data demonstrating genotoxicity of an impurity; the existence of structural alerts alone is considered insufficient justification to trigger follow-up measures. The USP have held similar discussions to discuss the issues of GIs.[41]

10.4   EPOXIDES AND HYDROPEROXIDES

The analytical approach for hydroperoxide impurities is typically based on a redox strategy; either oxidation to ketone or reduction to the corresponding alcohol. The sensitivity of the method is very dependent on the relative stability of the analyte, particularly in aqueous systems.[24] HPLC-ESI-MS has been used to analyze these analytes, and most MS-ionization techniques typically prompt condensation of the protonated molecule, with resultant loss of water.[42] The ability of these analytes to form adducts with mono-protonated cations, for example Li^+, Na^+, K^+, NH_4^+ or Ag^+ has facilitated the use of coordination ion-spray mass spectrometry via the formation of ammonium or silver adducts.[43]

In contrast, there appears to be no standard analytical approach for epoxide impurities. Some recent publications have utilized derivatization due to the relative hydroloytic instabilities of epoxides leading to ring opening. Liu et al.[24] utilized the dimethylamine (DMA) derivative of an epoxide VII to develop a method with an LOD of 1 ng/mL. This derivative can be used for ESI-MS analysis.

Liu et al.[24] also reported on a direct MS approach for an epoxide impurity (VIII) in an API, which was appropriately validated despite the potential instability issues. Due to the formation of multiple reaction products following derivatization using DMA, this approach was abandoned. Although epoxide VIII could not be protonated or deprotonated easily, it was found to be a good candidate for the coordination ion-spray MS approach previously described by Havrilla et al.[43] The [M + K]+ species with an m/z value of 266 was selected, and the LOQ was found to be 1.5 ppm. The method was linear and gave good precision (RSD 1.3%) and acceptable recoveries (87%) at 3 ppm.

HPLC remains a key separation technique for those analytes that are insufficiently volatile and/or too thermally labile to allow analysis directly by GC; this is the case for many compounds in this class, explaining the plethora of references to HPLC. Interestingly, virtually all of literature references accessed employed HPLC with either single or dual wavelength UV detection[44-46] or diode array UV detection.[44,47-51] There were surprisingly few reported usages of HPLC-MS.[52,53] There are single literature references to the use of other less common detection techniques, including evaporative light scattering detection (ELSD) detection[54] and fluorescence detection[55] and two literature references to the use of normal phase HPLC.[46,47]

A significant amount of the work reported in the literature relates to Chinese Herbal Medicines and the presence of epoxides therein. Due to the complexity of the sample a variety of extraction techniques and/or pre-concentration techniques, designed to improve matrix interference prior to analysis, were reported (Lin et al., 1998[56] Brinker and Raskin, 2005;[57] Kong et al., 2001;[54] Seger et al., 2003;[48] Kurzinski et al., 2005;[49] Ye et al., 2006;[50] Zhou et al., 2006[52] Zhau et al.,2008;[51] Mroczek et al., 2006.[58] Mroczek et al. (2006)[58] used both HPLC and HPTLC (high-performance thin layer chromatography) to analyze residual levels of scopolamine (a naturally occurring alkaloid containing a epoxide moiety that is used legitimately to treat motion sickness), extracted from *Datura stramonium* root extracts. The correlation between the two methods was excellent for both alkaloids (scopolamine (correlation coefficient 0.99995) and hyoscyamine (correlation coefficient 0.92086)). The authors tested extracts from 14 leaf and seed samples of different *Datura* species and varieties. They showed good correlations between the two analytical methods, with recoveries in the range of 0.04%–0.16% for HPTLC estimations, versus 0.04%–0.13%, respectively for HPLC determinations.

GC, while not seeing the same scale of renaissance as was observed for alkyl halides, is still well represented. GC-FID[59,60] and GC-MS with ESI detection[61-64] are the typical analytical approaches. As with HPLC, a variety of extraction techniques and/or preconcentration techniques, which are designed to improve matrix interference prior to analysis, were routinely used for traditional Chinese herbal medicines.[61-65]

Capillary zone electrophoresis (CZE) is also well represented in the trace level analysis of herbal products. The typical sensitivity deficiencies of capillary electrophoresis (CE) and CZE being addressed by hyphenated MS approaches,[53,66,67] including CE-MS-EI with time of flight (ToF) detection. Extraction and/or preconcentration techniques were less routinely applied presumably because of CE's enhanced selectivity compared with other separation techniques. There were also examples of the related technique of micellar electrokinetic chromatography (MEKC) with MS-ESI detection[53,68] being used for both traditional Chinese herbal medicines and standard medicinal products.[68]

Methodologies based on TLC and HPTLC separations followed by visualization were not used for any of the pharmacopoeial monographs reviewed. In contrast, their use as an adjunct to other chromatographic techniques was reported in conjunction with the quantitative analysis of traditional Chinese herbal medicines.[58,69]

Again, there are some differences seen between pharmacopoeial monographs and literature references. For instance, the latest pharmacopoeial monographs for stavudine[70] does not control the cyclic hydroperoxide reported by Kažoka and Madre.[47] Similarly, the monographs for dexamethasone,[71] nadalol,[72] norethisterone[73] do not control the epoxide impurities, in contrast to literature reports.[74–76]

10.5 HYDRAZINES AND HYDRAZIDES

Considering the huge challenges inherent in the determination of very low levels of volatile hydrazines and hydrazides in APIs, and, in particular, the lack of any meaningful chromophore, the breadth of analytical techniques utilized is very striking. Unlike alkyl halides, which typically utilize hyphenated GC or HPLC methodologies, derivatization has been utilized as one of the main analytical strategies toward enhancing sensitivity and addressing volatility. This has ensured that spectroscopic as well as chromatographic techniques have been applied.

HPLC, exclusively in reversed phase mode, remains a key separation technique, and the favored derivative using this approach has been benzalazine; formed via the reaction between hydrazine and benzaldehyde (see Fig. 10.5).

There is a single report of normal phase chromatography.[77] There are two very recent examples of nonderivatized hydrophilic interaction chromatography (HILIC), and this seems to be a promising approach that may be the favored approach in the future.[78,79]

A novel separation method for the impurities in mildronate API was recently reported by Hmelnickis et al.[78] The authors used a HILIC method with several different, polar, stationary phases (silica, cyano, amino, and the zwitterionic sulfobetaine) to separate the six polar impurities, including the hydrazine impurity, 1,1,1-trimethylhydrazinium bromide (impurity II). They demonstrated that HILIC was a useful alternative to reverse phase for IC. The impact of method separation conditions, including organic modifier content and pH, were studied. Finally, a HILIC method using the zwitterionic sulfobetaine stationary phase was developed and validated. Linearity of the method was established over the range of 50%–125% of the nominal 0.1% level, which was the proposed specification limit, and showed

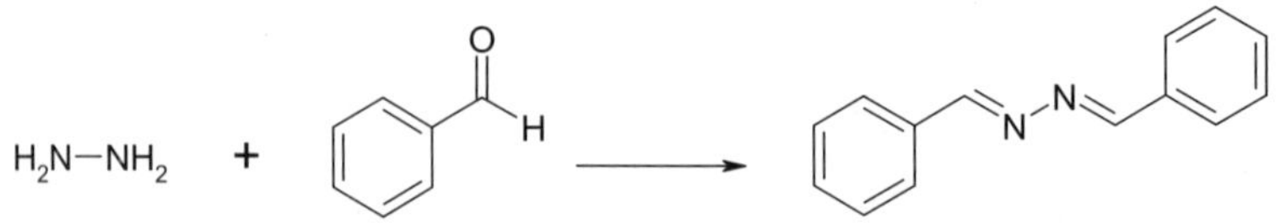

Figure 10.5 Derivatization of hydrazine residues with benzaldehyde.

good linearity for impurity II (correlation coefficient of 0.997), with an LOD of 0.0003% (3 ppm) and an LOQ of 0.001% (10 ppm). The accuracy of the method to determine recoveries of impurity II at levels of 0.05%, 0.075%, 0.100%, and 0.125% were assessed. The recoveries were in the range of 105.7%–114.0%, with RSDs of between 1.1% and 5.1%. The precision at the 0.1% level was 3.3%. The method was found to be robust and applied to two batches of mildronate API. In the technical batch, the levels of residual impurity II were high (3500 ppm), but in the commercial batch, the levels were much reduced, and only seen at levels equating to the LOQ of the method, that is 3 ppm. This demonstrates that greater understanding of the reaction chemistries typically leads to better control strategies and lowered levels of these reactive impurities.

A novel generic method for the direct determination of hydrazine and 1,1-dimethylhydrazine in a pharmaceutical intermediate was reported by Lui et al.[79] The method again used a HILIC approach with ethanol as a weak eluent and chemiluminescent nitrogen detection (CLND). The method is simple and reasonably sensitive (0.02%, 200 ppm, 2 μg/mL). The method was linear over the range of 0.01%–0.1% of both analytes. The precision of the standard solutions at 0.02% was 5.0 and 3.9%, respectively. The recoveries were excellent for 1,1-dimethylhydrazine at 0.02 and 0.04% (100.9 and 102.7%, respectively). However, in contrast, the recoveries for hydrazine were somewhat low at 0.02% (84.3%), but were satisfactory at the 0.04% level (102.7%).

All HPLC methods reported to date in literature have employed single wavelength UV/visible detection, preceded by derivatization. The greater sensitivity afforded by derivatization precludes the need for more sensitive detection approaches. There are also single reports of dual wavelength detection,[80] of combined diode array detection,[81] of CLND detection,[79] of ESI with an ion trap in the SIM mode,[81] of ESI with ToF detection,[82] of ESI[78], and two reports of quadrupole MS detection.[83,84]

Derivatization is routinely employed with GC, and as with HPLC, the favored derivative is benzalazine.[85,86] Several of the earlier research groups used nitrogen selective detection,[85,87] but Kirtley et al.[88] recently commented on the poor sensitivity of NPD (nitrogen phosphorous detection), and they found the LOD was inadequate to address the analytical issues.

Static headspace techniques, combined with quadrupole EI detection with SIM, have been routinely used by Sun et al.[84] These authors reported on a generic *in situ* derivatization headspace GC-MS method for the determination of hydrazine in API at low ppm levels. This general method has been utilized for the determination of residual hydrazine in a wide range of different API matrices. The method utilizes either acetone or the stable isotope analogue, acetone-d_6 as the derivatizing agent, yielding the corresponding azine (acetone-azine or acetone-azine-d_{12}) derivative. This volatile derivative can be analyzed by headspace GC-MS (Fig. 10.6).

The method is highly sensitive and is capable of detecting levels of hydrazine at 0.1 ppm in the presence of 10 mg of API. The method is linear over the range of 0.1–10 ppm, with a correlation coefficient of 0.999. The recoveries at the 1 ppm level were in the range of 79%–117%, and the precision at this level were ≤5.6% RSD. The recoveries were slightly impacted by the presence of interfering functional groups on the different APIs (e.g. ketone, primary amine, etc.) that could react with

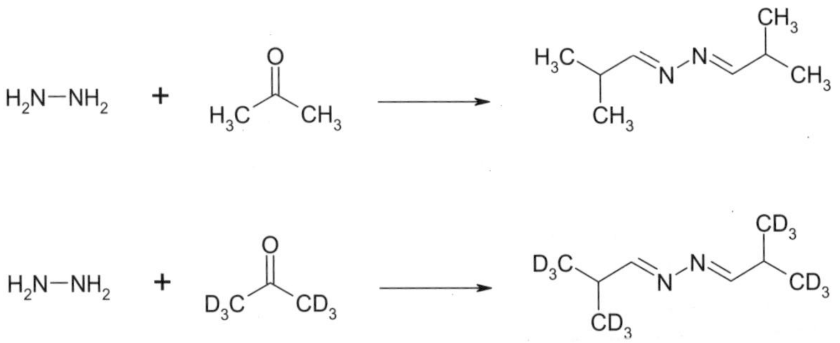

Figure 10.6   Derivatization of hydrazine residues with acetone or acetone-d6.

acetone or a weak Michael acceptor that could react with hydrazine. However, these interferences were fairly insignificant, considering the very low level of analyte, that is 0.1 ppm.

The generic method was successfully applied to the determination of residual hydrazine at 1 ppm in five different APIs and using the stable isotope alternative (acetone-d_6) for another 2 APIs where acetone was present as a residual solvent. The method was validated at slightly higher residual analyte levels (25 and 100 ppm hydrazine) for a further 2 APIs due to the higher control limits necessitated by these projects. The authors commented that instrument contamination was minimized, and that the method could be automated by using autosamplers with heating, stirring, and reagent addition facilities.

There are several literature references to the use of CE and related electrokinetic chromatography techniques (MEKC and MEEKC). There are two examples of CE for the determination of residual hydrazine and methylhydrazine in isoniazid.[89,90] In both cases, the authors utilized electrochemical detection with novel electrodes to overcome the intrinsic issue of the high overpotential of these analytes toward oxidation using standard electrodes. Liu et al.[89] used Pd modified carbon micro-disk array electrodes, whereas You et al.[90] utilized Pt-modified 4-pyridylhydroquinone micro-disk array electrodes. The sensitivity of both methods for detection of residual levels of these analytes was good. The LODs for hydrazine and methylhydrazine were 1.0 and 5.0 μM, respectively, for the former method. However, the sensitivity of the latter method was significantly enhanced, with LODs for hydrazine and methylhydrazine of 0.1 μM.

There was one reported example of MEKC for the determination of residual levels of 4-hydrazine benzene sulphonamide in celecoxib.[91] The LOD of this method was 3.5 μg/mL. In contrast, the same research group[92] had earlier demonstrated that the corresponding HPLC method had an LOD of 97 ng/mL. This highlights the continuing issue of CE, that of lack of sensitivity.

The use of IC is also widely reported[88,93–95] exclusively in the nonderivatized mode with amperometric detection. Most authors used amperometric detection because of the enhanced selectivity, increased sensitivity, and reduced matrix interference. Jagota et al.[95] reported on the development and validation of an IC method for residual hydrazine. Although the method sensitivity was lower than typically reported (50 ppm), it was fit for purpose as the substrate was the penultimate intermediate of a novel anti-infective API.

However, typically, most IC methods were significantly more sensitive. Researcher's from Merck[88] developed an IC method for the penultimate intermediate of a highly water soluble API, with an LOD of 0.05 ppm. The significantly enhanced sensitivity was attributed to the sample pretreatment. The authors used a strong cation exchange matrix to clean up the sample before running the assay on a weak cation exchange resin stationary phase. Similarly, researchers from Abbott[93] developed a generic method with LOQs for hydrazine and methylhydrazine of 0.5 and 1.2 ppm, respectively.

Kirtley et al.[88] reported that the advantages over the standard derivative HPLC procedure were increased selectivity and reduced matrix interference. Kean et al.[94] were able to show concordance of their IC method with the pharmacopoeial method (3.9 ppm vs. 3.2 ppm hydrazine, respectively), but lower levels than in the derivative HPLC method.

Considering the sensitivity requirements for these toxic analytes (ca. 1 ppm), TLC methods surprisingly still feature heavily and can generate equivalent data compared with more sensitive techniques, that is HPLC.[94] All of the methods reviewed for determination of residual hydrazine used derivatization, but here the favored derivatizing reagent was salicylaldehyde rather the benzaldehyde. In the majority of cases, the hydrazine was visualized with far-UV light and densitometry, but in a few cases, the pharmacopoeial method utilizes visualization with dimethylaminobenzaldehyde.[96–99] There were two reports of TLC methods for other analytes.[99,100] These methods were for various hydrazone degradation products of rifampicin, for example 1-amino-4-methylpiperazine, rifampicin quinone (RQU), and 25-desacetyl rifampicin (DAR).

There were two examples of spectroscopy methods, both of which assessed residual hydrazine levels in isoniazid and iponiazid[101] and isoniazid.[102] The former method utilized fluorescence spectroscopy and used 2-hydroxy-1-naphthaldehyde derivatization, whereas the latter utilized UV/visible spectroscopy and used 4-dimethyl aminobenzaldehyde (DMAB) derivatization. The fluorescence method was very sensitive with an LOD of 3.2 ppb. Interestingly, by fixing the DMAB derivatizing agent onto a cation exchange resin, the sensitivity of the UV/visible method was enhanced with an LOD 0.26 ng/mL.

Substrate interference, from the API or the formulation matrix, appears to be less of a restricting factor when derivative analysis is employed with HPLC techniques. However, there are still some reported examples of LLE techniques utilized for HPLC methods,[88,94] and one reported example of LSE techniques.[88] In contrast, extraction and/or preconcentration techniques, such as static head space analysis,[84] and, more particularly, LLE, are used routinely to reduce matrix interference in GC methodologies.[85–87] For IC, only one of the research groups cited utilized an extraction technique using strong cation exchange resins prior to running the chromatography on a weak cation exchange stationary phase.[88] TLC methods used extraction techniques almost exclusively; the only exceptions were the aryl hydrazones impurities of rifampicin (RQU and DAR). Typically, LLE alone was used, but in one example, both LLE and LSE were utilized.[103] Finally, none of the CE or electrokinetic methods used extraction techniques, perhaps a testament to the greater selectivity of these techniques.

10.6 N-NITROSO

The TTC concept typically excludes highly toxic compounds such as aflatoxins and N-nitroso compounds. These analytes are treated on a case-by-case basis by regulators and pharmacopoeias. From an analytical perspective, this can have a significant impact as it can result in detection limits being driven down to ppb levels.

References relating to N-nitrosamines in pharmaceuticals are relatively rare.

The Ph. Eur. established a specific limit for total N-nitroso groups (TNG) in nadroparin sodium[104] and dalteparin sodium,[105] which are low molecular weight heparins (LMWH), of 0.25 ppm. The method involves cleavage of the N-NO group by hydrobromic acid in ethyl acetate using a reflux condenser and detection of the liberated NO by chemiluminescence. Unfortunately, it is prone to interference from residual inorganic nitrite, which is not controlled in nadroparin, unlike in dalteparin, where there is a limit of 5 ppm. As a consequence of these limitations, Beretta et al.[106] published a simplified screening procedure for the determination of both TNG and residual nitrite in commercial LMWHs using selective chemical denitrozation followed by high sensitivity chemical luminescence detection using a NO analyzer. The proposed approach uses three sequentially connected purge vessels, where specific reagents are utilized for the separate conversion of nitrite and N-NO (as either volatile or nonvolatile fractions) to NO.

The method was shown to be selective over a linear range of 1–1000 ppb. The bias and intra- and inter-day precision were all <1%. The method was linear over the range of 1–1000 ppb ($R^2 = 0.9999$), with an LOD and LOQ of 0.2 and 0.6 pmol, respectively. The accuracy of the method was extremely good, and was in the range of 99.12–101.50% for both analytes. The method was assessed by critical comparison with an alternative chemical denitrosation method described by Wang et al.,[107] using a CuCl reagent. The methods were comparable ($P > 0.05$), but the method of Beretta et al.[106] was slightly more sensitive (LOD 0.2 pmol) than that of Wang et al.,[107] which had an LOD of 1 pmol.

Seven batches of commercial nadroparin injections and 11 batches of dalteparin injections were assessed for residual nitrite and TNG levels.[106] Whereas the nadroparin LMWH samples had low levels of residual nitrite (0.28–0.63 ppm) and TNG (ND-0.007 ppm), complying with the appropriate Ph. Eur limit (TNG <0.25 ppm), dalteparin had acceptable nitrite levels (0.98–3.23 ppm), but levels of TNG in all cases exceeded the proposed Ph. Eur. limit (0.25 ppm), in some cases by 60-fold (6.69–15.80 ppm). The authors indicated that this could be tentatively explained by differences in the processing conditions for the deploymerization of heparin by nitrous acid, for example pH, reaction temperatures, reagent volumes, etc., leading to differing levels of contamination.

The authors reported that their data were indicative of the fact that most of the denitrosable material may be either nonextractable N-NO material attributable to hydrophilic N-nitrosamines and N-nitrosamides, or due to the cleavage of the

N-NO groups covalently bonded to the LMWH backbone, probably *N*-(NO)-acetyl short side chains on the surface of the dalteparin structure. They considered that about 2% of the LMHW consisted of NO adducted molecules, and were in the process of utilizing high resolution MS to confirm these findings.

The authors indicated that their method was simpler and cheaper than the pharmacopoeial method together with the following specific benefits: (1) no requirements to add nitrite depleting agents, which can subsequently destabilize *N*-nitrosamides in aqueous media; (2) the equipment comprises of one piece, with no requirements for disassembly and cleaning when reagents are changed; (3) conditions for trapping of volatile *N*-nitroso compounds have been optimized; and (4) minimal cross-contamination arising from LMWH degradation.

Pötter and Hülm[108] investigated the photodegradation of nifedipine to form its nitroso derivative (impurity II). The authors developed a normal phase HPLC method with a silica stationary phase and an isocratic mobile phase comprising saturated formamide at 237 nm. The method was linear for the nitroso impurity over the range of 0.8–4.0 μg, with a correlation coefficient of greater than 0.98. The LOD of the nitroso compound was 8 ng (0.01%, 100 ppm).

Kawabe et al.[109] expanded on these photo-degradation investigations on dihydropyridine (DHP) calcium-channel blockers to include first generation (nifedipine), second generation (nilvadapine), and third generation (amlodipine) agents. The authors showed that DHP agents, which included the nitrophenyl moiety, for example nifedipine and nilvadapine, were commonly photolabile and converted into the corresponding dehydro (aromatization of dihydropyridine ring) or dehydronitroso (dehydration) degradation products. In contrast, those DHP agents without the nitrophenyl substitution, for example amlodipine, only formed the dehydro compound. The authors reported that the analytical conditions utilized to monitor the photodegradation reaction comprised of an octadecylsilyl stationary phase (Cosmoil C18), with an isocratic mobile phase comprising of water/methanol (35/65 v/v), with a detection wavelength of 234 nm. No validation details were reported for either DHP compound.

Walash and co-workers[110] reported on a simple HPLC method for the determination of dinitrosopiperazine in piperazine exposed to simulated gastric juice. The method was linear over the range of 0.072–2.88 μg/mL, with an LOD of 0.01 μg/mL. The method was accurate (100.17 ± 0.38) and precise, and the intra-day precision was in the range of 0.19%–0.25%. The authors assessed the robustness of the method to changes in pH, organic modifier, and ionic strength of the aqueous buffer. These changes had no affect on the capacity factor of the method.

Belal et al.[111] developed an alternative voltametric method for the determination of the same analyte (dinitrosopiperazine) in the same matrix. The method was linear over the range of 0.4–24 μg/mL ($r = 0.9999$), with an LOD of 0.007 μg/mL. The method was accurate (100.24 ± 0.80), but no precision data was reported.

10.7   AROMATIC AMINES

Aromatic amines, which include phenylamines, aminopyridines, and other heterocyclic amines, form a broad class of potential GIs. As a result, it might be expected that a considerable amount of information pertaining to their analysis would exist in the literature. Surprisingly, however, there is somewhat of a paucity of information that may well reflect the relatively low level of concerns as to toxicity prior to the advent of the EMEA guideline.

The most extensively studied of the aromatic amines is 4-aminophenol (4-AP), this being an intermediate used in the manufacture of paracetamol (acetaminophen) and also a degradation product. Interestingly, a variety of techniques, both chromatographic and spectroscopic, have been applied to the analysis of 4-AP.

An HPLC method using electrochemical detection (EC) has been developed by Wyszecka-Kaszuba and co-workers[112] for the determination of trace levels of 4-AP in multicomponent analgesic preparations containing paracetamol. The method was selective and could be used to assess residual 4-AP levels in preparations containing paracetamol, pseudoephedrine, dextromethorphan, guaiophenasin, chlorpheniramine, codeine, mepiramine, propyphenazone, and caffeine, but not in the presence of ascorbic or acetylsalicylic acids. The method was linear, with a correlation coefficient of 0.998, and demonstrated good precision: between-day precision of 0.99% RSD and a within-day precision of 0.49% RSD. The method could readily determine residual levels of 4-AP in API (LOD 1 ng/mL) or a multicomponent dosage form, for example a tablet or capsule (LOD 4 ng/mL). The method was used to assess residual levels of 4-AP in commercial multicomponent analgesic preparations and levels were in the range of 0.00019%–0.0015% (2–15 ppm).

García et al.[113] reported on the use of a novel poly(ethyleneglycol) (PEG) stationary phase for the determination of acetaminophen, phenylephrine, and chlorpheniramine and related compounds (including 4-AP) in pharmaceutical formulations. They were able to show the resolution and selectivity of the method and its ability to resolve 4-AP, but no validation details were provided for this analyte.

As well as HPLC, several methods for analysis of 4-AP based on CZE have been published. Chen and co-workers[114] developed a CZE method with EC detection (CZE-EC) for the determination of the hydrolysis rate constants and activation energy of paracetamol. This involved the simultaneous determination of 4-AP and paracetamol. The method showed good selectivity in test mixtures, resolving the two analytes within 6 min. The method showed good linearity for both analytes, with correlation coefficients in excess of 0.9996. The detection limit of 4-AP was 1.69×10^{-6} M. The RSDs for peak current and migration time for both analytes were good, and values of 2.85% and 0.79% for 4-AP and 1.65% and 1.33% for paracetamol, respectively, were reported.

Pérez-Ruiz and co-workers[115] developed a CZE method for the determination of 4-AP in drug products containing paracetamol. The method showed good selectivity in test mixtures containing amino acids, vitamins, and excipients, as well as of 4-AP and paracetamol. The method showed good linearity for both primary analytes, with correlation coefficients in excess of 0.9990. The repeatability at low levels of 4-AP was good showing RSDs of 1.90% and 1.57%, respectively, at levels of 0.5 and 1.0 μg/mL (ppm). The intra-day precision at levels of 4-AP equal to 0.5 μg/mL was 1.97%, whereas the inter-day precision at the same level was 2.31%. The LOQ of the method was 37.3 ng/mL, with a precision of 3.0%. Unfortunately, the LOQ could not be enhanced further due to problems with selectivity, as the paracetamol peak interfered with that of 4-AP at lower analyte levels. The accuracy was in the range of 97%–103.8% for both analytes, and the method was robust when variations in the electrophoretic parameters up to a maximum of ±10% of the optimum values were applied. None of the three commercial formulations showed residual levels of 4-AP above the method LOQ.

Recently, Németh et al.[116] reported on the use of MEKC to determine residual levels of 4-AP in analgesic preparations containing paracetamol. The method is specific and 4-AP elutes prior to the paracetamol peak with no formulation interference and a run time of only 10 min. The accuracy of the method was demonstrated by spiking paracetamol preparations with 0.3, 0.4, and 0.5% of 4-AP and recoveries were in the range of 99.9%–104.1%. The method was linear over the range of 0.1%–0.75% for 4-AP. The LOQ of the method for 4-AP was 6 µg/mL (0.03%, 300 ppm), and at that level, it showed appropriate precision (RSD 5.7%). The LOD is three times lower than the LOQ at 2 µg/mL (0.01%, 100 ppm), and in the three batches of product that were assessed, there was no 4-AP seen at or above the LOD value. The method was also shown to be robust and insensitive to sodium dodecylsulfate (SDS) and buffer pH changes in the range of ±10% of the stated conditions.

In contrast, the propacetamol (a pro-drug of paracetamol) monograph[117] describes a TLC related substances method for the same impurity (impurity A: 4-AP). The TLC method used a silica gel F_{254} TLC plate with a formic acid/water/methanol/methylene chloride (3/4/30/64 v/v) mobile phase. The analyte is visualized using dimethyl acetylenedicarboxylate and is observed as a yellow spot (not visible under ultraviolet light at 254 nm).

In a similar fashion, Gotti and co-workers[118] developed a MEKC method for the determination of residual 4-AP in mesalazine (5-aminosalicylic acid). The method was selective and could be used to resolve residual 4-AP levels from 3-aminosalicylic acid, sulfanilic acid, and mesalazine. The method was linear with a correlation coefficient of 0.998 over the concentration range of 0.7–14 µg/mL. The method demonstrated good precision; the migration time precision was 0.54% RSD, and the peak area precision was 3.21% RSD. The method could readily determine residual levels of 4-AP down to 0.02% (LOD, 200 ppm) and 0.05% (LOQ, 500 ppm). The method was used to assess residual levels in API, but no levels of 4-AP were seen in any of the batches tested.

As well as chromatographic techniques, spectroscopic techniques have also been employed. Forshed et al.[119] describe the use of NMR and a regularized neural network regression procedure for the impurity determination of 4-AP in paracetamol. The method was described as simple and relatively rapid (about 20 min); no pretreatment was required (simply dissolution of the sample) and the selectivity was good.

Recently, Vanhoenacker et al.[120] have described two generic HPLC-MS methods using a single quadrupole mass spectrometer with SIM detection. The first method used direct injection, whereas the second method utilized hexylchloroformate derivatization, with a reaction time of 30 min, to form amide derivatives (see Fig. 10.7).

The advantages of derivatization were described as being twofold. First, that the derivatized analyte had a higher molecular weight and hence a more specific ion

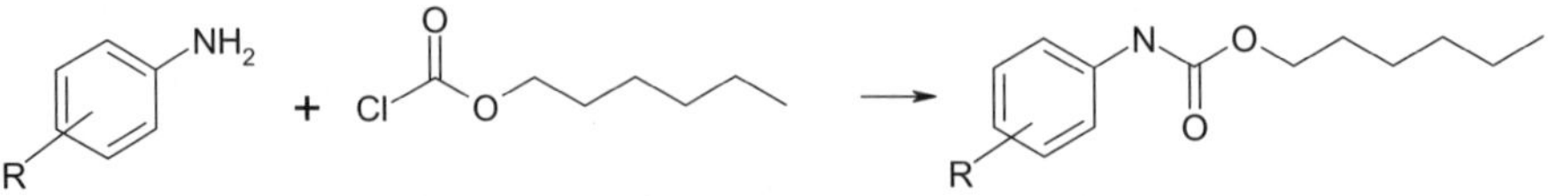

Figure 10.7 Derivatization of aniline residues with hexylchloroformate.

for SIM detection. Second, the chromatographic retention of the derivatized analyte was significantly enhanced, avoiding, in some cases, elution on the solvent front. Using these approaches, the authors claimed greater flexibility and the ability to be able to cover a wide range of analytes and different API matrices. The authors also claimed that selectivity could be enhanced by "fine-tuning" of stationary and mobile phases.

Both methods used a Zorbax Eclipse Plus C18 (Agilent Technologies Inc., Colorado Springs, CO) stationary phase held at 25°C and a gradient mobile phase comprising of 0.05% formic acid and water and acetonitrile. The direct injection method used a 5 µL injection volume, whereas the derivative method used a 50 µL injection volume, which, taking into account the one-tenth dilution for derivatization, equated to identical on-column concentrations. The MS was a single quadrupole with positive EI in the SIM mode using the M + 1 ion of the GI.

The authors assessed 13 analytes covering a wide range of polarities and volatilities. As neither volatility enrichment (static headspace) nor polarity enrichment (SPE) were achievable for all analytes in all matrices, the authors elected to use direct injection with MS-SIM detection (LOD <0.1 ppm). The supplementary derivatization method also typically ensured that problems of ionization suppression that arose due to co-elution of the API and some of the GIs studied could be addressed through the greater retention of the derivatized analyte.

10.8 ALDEHYDES

A number of low molecular weight aldehydes, for example formaldehyde, are considered to be of concern from a genotoxic perspective, and hence there is need to ensure control over their levels. This has subsequently led to the need to develop suitable analytical methods. However, the determination of very low levels of volatile alkyl aldehydes as potential impurities in APIs presents very real analytical challenges. In common with hydrazines, reported methods for aldehydes are typically based on derivatization. Derivatization is employed to both stabilize the analyte and modify its physicochemical properties. On consequence of this is that it has ensured that spectroscopic and polagraphic, as well as chromatographic methods (HPLC and GC), have been applied.

HPLC, almost exclusively in reverse phase mode, remains a key separation technique, and the favored derivative using this approach has been 2, 4-dinitrophenylhydrazone (2, 4-DNPH), see Figure 10.8.

There are also reports of other potentially more sensitive derivatives formed with s-triazolo-[3, 4, a]-phthalazines,[121] acetylacetone,[122,123] or o-(2,3,4,5,6-pentafluorobenzyl)oxime derivatives,[124] but their utilization appears to be limited.

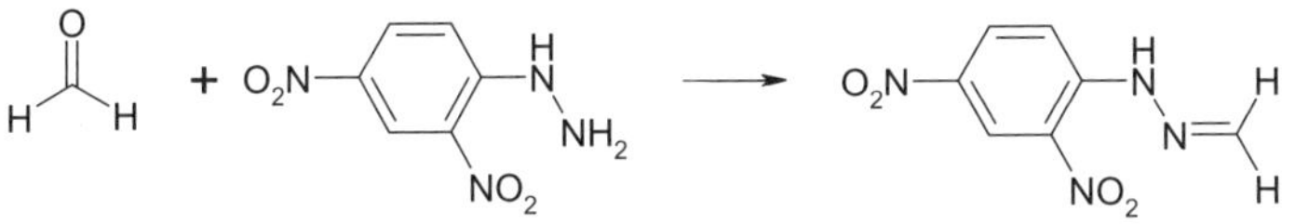

2,4 dinitrophenylhydrazine

Figure 10.8   Derivatization of formaldehyde residues with 2,4 dinitrophenylhydrazine.

Argentine et al.[123] reported on the utility of the 3,5-deacteyl-1,4-dihydrolutidine derivative followed by HPLC-UV at 412 nm for the determination of residual formaldehyde in intermediates and API. The LOD was reported to be 1 ppm. There was some substrate interference at these lower levels, and recoveries were slightly elevated at 10 ppm (113%).

All of the described references to HPLC employ single wavelength UV/visible detection. The greater sensitivity afforded by these derivatization techniques typically precludes the need for more sensitive detection approaches, for example MS. There is one report of combined UV/visible and fluorescence detection,[122] and one report of APCI MS detection. This latter method also utilized CAD (charged aerosol detection) to ascertain the retention times of the matrix peaks (glycerol and propylene glycol) so that they can be eluted to waste, thereby reducing matrix interference and improving accuracy and precision of the APCI MS detector.

In contrast, the literature shows slightly different emphasis when using GC as the detection technique. Direct analysis with static headspace techniques, using either FID or MS detection, have been routinely used by several groups.[125–129]

Derivatization has also been employed with GC, but in contrast, with HPLC, there appears to be no favored approach. Del Barrio et al.[130] reported on a static headspace method employing ethyl ester derivatization. In contrast, Manius et al.[128] utilized the oxime derivatives, whereas Martos and Pawliszn[131] used the more volatile o-(2,3,4,5,6-pentafluorobenzyl)oxime derivatives. Manius et al.[128] utilized FID, with the option of using a nitrogen-sensitive detector for enhanced sensitivity, whereas both Del Barrio et al.[130] and Martos and Pawliszn[131] used MS detection with SIM detection.

There is one report of ion chromatography[128] where the volatile formaldehyde analyte is oxidized to the corresponding formate ion. This method suffered from matrix interference from other anions, such as hydroxide and chloride anions, and appears to have limited utility.

There is a single literature reference to the use of CE,[132] which again relied on derivatization, this time using the charged aldehyde dansylhydrazone complex, which is detected at 214 nm. These authors reported exquisite sensitivity from this method, with an LOD of 200 ppb for the named aldehydes, including formaldehyde.

Substrate interference, from the API or the formulation matrix, does not appear to be to be a significant factor with HPLC techniques where derivatization is employed. As a result, there is only one reported example of the application of LLE.[122] In contrast, extraction and/or preconcentration techniques, such as static HS analysis[125,127,128] or SPME,[126,131] are used routinely to reduce matrix interference in GC methodologies.

Methodologies based on TLC separations followed by visualization do not appear to play a role in the detection of residual levels of volatile aldehydes. None of the pharmacopoeial monographs used TLC for the determination of residual volatile aldehydes. In contrast, spectrophotometric methods feature extensively. They are sometimes used as a fast-screening method prior to chromatographic analysis,[133] but more often than not they are used as sensitive analytical techniques in their own right. Most of the reported methods utilize the chromotropic colourimetric test,[128,133,134] but there are also reports of other derivatives, for example N-methylbenzo-thiazolon-2-hydrazone (MBTH) and 4-amino-5-mercapto-1,2,4-triazole (Purpald reagent).[135]

10.9 TECHNOLOGY TRANSFER

The transfer of analytical methodologies into different laboratories or into a routine production environment is often a challenging undertaking. Where, as is often the case in the analysis of GIs, the procedure entails both sample pretreatment and the use of nonroutine sensitive detection techniques, the challenge is significantly increased.

In their recent paper on the trace analysis of reactive organohalides, Elder et al.[136] reflected that in many cases, this required the application of techniques that although common in a development environment are not well established in QC laboratories. This may also be true in terms of the laboratories of the worldwide regulatory agencies. Moreover, the techniques often require not only specialized equipment, but also specialized expert analytical scientists with extensive knowledge of the techniques and procedures concerned. This is particularly true where sample pretreatment (extraction, derivatization, etc.) is required. While most/all literature references include extensive method validation data, there are few reports[19,24] of interlaboratory studies, the true test of the method robustness.

In terms of the technology transfer of complex trace analysis methods analogous to GI methodology, Borman et al.[137] reported on the transfer of the method for the determination of residual FMTP (4-(4-fluorophenyl)-1-methyl-1,2,3,6-tetrahydropyridine) in paroxetine API at the 10 ppb level. The authors assessed the reproducibility (ruggedness) of the method transfer using a fully nested design assessing instrument, sample preparation, analyst, and day. The variation of each factor and the total variation were all assessed. It was seen that analyst (63%) and sample preparation (27%) contributed toward the largest sources of error during the method transfer, whereas neither day nor instrument contributed significantly toward the total error. The RSD for the method performed on the same day by the same analyst on the same equipment was 12%. This increased to 20% when allowance was made for changes in preparation, day, analyst, and instrument.

Variability plots showed a much larger variability in results from within the factory environment (instrument 2) compared with within the development environment (instrument 1). The authors felt that this could be attributed to a number of different factors relating to different ways of working within the two environments, but commented that as with environmental analysis, that technique is paramount and that even the most robust methods struggle to overcome problems of poor technique, transient contamination, etc. However, as this was a 10 ppb limit test, as long as the LOQs of the method at the two different sites were less than this value, then these differences in method variance were deemed to be acceptable. Interestingly, at these very low analyte levels, the absolute detection limits are dependent on the instrument response (i.e. sensitivity). The two different instruments used in the study described give different absolute responses, but it was stressed that this was not important as long as the 10 ppb limit can be reproducibly attained. The more sensitive instrument was that used in the factory environment (instrument 2), which gave an LOQ of 0.5 ppb, whereas the development instrument gave an LOQ of 7.7 ppb. The recoveries of the method were in the range of 115.4%–112.2% over the range of 10–20 ppb, which was within the range of 4× the average standard deviation for the repeatability of the method, and deemed to be acceptable for a method operating at the 10 ppb level. In addition, a positive bias for a limit test is acceptable as the method always "fails safe," that is calculated levels are always slightly higher than actual levels. Five paroxetine API batches manufactured within the factory were tested for residual levels of FMTP, and in all cases, no FMTP was detected (<LOQ).

The authors showed surprisingly that the method transfer could be approached in a similar fashion to a standard ICH Q3A method. The method showed acceptable repeatability and linearity, and could be used as a limit test for the detection of residual FMTP levels in excess of 10 ppb in production batches of paroxetine API. The validation was reported for a specific model of a triple quadrupole MS, and the authors cautioned that revalidation would be required for different instruments, and there was a critical need to assess and optimize tuning parameters of the new instrument. This test was added to the specification as a skip lot test, and is performed on an annual basis. The authors also indicated their concerns that neither they nor the industry had any long-term experience of usage of these methods within a factory environment. They cautioned that without significant investment in technology and analytical skill sets, it might not be a viable long term option.

Subsequently, Elder[138] reported that the long-term use of this method in the pharmacopoeial arena had proved to be challenging, which had prompted significant changes. The current USP limit is 0.0001%, that is 1 ppm, and the changes were made in USP 28 (2002) at the behest of the EDQM. The current USP uses an HPLC-UV method with an L1 (Purospher RP-18e, 5 μm; Agilent Technologies, Inc., Colorado Springs, CO) stationary phase at 30°C, and a gradient mobile phase comprising eluant A (pH 2.0 perchlorate buffer and triethylamine) and eluant B (acetonitrile). The flow rate is 1.5 mL/min, and the detection wavelength is 242 nm. The changes were made in USP 31 (2005) on the basis of simplifying a complex method.

The current limit in Ph. Eur. is also 1 ppm,[139,140] but interestingly, no method is specified. There is a Production Statement for Impurity G (FMTP), stating that "Maximum 1 ppm, determined by a suitable, validated method."

Liu et al.[24] reflected that the development of an analytical strategy for later phase new chemical entities (NCEs), which utilizes simplified analytical hardware with commensurately higher detection limits, for example HPLC-UV, significantly improves the potential of an issue-free technology transfer exercise. However, they cautioned that such a simplification exercise must be based on extensive process understanding and is predicated on the ability of the GIs to be controlled by upstream chemistries, and that the testing strategy is based on control of starting materials and intermediates, rather than testing for absence of GI in the final API. They reported on the extensive process understanding and control of five GIs in the anticancer drug, pazopanib HCL. They utilized state-of-the-art mass spectrometry-based techniques during early development, but transferred conventional HPLC-UV methodology, with standard ICH Q3A sensitivity, that is 0.05% (500 ppm). They commented that these standard HPLC-UV methods are much more robust and better aligned with transfer into a production environment. They did add the caveat that many production laboratories are suitably equipped with single quadrapole HPLC-MS or GC-MS instrumentation, and that transfer exercises utilizing these more complex techniques could be anticipated in the future.

10.10   GENERAL DISCUSSION

The regulatory challenges associated with the analysis and control of GIs has seen a rich flowering of the analytical sciences within the pharmaceutical industry. The analysis of very low levels (ppm or even lower) of reactive, often volatile analytes, frequently lacking any meaningful chromophore, is a difficult, challenging undertaking, which has necessitated the use of many different analytical approaches often borrowed from environmental science. These include both preconcentration, derivatization, stabilizing the analyte, and column switching to enhance the analyte concentration and/or sensitivity, while in parallel reducing matrix (particularly API) interference.

Preconcentration strategies have covered most of the common extraction techniques, for example LLE, LPME, SPE, and SPME. Colon and Richoll[8] assessed all of these approaches to reduce matrix interference, which allowed the development of a reproducible GC-MS method for sulfonate esters. Similarly, a variety of extraction and/or preconcentration techniques are routinely used for traditional Chinese herbal medicines. Static headspace approaches in combination with GC and appropriate detection methods, for example FID, ECD, or MS, have been routinely used, for example Jacq et al.[12] or Sun et al.[84] for a wide range of different analytes.

Several research groups have utilized column switching to reduce matrix interference. Kirtley et al.[88] utilized a strong cation exchange column in series with a weak cation exchange column to address API interference in the analysis of residual hydrazine, whereas Lee et al.[9] used a reverse phase C18 stationary phase stationary phase in series with an ion exchange stationary phase to assess residual levels of an alkylating agent. In contrast, many researchers have developed methods utilizing early elution of the analyte of interest, followed by column switching to waste of the later eluting API. This is exemplified, by the exquisitively sensitive method (10 ppb) for the determination of residual FMTP in paroxetine API. The FMTP elutes rapidly after 3.5 min, and then the gradient is altered after 10 min to elute off to waste the API.[137] This ensures that residual API does not contaminate the MS ion source.

The issue of stabilizing these very reactive analytes has received surprisingly little in-depth focus. Clarke[23] utilized reduced energy sample mixing (vortexing vs. the more common sonication) and refrigerated autosampler storage to maximize stability of the analyte, and allow analysis to proceed in a reasonable time frame. Liu et al.[24] recently described a variety of matrix deactivation approaches to stabilize reactive electrophiles. The great irony is that this self-same reactivity that bedevils the analytical procedure also almost certainly ensures that downstream chemistries will effectively purge the GI from the synthetic process and ensure absence from the API.

Derivatization has been widely utilized across the whole field of GI analysis. Historically, it has been utilized much more for GC analysis to ensure greater volatility of the analyte. However, derivatization has seen wide-spread applicability in the analysis of GIs across all of the major chromatographic techniques, GC, HPLC, TLC, IC, CE, and within all spectroscopic applications. The analytical approach is governed by the structure of the GI, as well as both the separation and detection methodologies. Sulfonate esters provide a good example of this; although direct analysis has been shown to be feasible both by GC and HPLC, derivatization has now largely superseded this as the preferred approach. Derivatization using pentafluorothiophenol has seen extensive utility,[10,12] particularly in conjunction with HS-GC-MS with SIM detection. Other derivatives, for example alkylthiocyanates[9] and more recently triethylamine,[24] have also been used. An added benefit of such approaches is also that the derivative is generally more stable than the GI, although interestingly, this point is not generally emphasized in the publications.

Hydrazine and related alkyl hydrazides have historically utilized derivatization, benzaldehyde being the most common reagent used to yield the corresponding benzalazine derivative.[85–87] More recently, other derivatization procedures have been developed. A novel generic method generally applicable to the determination of residual hydrazine at low ppm levels in many different APIs was developed by Sun et al.[84] They utilized acetone to yield the corresponding acetone-azine derivative, together with an internal standard comprising of the corresponding stable isotope analogue, acetone–d_6. This volatile derivative can be readily analyzed by HS-GC-MS.

Analysis of hydrazine itself has seen the greatest applicability of broad spectrum analytical techniques including, somewhat surprisingly HPTLC. In this case the preferred derivative is salicylaldehyde, in combination with either far-UV visualization, or spraying with DMAB.[94] DMAB has also been used for the UV spectroscopic analysis of residual hydrazine in isoniazid.[102] Interestingly, the sensitivity can be enhanced by fixing the DMAB derivatizing agent onto a cation exchange resin. Alternatively, another very sensitive approach is to utilize 2-hydroxy-1-naphthaladehyde as the derivatization agent for the fluorimetric determination of residual hydrazine in isoniazid and iponiazid.[101]

Derivatization has been also utilized as the main analytical strategy toward enhancing sensitivity of the volatile aldehydes. For HPLC, the favored derivative is 2,4-DNPH, but there are also some reports of potentially more sensitive derivatives, for instance, *s*-triazolo-[3,4a]-phthalazine,[121] acetylacetone,[122,123] or *o*-pentafluorobenzyl)oxime,[124] but their utilization appears limited. In contrast, GC appears to have no favored derivatization approach. Ethyl esters were used by Del Barrio et al.,[130] oximes were utilized by Manius et al.,[128] whereas the more volatile o-pentafluorobenzyl)oxime derivative were used by Martos and Pawliszn.[131]

Derivatization of aldehydes for the spectroscopic applications is also very common. Most of the reported methods utilize the chromotropic colourimetric test,[128,133,134] but there are also reports of other approaches, for example MBTH and the Purpald reagent.[135] Derivatization is generally not applied to CE or related electrochromatographic techniques. One notable exception was the application of a charged aldehyde-dansylhydrazone complex with UV detection at 214 nm for the CE determination of volatile aldehydes, including formaldehyde. The method has exquisite sensitivity, with an LOD of 200 ppb.[132]

In some cases, the derivatization strategy is based on the need to enhance the retention of the analyte. Such a strategy was employed by Vanhoenacker et al.,[120] who used hexylchloroformate to derivatize a wide range of aromatic amines, aminopyridines, and other heterocyclic amines to form the corresponding amides. As neither volatility enrichment (static HS) nor polarity enrichment (SPE) were achievable across all of the analytes in all of the matrices, the authors elected to use direct injection with MS-SIM detection. Another benefit of this derivatisation approach was that the increased molecular weight provided a more specific ion for subsequent MS-SIM detection.

Overall, GC and HPLC, typically with either derivatization and/or sample pretreatment, are the main analytical approaches utilized to assay and control GIs. MS, in both single[10,120] and quadrupole modes,[13,82,83,137] remains the detection strategy of choice for both GC and HPLC. In addition, SIM,[10,19,81,120] and, occasionally, SRM,[137] have been utilized to enhance specificity and attain the required sensitivity. EI still remains a popular choice of MS ionization, particularly for traditional Chinese herbal medicines,[61–65] but there are reports of this being supplemented with an ion trap.[81] or a TOF.[82] There are some limited reports of other detection approaches, for example CLND,[79] ELSD,[54] and fluorescence.[55,122]

There is some evidence that novel HPLC stationary phases tailored to the polar nature of GIs are seeing increased usage and may be useful alternatives to both reverse phase and ion chromatography. This is exemplified by the use of HILIC columns for the analysis of alkyl esters of sulfonates and sulfates[16] and hydrazine.[78,79] There appears to be adequate molecular diversity in these novel stationary phases. Hmelnickis et al.[78] evaluated four different types: silica, nitrile, amino, and zwitterionic sulfobetaine before selecting the latter phase based on greater robustness and selectivity. Lui et al.[79] also utilized HILIC stationary phases with ethanol as the eluant, and CLND detection for the assessment of residual hydrazine and 1,1-dimethylhydrazine in a pharmaceutical intermediate.

Ion chromatography has seen widespread use in the analysis of hydrazines,[88,93–95] typically in the nonderivatized mode with amperometric detection. It has also been used less extensively for volatile aldehydes.[128] Electrochemical detection is utilized, as it ensures enhanced selectivity, increased sensitivity, and reduced matrix interference. Typically, these methods are very sensitive with LODs in the region of 0.05 ppm.[88]

TLC and the related HPTLC techniques are encountered mostly as pharmaco-poeial methods. They typically suffer from poor sensitivity and are not well suited to the task of analysis of GIs. However, in certain isolated situations, they have shown equivalent data to orthogonal HPLC techniques. Mroczek et al.[58] used both techniques for the analysis of residual levels of the tropane alkaloid, scopolamine and hyoscyamine, in traditional Chinese herbal medicines, and showed good correlation between the two techniques (correlation coefficients of mean values were 0.9995 and 0.92086, respectively, for the two analytes).

There is only one reported reference to the use of SFC-MS in this review. This approach was used as an orthogonal method to the preferred HPLC technique.[19] Both methods had the same reporting threshold (0.5 ppm), and both were claimed to be "QC-friendly."

Spectroscopic approaches are widely used for both hydrazines and volatile aldehydes. They are sometimes used as fast screening methods prior to HPLC, but typically are used as sensitive analytical techniques in their own right. Like TLC, they do suffer from sensitivity issues, but tend to be more aligned to rapid through-put, automated (or semi-automated) screens.

CE and the related electrochromatographic techniques (MEKC and MEEKC) show good selectivity but poorer sensitivity than other mainstream chromatography techniques, for example HPLC, GC, IC, etc. This has seen their use restricted to certain types of GI, for example hydrazines,[89,90] or with certain types of samples, for example traditional Chinese herbal medicines, where the matrix is complex and selectivity is the most important variable.[53,66,67] In the latter case, the issue of poor sensitivity is addressed using hyphenated MS approaches, for example MS-EI.[53,66,67] In addition, electrochemical detection has been extensively used.[89,90]

Alongside the development of suitable methodology, the technology transfer into a QC/production environment is also a critical aspect of the overall process. Information relating to such transfers is scant; however, the transfer of a method for residual FMTP in paroxetine API has been described.[137] Elder[138] subsequently reported on longer term issues with the method in the pharmacopoeial arena, and it has been subsequently markedly modified (HPLC-UV) to make it amenable to use in a worldwide environment, indicating the difficulties in establishing complex methods such as those necessary for GI related analysis within a QC environment and within multiple labs.

Indeed, with the issues associated with the transferring of such methods in mind, Liu et al.[24] reflected that the development of an analytical strategy for later phase new chemical entities (NCEs), which utilizes simplified analytical hardware with commensurately higher detection limits, for example HPLC-UV, significantly improves the potential of an issue-free technology transfer exercise. They utilized state-of-the-art mass spectrometry-based techniques during early development, but transferred conventional HPLC-UV methodology, with standard ICH Q3A sensitivity, that is 0.05% (500 ppm). They commented that these standard HPLC-UV methods are much more robust and better aligned with transfer into a production environment.

ACKNOWLEDGMENTS

Andrew Teasdale (AstraZeneca) and Andrew Lipczynski (Pfizer) for permission to use various extracts from our joint publications. The editors of the *Journal of Pharmacy and Biomedical Analysis* for their permission to reproduce various graphs, tables, and text from the authors' own publications.

REFERENCES

1. Committee for Medicinal Products (CHMP), European Medicines Agency. 2006. *Guideline on the limits of genotoxic impurities*. London, June 28, 2006. (CPMP/SWP/5199/02, EMEA/CHMP/QWP/251344/2006).
2. U.S. Department of Health and Human Services, Food and Drug Administration, Center for Drug Evaluation and Research (CDER). 2008, December. *Guidance for industry. Genotoxic and carcinogenic impurities in drug substances and products: Recommended approaches.*
3. EDQM. 2000. Enquiry: Alkyl mesilate (methanesulfonate) impurities in mesilate salts. *PharmEuropa* 12(1):27.
4. Anon. 2009. Dihydroergocristine mesilate monograph. Ph. Eur. Monograph 1416. *European Pharmacopoeia*, 6th ed., as amended by Supplements 6.1 and 6.2. Council of Europe, Strasbourg.
5. European Medicines Agency. 2007. *European Medicines Agency announces recall of Viracept*. Press release. EMEA/251283/2007, June 6.
6. European Medicines Agency. 2007. *Agrees on action plan following the recall of viracept and recommends suspension of the marketing authorization*. London. EMEA /275367/2007.
7. European Medicines Agency 2007. *CHMP assessment report for Viracept*. London. EMEA/H/C/164/Z/109. Press Release, September 20.
8. Colon I, Richoll SM. 2005. Determination of methyl and ethyl esters of methanesulfonic, benzenesulfonic and *p*-toluenesulfonic acids in active pharmaceutical ingredients by solid-phase microextraction (SPME) coupled to GC/SIM-MS. *J. Pharm. Biomed. Anal.* 39:477–485.
9. Lee CR, Guivarch F, Van Dau CN, et al. 2003. Determination of polar alkylating agents as thiocyanate/isothiocyanate derivatives by reaction headspace gas chromatography. *Analyst* 128:857–863.
10. Alzaga R, Ryan RW, Taylor-Worth K, Lipczynski AM, Szucs R, Sandra P. 2007. A generic approach for the determination of of residues of alkylating agents in active pharmaceutical ingredients by *in situ* derivatization-headspace–gas chromatography-mass spectrometry. *J. Pharm. Biomed Anal.* 45:472–479.
11. Teasdale A, Eyley S, Delaney E, et al. 2009. Mechanism and processing parameters affecting the formation of methyl methanesulfonate from methanol and sulfonic acid: An illustrative example for sulfonate ester impurity formation. *Org. Process Res. Dev.* 13:429–433.
12. Jacq K, Delaney E, Teasdale A, et al. 2008. Development and validation of an automated static headspace gas chromotography-mass spectrometry (SHS-GC-MS) method for monitoring the formation of ethyl methane sulfonate from ethanol and methane sulphonic acid. *J. Pharm. Biomed. Anal.* 48:1339–1344.
13. Ramakrishna K, Raman NVVSS, Narayana KMV, et al. 2008. Development and validation of a GC-MS method for the determination of methylmethanesulfonate and ethylmethanesulfonate in imatinib mesylate. *J. Pharm. Biomed. Anal.* 46:780–783.
14. Zheng J, Pritts WA, Zhang S, et al. 2009. Determination of low ppm levels of dimethyl sulphate in an aqueous soluble API intermediate using liquid-liquid extraction and GC-MS. *J. Pharm. Biomed. Anal.* 50:1054–1059.
15. Taylor GE, Gosling M, Pearce A. 2006. Low level determination of *p*-toluenesulfonate and benzenesulfonate esters in drug substance by high performance liquid chromatography/mass spectrometry. *J. Chromatgr. A.* 1119:231–237.

16. An J, Sun M, Bia L, et al. 2008. A practical derivatization LC/MS approach for the determination of trace level alkyl sulfonates and di-alkyl sulfonates genotoxic impurities in drug substances. *J. Pharm. Biomed. Anal.* 48: 1016–1010.

17. Skett P. 2007. Low-level measurement of potent toxins. In: *Analysis of Drug Impurities*, edited by RJ Smith, ML Webb. Blackwell Publishing, Oxford, pp. 82–123.

18. Görög S, Balogh G, Csehi A, et al. 1993. Estimation of impurity profile in drugs and related materials. Part 11—the role of chromatographic and spectroscopic methods in the estimation of side-reactions in drug syntheses. *J. Pharm. Biomed. Anal.* 11:1219–1226.

19. Huybrechts T. 2007. Successfully developing and validating methods for the quantification of genotoxic impurities in APIs. Informa Genotoxic Impurities Meeting, Hilton Prague, 24th September, 2007.

20. Lee CB, Hubert M, Nguyen Van Dua C, et al. 2000. Determination of N,N-dimethylaminoethyl chloride and the dimethylaziridinium ion at sub-ppm levels in diltiazem hydrochloride by LC-MS with electrospray ionization. *Analyst* 125:1255–1259.

21. Hansen SH, Sheribah ZA. 2005. Comparison of CZE, MEKC, MEEKC and non-aqueous capillary electrophoresis for the determination of impurities in bromazepam. *J. Pharm. Biomed. Anal.* 39:322–327.

22. Ellison GK. 2006. Development of a general headspace GC-ECD method for genotoxic alkyl halides at trace levels in API—The challenge of genotoxic impurities and their analysis. Pharmaceutical Analysis Science Group (PASG) Autumn Meeting, October 2, 2006, Milton Keynes, UK.

23. Clarke C. 2004. Development and validation of LC-MS methods that demonstrate the control of toxic impurities at the low ppm levels in drug substance. *Proceedings of the International Separations Conference*.

24. Liu DQ, Sun M, Korda AS. 2010. Recent advances in trace analysis of pharmaceutical genotoxic impurities. *J. Pharm. Biomed. Anal.* 51:999–1014.

25. Anon. 2009. Amiodarone HCL monograph. Ph. Eur. Monograph 0803. *European Pharmacopoeia*, 6th ed., as amended by Supplements 6.1–6.3. Council of Europe, Strasbourg.

26. Lacroix PM, Curran NM, Sy WW, Gorecki DKJ, Thibault P, Blay BKS. 1994. Liquid chromatographic determination of amiodarone hydrochloride and related compounds in raw materials and tablets. *J. AOAC Int.* 77:1447–1453.

27. Anon. 2009. Tolnaftate monograph. Ph. Eur. Monograph 1158. *European Pharmacopoeia*, 6th ed., as amended by Supplements 6.1 and 6.2. Council of Europe, Strasbourg.

28. Vaidya VV, Khanolkar M, Gadre JN. Generation of trace impurity profiles for Tolnafate by reverse phase high performance liquid chromatography. *Indian Drugs* 2000, 37 521–523.

29. Anon. 2009. Verapamil hydrochloride monograph. Ph. Eur. Monograph 0573. *European Pharmacopoeia*, 6th ed., as amended by Supplements 6.1 and 6.2. Council of Europe, Strasbourg.

30. Lacroix PM, Gragham SJ, Lovering EG. 1991. High-performance liquid chromatography method for the assay of verapamil hydrochloride and related compounds in raw material. *J. Pharm. Biomed. Anal.* 9:817–822.

31. Valvo L, Alimenti R, Alimonti S, et al. 1997. Development and validation of a liquid chromatographic method for the determination of related compounds of verapamil hydrochloride. *J. Pharm. Biomed. Anal.* 15:989–996.

32. Anon. 2009. Famotidine monograph. Ph Eur Monograph 1012. *European Pharmacopoeia*, 6th ed., as amended by Supplements 6.1 and 6.2. Council of Europe, Strasbourg.

33. Anon. 2009. Famotidine tablets monograph. BP Online Monograph, Market Towers, The Stationary Office, London.

34. Helali N, Dargouth F, Monser L. 2004. RP HPLC determination of famotidine and its potential impurities in pharmaceuticals. *Chromatographia* 60:455–460.

35. Lambropoulis J, Spanos GA, Lazaridis NV, et al. 1999. Development and validation of an HPLC assay for fentanyl and related substances in fentanyl citrate injection, USP. *J. Pharm. Biomed. Anal.* 20:705–716.

36. Anon. 2009. Fentanyl citrate injection monograph. BP Online Monograph, Market Towers, The Stationary Office, London.

37. Anon. 2009. Fentanyl monograph. Ph. Eur. Monograph 1210. *European Pharmacopoeia*, 6th ed., as amended by Supplements 6.1 and 6.2. Council of Europe, Strasbourg.

38. Anon. 2009. Fentanyl citrate monograph. Ph. Eur. Monograph 1103. *European Pharmacopoeia*, 6th ed., as amended by Supplements 6.1 and 6.2. Council of Europe, Strasbourg.

39. EDQM. 2007. Potentially genotoxic impurities and European Pharmacopeia monographs. Summary and conclusions of meeting held at the EDQM on July 4, 2007, European Directorate for the Quality of Medicines and Healthcare, European Pharmacopeia Commission, PA/PH/SG (07) 52 Com, Strasbourg, November 2007.

40. EDQM. 2008. Potentially genotoxic impurities and European pharmacopeia monographs on substance for human use. *PharmEuropa* 20(3):426.

41. Olsen BJ (chair). 2006. Impact the future of pharmacopoeial standards. USP Annual Scientific Meeting 2006. Session IV: Impurities in Drug Substances and Products. Genotoxic Impurities. September 29, 2006, Marriott Denver City Center, Denver, Colorado.

42. Lee SH, Oe T, Arora JS, Blair IA. 2005. Analysis of Fe^{II}-mediated decomposition of a linoleic acid-derived lipid hydroperoxide by liquid chromatography/mass spectrometry. *J. Mass. Spectrom.* 40:661–668.

43. Havrilla CM, Hachey DL, Porter NA. 2000. Coordination (Ag$^+$) ion spray–mass spectrometry of peroxidation products of cholesterol linoleate and cholesterol arachidonate: High-performance liquid chromatography-mass spectrometry analysis of peroxide products from polyunsaturated lipid autoxidation. *J. Am. Chem. Soc.* 122:8042–8055.

44. Andrisano V, Bertucci C, Battaglia A, et al. 2000. Photostability of drugs: Photo-degradation of melatonin and its determination in commercial formulations. *J. Pharm. Biomed. Anal.* 23:15–23.

45. Won CH, Tang S-Y, Strohbeck CL. 1995. Photolytic and oxidative degradation of a photolytic agent, RG 12915. *Int. J. Pharm.* 121:95–105.

46. Bempong DK, Honigberg IL, Meltzer NM. 1995. Normal-phase LC-MS determination of retinoic acid degradation products. *J. Pharm. Biomed. Anal.* 13:285–291.

47. Kažoka H, Madre M. 2005. Isocratic simultaneous normal-phase LC separation of four impurities for a stavudine synthesis control. *Talanta* 67:98–102.

48. Seger C, Römpp H, Sturm S, et al. 2004. Characterization of supercritical fluid extracts of St. John's Wort (*Hypericum perforatum* L.) by HPLC-MS and GC-MS. *Eur. J. Pharm. Sci.* 21:453–463.

49. Kursinzki L, Hank H, László I, et al. 2005. Simultaneous determination of hyoscyamine, scopolamine, 6-ß-hydroxy hyoscyamine, and apoatropine in Solanaceous hairy roots by reversed-phase high-performance liquid chromatography. *J. Chromatographr. A.* 1091:32–39.

50. Ye M, Guo H, Guo H, et al. 2006. Simultaneous determination of cytotoxic bufadienolides in the Chinese medicine ChanSu by high performance liquid chromatography coupled with photodiode-array and mass spectrometry detections. *J. Chromatographr. B* 838:86–95.

51. Zhau Y, Li Z, Zhou X, et al. 2008. Quality evaluation of Evodia rutaecarpa (Juss) Benth by high performance liquid chromatography with photodiode-array detection. *J. Pharm. Biomed. Anal.* 48: 1230–1236.

52. Zhou Y, Li S-H, Jiang R-W, et al. 2006. Quantitative analysis of indoloquinazoline alkoloids in Fructus Evodiae by high-performance liquid chromatography with atmospheric pres=ure chemical ionization tandem mass spectrometry. *Rapid Commun. Mass. Spectrom.* 20:3111–31118.

53. Bempong DK, Honigberg IL, Meltzer NM. 1993. Separation of 13-cis and all-trans retinoic acid and their photo-degradation products using capillary zone electrophoresis and micellar electrokinetic chromatography (MEC). *J. Pharm. Biomed. Anal.* 11:829–833.

54. Kong L, Li X, Zou H, et al. 2001. Analysis of terpene compounds in *Cimicifuga foetida* L. by reversed-phase high-performance liquid chromatography with evaporative light scattering detection. *J. Chromatographr. A* 936:111–118.

55. Quaglia MG, Farin A, Bossu E. 1992. Analysis of ICI 118551, a new ß2 blocking drug, and related compounds by RP-HPLC-DAD. *J. Pharm. Biomed. Anal.* 10:1081–1084.

56. Lin L-Z, He X-G, Lian L-Z, et al. 1998. Liquid chromatographic-electrospray mass spectrometric study of the phthalides of *Angelica sinensis* and chemical changes of Z-ligustilide. *J. Chromatographr. A.* 810:71–79.

57. Brinker AM, Raskin I. 2005. Determination of triptolide in root extracts of *Triptrygium wilfordii* by solid-phase extraction and reverse-phase high-performance liquid chromatography. *J. Chromatographr. A.* 1070:65–70.

58. Mroczek T, Glowniak K, Kowalska J. 2006. Solid-liquid extraction and cation-exchange solid-phase extraction using a mixed mode polymeric sorbent of *Datura* and relate alkaloids. *J. Chromatographr. A* 1107:9–18.

59. Klick S. 1995. Evaluation of different injection techniques in the gas chromatographic determination of thermo-labile trace impurities in a drug substance. *J. Pharm. Biomed. Anal.* 13:563–566.

60. Klick S. 1995. Evaluation of different injection techniques in the gas chromatographic determination of thermo-labile trace impurities in a drug substance. *J. Chromatographr. A* 689:69–76.

61. Xiao KP, Xiong Y, Liu FZ, et al. 2007. Efficient method development strategy for challenging separation of pharmaceutical molecules using advanced chromatographic techniques. *J. Chromatographr. A.* 1163:145–156.

62. Guo F-Q, Liang Y-Z, Xu C-J, et al. 2003. Determination of the volatile chemical constituents of *Notoptergium incium* by GC-MS and iterative or non-iterative chemometrics resolution methods. *J. Chromatographr. A.* 1016:99–110.

63. Cao J, Qi M, Zhang Y, et al. 2006. Analysis of volatile compounds in *Curcuma wenyujin* by headspace solvent micro-extraction-gas chromatography-mass spectrometry. *Anal. Chim. Acta* 561:88–95.

64. Lao SC, Li SP, Kan KKW, et al. 2004. Identification and quantification of 13-components in *Angelica sinensis* (Danggui) by gas chromatography-mass spectroscopy coupled with pressurized liquid extraction. *Anal. Chim. Acta* 526:131–137.

65. Guo F-Q, Liang Y-Z, Xu C-J, et al. 2004. Analyzing of the volatile chemical constituents of *Arteisi capillaries* herba by GC-MS and correlative chemometric resolution methods. *J. Pharm. Biomed. Anal.* 35:469–478.

66. Mateus L, Cherkaoul S, Christen P, et al. 1998. The use of a Doehlert design in optimizing the analysis of selected tropane alkaloids by micellar electrokinetic capillary chromatography. *J. Chromatographr. A* 829:317–325.

67. Eeva M, Salo J-K, Oksman-Caldentey K-M. 1998. Determination of the main tropane alkoloids from transformed Hyoscyamus muticus by capillary zone electrophoresis. *J. Pharm. Biomed. Anal.* 16:717–722.

68. Mateus L, Cherkaoul S, Christen P, et al. 1999. Capillary electrophoresis-diode array detection—electrospray mass spectrometry for the analysis of selected tropane alkaloids in plant extracts. *Electrophoresis* 20:3402–3409.

69. Monforte-González M, Ayora-Talavera T, Maldonado-Mendoza IE, et al. 1992. Quantitative analysis of serpentine and ajmalicine in plant tissues of *Catharanthus roseus* and hyoscyamine and scopolamine in root tissues of *Datura stramonium* by thin layer chromatography-densitometry. *Phytochem. Anal.* 3:117.

70. Anon. 2009. Stavudine monograph. Ph. Eur. Monograph 2130. *European Pharmacopoeia*, 6th ed., as amended by Supplements 6.1 and 6.2. Council of Europe, Strasbourg.

71. Anon. 2009. Dexamethasone monograph. Ph. Eur. Monograph 0388. *European Pharmacopoeia*, 6th ed., as amended by Supplements 6.1 and 6.2. Council of Europe, Strasbourg.

72. Anon. 2009. Nadolol monograph. Ph. Eur. Monograph 1789. *European Pharmacopoeia*, 6th ed., as amended by Supplements 6.1 and 6.2. Council of Europe, Strasbourg.

73. Anon. 2009. Norethisterone monograph. Ph. Eur. Monograph 0234. *European Pharmacopoeia*, 6th ed., as amended by Supplements 6.1 and 6.2. Council of Europe, Strasbourg.

74. Spangler M, Mularz E. 2001. A validated, stability-indicating method for the assay of dexamethasone in drug substance and drug product analyses, and the assay of preservatives in drug product. *Chromatography* 54:329–334.

75. Lacroix PM, Curran NM, Lovering EG. 1992. Nadolol: High-pressure liquid chromatographic methods for assay racemate composition and related compounds. *J. Pharm. Biomed. Anal.* 10:917–924.

76. Sedee AGJ, Beijersbergen GMJ, Blauwgeer HJA. 1983. Isolation, identification and densitometric determination of norethisterone-4/gb,5/gb-epoxide after photochemical decomposition of norethisterone. *Int. J. Pharm.* 15:149–158.

77. Butterfield AG, Lovering EG, Sears RW. 1979. High-performance liquid chromatographic determination of isoniazid and 1-isonicotinyl-2-lactosyl hydrazine in isoniazid tablet formulations. *J. Pharm. Sci.* 69:222–224.

78. Hmelnickis J, Pugovičs O, Kažoka H, et al. 2008. Application of hydrophilic interaction chromatography for the simultaneous separation of six impurities of mildronate substance. *J. Pharm. Biomed. Anal.* 48:649–656.

79. Liu M, Ostovic J, Chen EX, et al. 2009. Hydrophilic interaction liquid chromatography with alcohol as a weak eluent. *J. Chromatographr. A* 1216:2362–2370.

80. Kovaříková P, Mokrý M, Klimeš J, et al. 2006. HPLC study on stability of pyridoxal isonicotinoyl hydrazone. *J. Pharm. Biomed. Anal.* 40:105–112.

81. Kovaříková P, Vávrová K, Tomalová K, et al. 2008. HPLC-DAD and MS/MS analysis of novel drug candidates from the group of aromatic hydrazones revealing the presence of geometrical isomers. *J. Pharm. Biomed. Anal.* 48:295–302.

82. Bhutani H, Singh S, Vir S, et al. 2007. LC and LC-MS study of stress decomposition behaviour of isoniazid and establishment of validated stability-indicating assay method. *J. Pharm. Biomed. Anal.* 43:1213–1220.

83. Satyanarayana U, Rao DS, Kumar YR, et al. 2004. Isolation, synthesis and characterization of impurities in Celecoxib, a cox-2 inhibitor. *J. Pharm. Biomed. Anal.* 25:951–957.

84. Sun M, Bai L, Lui DQ. 2008. A generic approach for the determination of trace hydrazine in drug substances using in situ derivatization-headspace-GC-MS. *J. Pharm. Biomed. Anal.* 49:529–533.

85. Glyenhaal O, Grönberg L, Vessman J. 1990. Determination of hydrazine in hydralazine by capillary gas chromatography with nitrogen-selective detection after benzaldehyde derivatization. *J. Chromatographr. A* 511:303–315.

86. Carlin J, Gregory N, Simmons J. 1998. Stability of isoniazid in isoniazid syrup: Formation of hydrazine. *J. Pharm. Biomed. Anal.* 17:885–890.

87. Matsui F, Robertson DL, Lovering EG. 1983. Determination of hydrazine in pharmaceuticals III. Hydralazine and isoniazid using GLC. *J. Pharm. Sci.* 72:948–951.

88. Kirtley A, Strickfuss S, Yehl PM. 2006. Determination of Residual Hydrazine in a High Dose Drug presented at PASG Annual meeting in 2006, Bedfordshire, UK.

89. Liu J, Zhou W, You T, et al. 1996. Detection of hydrazine, methylhydrazine, and isoniazid by capillary electrophoresis with a palladium-modified microdisk array electrode. *Anal. Chem.* 68:3350–3353.

90. You T, Niu L, Gui JY, et al. 1999. Detection of hydrazine, methylhydrazine and isoniazid by capillary electrophoresis, with a 4-pyridylhydroquinone self-assembled microdisk platinum electrode. *J. Pharm. Biomed. Anal.* 19:231–237.

91. Srinivasu MK, Rao DS, Reddy O. 2002. Determination of Celecoxib, a COX-2 inhibitor, in pharmaceutical dosage forms by MEKC. *J. Pharm. Biomed. Anal.* 28:493–500.

92. Srinivasu MK, Narayana CL, Rao DS, et al. 2000. A validated LC method for the quantitative determination of Celecoxib in pharmaceutical dosage forms and purity evaluation in bulk drugs. *J. Pharm. Biomed. Anal.* 22:949–956.

93. Wang W, Bavda L, Benz N, et al. 2008. Analytical methodologies for Detection and Quantitation of Genotoxic Impurities, presentation at Informa Genotoxic Impurities Meeting, Philadelphia, 2–4th December, 2008.

94. Kean T, Miller JH, Skellern GG, Snodin DS. 2006. Acceptance criteria for levels of hydrazine in substances for pharmaceutical use and analytical methods for its determination. *Pharmeur. Sci. Notes* 2:23–33.

95. Jagota NK, Chetram AJ, Nair JB. 1998. Determination of trace levels of hydrazine in the penultimate intermediate of a novel anti-infective agent. *J. Pharm. Biomed. Anal.* 16:1083–1087.

96. Anon. 2009. Hydralazine tablets monograph. BP Online Monograph, Market Towers, The Stationary Office, London.

97. Anon. 2009. Hydralazine injection monograph. BP Online Monograph, Market Towers, The Stationary Office, London.

98. Anon. 2009. Isoniazid monograph. Ph. Eur. Monograph 0146. *European Pharmacopoeia*, 6th ed., as amended by Supplements 6.1 and 6.2. Council of Europe, Strasbourg.

99. Anon. 2008. Rifampicin tablets monograph. *International Pharmacopoeia*, 4th ed. WHO, Geneva, Switzerland.

100. Jindal KC, Chaudhary RS, Gangwal SS, et al. 1994. High performance thin-layer chromatographic method for monitoring of the degradation products of rifampicin in drug excipient interaction studies. *J. Chromatographr. A* 685:195–199.

101. Mañes J, Gimeno MJ, Moltó JC, et al. 1988. Fluorimetric determination of hydrazine in isoniazid formulations with 2-hydroxy-1-naphathaldehyde. *J. Pharm. Biomed. Anal.* 6:1023–1027.

102. Ortega-Barrales P, Molina-Díaz A, Pascual-Reguera MI, et al. 1997. Solid phase spectrophotometric determination of trace amounts of hydrazine at sub ng. ml^{-1} levels. *Anal. Chimica Acta* 353:115–122.

103. Anon. 2009. Carbidopa monograph. Ph. Eur. Monograph 0755. *European Pharmacopoeia*, 6th ed., as amended by Supplements 6.1 and 6.2. Council of Europe, Strasbourg.

104. Anon. 2009. Nadoparin calcium monograph. Ph. Eur. Monograph 1134. *European Pharmacopoeia*, 6th ed., as amended by Supplements 6.1 and 6.2. Council of Europe, Strasbourg.

105. Anon. 2009. Dalteparin sodium monograph. Ph. Eur. Monograph 1195. *European Pharmacopoeia*, 6th ed., as amended by Supplements 6.1 and 6.2. Council of Europe, Strasbourg.

106. Beretta G, Gelmini F, Merlino M, et al. 2009. A simplified screening procedure for the determination of total N-NO groups (TNG) and nitrite (NO2-) in commercial low-molecular-weight heparins (LMWH) by selective chemical denitrosation followed by high-sensitivity chemiluminescence detection (NO-analyzer, NOA). *J. Pharm. Biomed. Anal.* 49:1179–1184.

107. Wang J, Chan G, Haut SA, et al. 2005. Determination of total *N*-nitroso compounds by chemical denitrosation Using CuCl. *J. Agric. Food Chem.* 53:4686–4691.

108. Pötter H, Hülm M. 1988. Assay of nifedipine and its by- and degradation products in the drug substance by liquid chromatography on formamide-saturated silica gel columns. *J. Pharm. Biomed. Anal.* 6:115–119.

109. Kawabe Y, Nakamura H, Hino E, et al. 2009. Photochemical stabilities of some di-hydropyridine calcium-channel blockers in powdered pharmaceutical tablets. *J. Pharm. Biomed. Anal.* 47:618–624.

110. Walash MI, Belal F, Ibrahim F, et al. 2001. LC determination of di-nitrosopiperazine in simulated gastric juice. *J. Pharm. Biomed. Anal.* 26:1003–1008.

111. Belal F, Walash MI, Ibrahim F, et al. 2000. Voltametric determination of N,N-di-nitrosopiperazine in simulated gastric juice. *Il Farmaco* 55:694–699.

112. Wyszecka-Kaszuba E, Warowna-Grezskiewicz M, Fijalek Z. 2003. Determination of 4-aminophenol impurities in multi-component analgesic preparations by HPLC with amperometric detection. *J. Pharm. Biomed. Anal.* 32:1081–1086.

113. Garćia A, Ruperez FJ, Marin A, et al. 2003. Poly(ethylene glycol) column for the determination of acetaminophen, phenylephrine and chlorpheniramine in pharmaceutical formulations. *J. Chromatogr. B.* 785:237–243.

114. Chen G, Ye J, Bao H, et al. 2002. Determination of the rate constants and activation energy of acetaminophen hydrolysis by capillary electrophoresis. *J. Pharm. Biomed. Anal.* 29:843–850.

115. Pérez-Ruiz T, Martinéz-Lozano C, Tomás V, et al. 2005. Migration behavior and separation of acetaminophen and p-aminophenol in capillary zone electrophoresis: Analysis of drugs based on acetaminophen. *J. Pharm. Biomed. Anal.* 38:87–93.

116. Németh T, Jankovics P, Németh-Palotás J, et al. 2008. Determination of paracetamol and its main impurity 4-aminophenol in analgesic preparations by micellar electrokinetic chromatography. *J. Pharm. Biomed. Anal.* 47:746–749.

117. Anon. 2009. Propacetamol hydrochloride monograph. Ph. Eur. Monograph 1366. *European Pharmacopoeia*, 6th ed., as amended by Supplements 6.1 and 6.2. Council of Europe, Strasbourg.

118. Gotti R, Pomponio R, Bertucci C, et al. 2001. Determination of 5-aminosalicylic acid related impurities by micellar electrokinetic chromatography with an ion-pair reagent. *J. Chromatogr. A.* 916:175–183.

119. Forshed J, Andersson FO, Jacobsson SP. 2002. NMR and Bayesian regularized neural network regression analysis for impurity determination of 4-aminophenol. *J. Pharm. Biomed. Anal.* 29:495–505.

120. Vanhoenacker G, Dumont E, David F, et al. 2009. Determination of arylamines and aminopyridines in pharmaceutical products using in-situ derivatization and liquid chromatography-mass spectrometry. *J. Chromatographr. A.* 1216:3563–3570.

121. Cohen HP, Tway PC. 1993. High performance liquid chromatographic detection of residual formaldehyde in hepatitisa vaccine by use of hydralazine. *J. Liq. Chromatograpr. Rel. Tech.* 16:1667–1684.

122. Engelhardt H, Klinkner R. 1985. Determination of free formaldehyde in the presence of donators in cosmetics by HPLC and post-column derivatization. *Chromatographia* 20:559–565.

123. Argentine MD, Owens PK, Olsen BA. 2007. Strategies for the investigation and control of process-related impurities in drug substances. *Adv. Drug. Deliv. Rev.* 59:12–28.
124. Beilin E, Baker LJ, Culbert P, et al. 2008. Quantitation of acetol in common pharmaceutical excipients using GC-MS. *J. Pharm. Biomed. Anal.* 46:316–321.
125. Yarramraju S, Akurathi V, Wolfs K, et al. 2008. Investigation of sorbic acid volatile degradation products in pharmaceutical formulations, using static headspace gas chromatography. *J. Pharm. Biomed. Anal.* 44:456–463.
126. Rivero RT, Topiwala V. 2004. Quantitative determination of formaldehyde in cosmetics using a combined solid-phase micro-extraction-isotope dilution mass spectroscopy method. *J. Chromatographr. A* 1029:217–222.
127. Barbarin N, Rollman B, Tilquin B. 1999. Role of residual solvents in formation of volatile compounds after radio-sterilization of cefotaxime. *Int. J. Pharm.* 178:203–212.
128. Manius GJ, Wen L-FL, Palling D. 1993. Three approaches to the analysis of trace formaldehyde in bulk and dosage form pharmaceuticals. *Pharm. Res.* 10:449–453.
129. Dahlquist I, Fregert S, Gruvberger B. 1980. Detection of formaldehyde in corticoid creams. *Contact Derm.* 6:494–494.
130. Del Barrio M-A, Hu J, Zhou P, et al. 2006. Simultaneous determination of formic acid and formaldehyde in pharmaceutical excipients using GC/MS. *J. Pharm. Biomed. Anal.* 41:738–743.
131. Martos PA, Pawliszyn J. 1998. Sampling and determination of formaldehyde using solid-phase micro-extraction with on-fiber derivatization. *Anal. Chem.* 70:2311–2320.
132. Feige K, Ried T, Bachmann K. 1996. Determination of formaldehyde by capillary electrophoresis in the presence of a dihydroxyacetone matrix. *J. Chromatographr. A* 730:333–336.
133. Teik-Jin Goon A, Gruvberger B, Persson L, et al. 2003. Presence of formaldehyde in topical corticosteroid preparations available on the Swedish market. *Contact Dermat.* 48:199–203.
134. Desai DS, Rubitski BA, Varia SA, et al. 1994. Effect of formaldehyde formation on dissolution stability of hydrochlorothiazide bead formulations. *Int. J. Pharm.* 107:141–147.
135. Zurek G, Karst U. 1997. Microplate photometric determination of aldehydes in disinfectant solutions. *Anal. Chim. Acta* 351:247–257.
136. Elder DP, Lipczynski AM, Teasdale A. 2008. Control and analysis of alkyl and benzyl halides and other related organohalides as potential genotoxic impurities in active pharmaceutical ingredients (API). *J. Pharm. Biomed. Anal.* 48:497–507.
137. Borman PJ, Chatfield MJ, Crowley EL, et al. 2008. Development, validation and transfer into a factory environment of a liquid chromatography tandem mass spectrometry assay for the highly neurotoxic impurity FMTP (4-(4-fluorophenyl)-1-methyl-1,2,3,6-tetrahydropyridine) in paroxetine active pharmaceutical ingredient (API). *J. Pharm. Biomed. Anal.* 48:1082–1089.
138. Elder DP, Borman PJ, Chatfield MJ, et al. 2009. Experiences of developing, validation and routine use of a gri analytical method in a production environment. Informa Genotoxic Impurities Conference, Hotel Danubius, London, June 16, 2009.
139. Anon. Paroxetine hydrochloride hemihydrate monograph. Ph. Eur. Monograph, *European Pharmacopoeia*, 6th ed., as amended by Supplements 6.1 and 6.2. Council of Europe, Strasbourg.
140. Anon. Paroxetine hydrochloride anhydrous monograph. Ph. Eur. Monograph, *European Pharmacopoeia*, 6th ed., as amended by Supplements 6.1 and 6.2. Council of Europe, Strasbourg.

CHAPTER 11

DEVELOPMENT OF A STRATEGY FOR ANALYSIS OF GENOTOXIC IMPURITIES

Andrew Baker

11.1 INTRODUCTION

The EMEA guideline relating to control of genotoxic impurities has undoubtedly presented analytical chemists within the pharmaceutical industry with a significant challenge. Upon its implementation, the analysis of such compounds came under close scrutiny, and the ability of organizations to develop suitable methods of analysis was severely tested.

It became quite clear at an early stage that analysis of genotoxic impurities would require a different approach and potentially a new skill set to that commonly in place within the pharmaceutical industry. The challenges that the analysis of genotoxic impurities poses are significant and include, for example:

- The active pharmaceutical ingredient (API), which is usually the focus of attention, suddenly becomes an interfering matrix that hinders the ability to observe and quantify the genotoxic analyte.

- Unlike other, well-established, fields where trace analysis is employed, for example pesticide residue analysis, the matrix properties of genotoxic impurities can often be similar to that of the analyte; this is particularly true for "API-like" genotoxic compounds, such as late-stage intermediates.

- Certainly, in terms of pharmaceuticals, the limits associated with genotoxic impurities are often significantly lower than anything previously measured, by up to three orders of magnitude.

- Finally, by their very nature, many of the (very diverse range of) genotoxic analytes are highly reactive and thus prone to degradation during the analysis, making analysis and particularly quantification, challenging in many instances.

In reaction to this, the approach taken within many pharmaceutical organizations has been to establish or utilize specialist groups of highly skilled and experienced analytical chemists. It was from these groups that many of the key methodologies and practices have emerged; these helped to gain insight into the true nature of the genotoxic impurity analysis challenge and also started to identify many of the common criteria and considerations that are vital to achieving successful methodologies and analyses.

Initially, many methods were developed on a case-by case-basis, often being analyte/matrix specific. However, as the understanding of analysis developed alongside an understanding of the developing business requirements, a sufficient picture started to emerge, which has allowed more formal strategies to be built. The following chapter explores the approach taken by AstraZeneca to develop such a strategy.

Prior to developing the strategy, it was commented that the first, and possibly most important step in designing a strategy, is to fully understand the problem and also to define what your goals and objectives are.

11.1.1 Problem Definition

Prior to the development of a formal strategy, the approach taken within AZ in respect to such analysis was not only analyte/matrix specific, it was also often site, and even group specific. This often meant that methods were developed for common analytes simultaneously within individual groups, resulting in significant inefficiencies. Not only was this inefficient in terms of time/resource, it also often meant that knowledge sharing in terms of technical experience and "know-how" was poor. This could and did lead to approaches being taken, which constituted a technical "blind alley," as techniques were explored that offered little chance of success, and, worse still, had already been tried and shown to be ineffective within other groups. Thus, the problem could be succinctly defined in four simple statements:

1. Methods were compound/matrix specific.
2. There was significant duplication of effort across sites/groups.
3. Best practice was not properly recognized and effectively shared.
4. Development of methods often required a high level of expertise, placing a heavy reliance on technical experts.

11.1.2 Definition of Key High-Level Requirements of the Strategy and Intended Benefits

Having identified the problem, the next step was to define in detail what was required in terms of the solution. The primary objective at the onset of the development of the strategy was to deliver a flexible yet systematic approach to the analysis of genotoxic impurities that was understood and applicable within all groups within the AZ organization. It was anticipated that by utilizing such an approach, there would be a higher level of consistency across projects that would in turn result in both efficiencies, and, equally importantly, an overall improvement in the effectiveness of genotoxic impurity analysis within the organization. It also had to be flexible enough to meet the specific needs of such analysis across the full R&D lifecycle from early preclinical development through product launch.

Any approach also had to be able to address the diverse range of analytes that constitute genotoxic impurities and the diverse range of samples that they may reside in. Thus, another goal of the strategy was to be able to utilize techniques that would, wherever possible, be unaffected by the matrix concerned, and thus be applicable to a class or range of analytes rather than an individual analyte/matrix combination. That would also, through appropriate sample preparation, render the analysis as close to routine as practically possible. Another goal was to eliminate the need for specific expertise, at least once the method has been developed, and finally to develop an approach allowing methods to be developed far more quickly than would be possible than if in each instance it were developed on a compound-specific basis.

The strategy also had to take into consideration the technical capabilities of the organization and the availability of equipment.

Condensed into a single statement, the objective of the strategy will ultimately defined to be to be to:

> Provide analytical chemists within AstraZeneca with a framework that would assist them in the development a suitable method for Genotoxic Impurity (GI) analysis for use within a timeframe acceptable to the project. This should be applicable across all stages of development and should take into account the technical capabilities of the organisation.

The strategy herewith described in detail is thus one that represented the best fit for AstraZeneca. In this context, the factors discussed in this chapter may differ in terms of their criticality from the readers' own perspective and that of their own organization, for example based on access to equipment or other preferences. Nevertheless, it is hoped that they should be comprehensive and flexible enough to provide a framework that it is possible for anybody involved in this field to utilize.

11.1.3 The Concept of Strategy

Before progressing any further, the concept of strategy should be considered. There can be a common misconception that a strategy is a rigid set of one-dimensional instructions or guidance that must be adhered to. However, most scenarios that require strategy are, by definition, complex (otherwise, a strategy would not be required), and analysis of genotoxic, as will be discussed, clearly falls into this category. Rigid and prescriptive instructions do not readily work in such circumstances, since they are either too simplistic to deal with the complexity and diversity encountered, or alternatively are so complex in themselves as to be restrictive and prohibitive.

Good strategies, although premeditated and designed to produce a specified outcome, need to make a complex problem easier to understand and solve in a simple way. Strategy should be about choice, that is maximizing the chance of success, which is very different to minimizing the routes by which it can be achieved.

11.1.4 Components of the Strategy

There are a number of separate and yet intrinsically linked components to the genotoxic impurity analytical strategy outlined below. Many will be common to other organizations strategies, other less so. The unique aspect of this strategy is perhaps its wide scope from a technique perspective, and also that it goes wider than just analytical methodology. Initially, when the concept of developing a genotoxic impurity analysis strategy was first discussed, it was entirely centered on understanding and describing the chromatographic techniques that would be suitable for different analytes. This is a key part of the strategy, and indeed, Chapter 12 describes this arm of the strategy in detail. However, as knowledge and understanding in this area increased, the reality has been (as will be shown further on) that in many scenarios, there are actually choices of which technique to use. In some instances, this involves nonchromatographic techniques, particularly NMR. In this context, the concept of strategy has developed to include ensuring that the techniques and approaches used are not only capable of doing the job, but are optimized against the external requirements, for example the activities being supported and the stage within the product development lifecycle a method is employed.

The AstraZeneca Strategy consists of five main areas, these are:

1. access to knowledge and information;
2. technical understanding;
3. a full understanding of business needs;
4. ready to use technology platforms; and
5. definition of quantitative processes.

Each of these will be discussed in detail before finally discussing how they might be brought together into a concerted analytical strategy for the analysis of genotoxic impurities.

11.2   ACCESS TO KNOWLEDGE AND INFORMATION

Strategies, as already described, should be about making a problem simpler and easier to solve, and one of the key aspects to achieving this is to make effective use of existing sources of information. There is a wide range of experience of analysis of genotoxic impurities across the AZ organization, both documented and held "*in cerebro*" by technical experts. Furthermore, as shown in Chapter 10, there is a wealth of data relating to the analysis of genotoxic impurities in the public domain. For example, several general methods for sulfonate esters[1] and alkyl halides[2] in particular are now very commonly run, and examples of methods for many different types of genotoxic compounds are widely available.

Within the AstraZeneca strategy, it is strongly recommended that the start point for any new analysis should always be to look to make use of any existing knowledge or practical experience that is relevant to the task in hand. Since its inception, this has shown to be an invaluable component of the strategy, many problems, certainly for common analyses, have been solved from utilizing existing methods.

A final key part of this aspect of the strategy was the development of a comprehensive internal database that contains information on analyses conducted throughout the organisation, both successful and unsuccessful.

11.3 TECHNICAL UNDERSTANDING

The technical understanding of the challenges faced in analysis of genotoxic impurities is ultimately the single most important element of the strategy. Key elements within this are:

1. Understanding the interrelationship between the analytes involved and the analytical techniques employed.

2. Understanding how through sample preparation the physicochemical properties of the analyte can be effectively manipulated in order to render them amenable to analysis using specific techniques.

This section therefore looks to explore both of these critical aspects, and how the interrelationship between these can be successfully managed in such a way as to maximize the chances of developing effective solutions to complex genotoxic impurity-related problems.

11.3.1 Overall Fit of Techniques

In order to understand the interrelationship between the analyte and the analytical technique, a technique map, based on analyte properties, was developed, see Figure 11.1. Using this map, it is possible to select the start point for a method that, in advance, gives the highest probability of success. This is critical when working in an environment where you are often faced with significant time pressure, for example supporting chemical development work. Here, the key requirement is often to be able to generate a "fit-for-purpose" method, which can facilitate high-quality data in very short timeframes.

In order to quickly and effectively identify which techniques might be suitable to perform a particular analysis, it is important to understand how they fit together for different applications.[3]

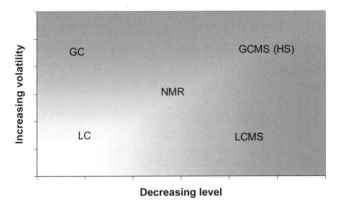

Figure 11.1 Technique map exploring the relationship between analyte properties and instrument capabilities.

One of the most important analyte characteristics to assess when determining which is the most appropriate analytical technique to employ is the difference in volatility between the analyte and matrix (although, as most active pharmaceutical ingredients [APIs] are nonvolatile, this will usually equate to the volatility of the analyte). This attribute is critical when assessing the suitability of chromatographic technology platforms.

A thorough review of analysis performed within the organization identified five key techniques that would, if employed as core techniques, deliver the majority of technical solutions required for routine analysis of GIs.

The five analytical techniques identified were:

1. liquid chromatography (LC, including ultra-high pressure liquid chromatography [UPLC]) with UV detection;
2. Liquid chromatography with mass spectrometery detection (LC-MS);
3. gas chromatography (GC), with flame ionization detection (FID);
4. GCMS with headspace extraction; and
5. NMR.

Other techniques were, however, also considered, and there have been important applications of other techniques, including ion chromatography and inductively coupled plasma (ICP) employed within the AZ organization.

The chromatographic techniques fit together in a very complimentary way; however, when NMR is considered, there are areas of quite significant overlap with the chromatographic techniques. This is where the opportunity for choice between techniques is most likely to present itself.

The general fit of where the different chromatographic techniques and NMR have most applicability is represented in the Figure 11.1, and each is discussed in further detail later within this chapter.

11.3.2 Individual Techniques

Within the AstraZeneca strategy, each of the five individual techniques is described in terms of:

1. applicability of the technique;
2. limitations of the technique; and
3. experimental application.

The purpose of this to provide the reader with the key information that will (using the applicability and limitations sections) enable them to identify from a technical perspective the technique most likely to deliver a successful method.

As already outlined, prior to the advent of the strategy, significant amounts of time could often be spent trying to develop methods on techniques that were not suitable for the analyte in question. Thus, for each technique, the Experimental section seeks to define a series of simple experiments that enable one to quickly determine as to whether of not the technique in question will deliver a suitable method.

11.3.2.1   Critical   Considerations:Chromatographic   Techniques   In the chromatographic analysis of genotoxic impurities, there are series of common principles that, when applied, can greatly increase the success rate of an analytical method. Typically, a chromatographic method can be considered as containing three components.

1. sample preparation;
2. chromatographic separation; and
3. detection component.

Generally, the key is to maximize as many and much of these as possible.

Sample preparation and introduction can be used very effectively to remove interfering matrices, concentrate analytes, and to optimize the amount of analyte being introduced to the instrument.

The chromatographic component can be used to further resolve the analyte from any matrix or undesired species. Chromatographic parameters are also important to optimize peak shape and therefore sensitivity.

The detection element is vital, not only to be able to detect at the appropriate levels, but many detectors also have elements of selectivity that can be used to focus specifically on the analyte(s) of interest.

It is by effectively combining these components that a sound analytical method can be achieved.

11.3.2.2   LC: UV Detection

Application   LC is typically applied to nonvolatile analytes or ones that are thermally unstable. In many cases, overlap with other chromatographic techniques exists, particularly GC. Thus, it is often appropriate to examine both potential techniques in parallel. Where this is the case, careful examination of both the analyte and matrix properties is required.

Recently, liquid chromatography has undergone a considerable transformation as traditional HPLC based on 3 or 4.6 mm id. columns, and 3–5 μm particles has started to be superseded by ultra high-pressure liquid chromatography (UHPLC). UHPLC utilizes narrower columns that contain particles of <2 μm; this results in improvements in terms of efficiency, resulting in improved resolution and sharper and more intense peaks, and thus improved detection and quantification limits. In addition, analysis times may be reduced significantly, typically three- to fivefold. The benefits of reduced particle sizes have been known about for many years; however, until recently, the use of such small particles was impractical both from a stationary phase perspective and in terms of instrumentation that would be able to manage the extremely high back pressures created by such small particles. This has been resolved by the introduction of the Waters Acquity® (Waters Corp., Milford, MA) UPLC and similar systems UHPLC systems. The use of UHPLC, in preference to HPLC, is an integral part of AstraZeneca's strategy.

In terms of detection, UV detection is typically less sensitive than MS, and also less specific. However, for compounds with a strong chromophore, UV detection is advantageous in terms of robustness, ease of use, low cost, and transferability.

From a technical perspective, gradient elution is recommended, since it is designed for the elution of a wide range of analyte properties, and peaks are typically focused (peak compression), giving improved detection. Furthermore gradient elution also often facilitates the use of large volume injections, leading to improved sensitivity (provided the eluotropic strength of the sample diluent is compatible with that of the mobile phase).

Reversed-phase (RP) LC is normally preferred, but to retain polar analytes, hydrophilic interaction liquid chromatography (HILIC) can be employed and may be preferable for MS detection.

Limitations   Naturally, the analyte must give a response with the detector of choice; this is a particular limitation in terms of LC-UV, where the analyte in question may not contain a suitable chromophore. Even where there is a chromophore present, the UV response at the optimal detection wavelength may not be sufficiently strong to allow detection at the levels required, dictated by limits for the genotoxic impurity in question. This often applies to low molecular weight, volatile alkylating reagents used in the synthesis of the API; in such instances, GC is often the preferred technique.

Another issue faced with the use of reverse phase LC is sample stability. Reverse phase LC requires the use of aqueous conditions both in terms of the chromatographic mobile phase and in terms of the sample diluent. Many highly reactive genotoxic compounds, for example epoxides, are unstable under aqueous conditions, or may react with the stationary phase and thus analysis by Reverse phase LC may be unsuitable. In such cases, sample pretreatment, for example derivatization, may be required in order to stabilize the analyte.

Another recently presented approach is sample or matrix deactivation to prevent formation of the GIs during analysis.[4]

Experimental   Prior to the analysis of a specific genotoxic impurity a general method is often developed to determine the organic impurities in the intermediate/API. The simplest and quickest way to analyse the genotoxic impurity of concern is firstly to simply check if the method applied for organic impurities can be used for analysis of the genotoxic impurity. Selectivity detection/quantification limit, recovery, and solution stability should be evaluated.

If the method for organic impurities does not apply, the following steps can be used to decide if LC UV is appropriate for the given application. Where appropriate, MS compatible mobile phase additives should be employed in order that MS detection can be investigated simultaneously:

1. Screen mobile phase and columns to develop a suitable separation. Key factors are:
   a. That there is suitable separation between the genotoxic analyte and other, larger components. Without chromatographic resolution, UV detection would be unsuitable, as would in many cases MS, owing to issues with ion suppression. Resolution of peaks other than the genotoxic impurity is of minor importance.

b. Another important factor is retention (K′), retention factors of between 3 and 10 are recommended, in order to ensure that components are separated from unretained peaks and the solvent front.

2. The use of short columns with small particles (<2 μm) at elevated pressures (>400 bar) is recommended where practically possible, due to the increased efficiency and improved detection/quantification limits that result from this. Increase the flow rate as much as possible to obtain a fast and efficient separation. If the genotoxic impurity is thermally stable, elevated temperatures will often improve efficiency and speed.

3. Where UV detection is employed, optimise the wavelength for maximal signal-to-noise ratio (S/N). It may also be possible to utilize longer flow cell path lengths to improve sensitivity further.

4. Determine the detection/quantification limits for a pure dissolved standard of the genotoxic analyte and calculate the required sample concentration and injection volume in order to meet target analyte levels.

5. Ideally, dissolve the sample at the required concentration in a solvent with an appropriate (elutropic) strength to that of the mobile phase.

6. Finally, check the detection/quantification limit for a dissolved standard spiked into the sample matrix, and also conduct recovery experiments spiking the genotoxic impurity into the matrix at appropriate levels (50%–150% of the limit), and ensuring that a satisfactory recovery and stability is achieved (see later validation section for details of typical validation criteria).

11.3.2.3 LC-MS

Application LCMS is typically applicable for scenarios where increased sensitivity or selectivity is required compared with liquid chromatography employing simple UV detection.

Limitations Although several ionization techniques exist that are applicable to LC/MS, for example electrospray Ionization (ESI), atmospheric pressure chemical ionization (APCI), and atmospheric pressure photoionization (APPI), none are as universal as electron ionization (EI) used for gas chromatography (GCMS). Matrix interference is often a higher risk than GCMS (since GCMS is usually used in conjunction with a sampling technique, such as headspace, that eliminates a large proportion of matrix interference), this may cause analyte ion suppression or enhancement. Such factors are very difficult to predict. Eluent composition (organic modifier and pH modifier) can also affect analyte response, sometimes dramatically; hence, gradient analysis may cause greater variation than isocratic analysis. Use of appropriate internal standards may compensate for these effects (see Section 11.3.3.3). Another factor in LC/MS can be the build up of nonvolatiles (predominantly the sample matrix) within the detector itself. This can also affect the detector performance, resulting in a diminished response. In order to avoid this, sample pretreatment to remove the matrix may be required.

Experimental The following experiments may be used to determine whether LCMS is appropriate for a given application.

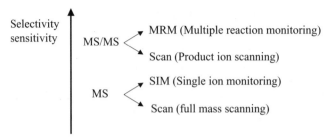

Figure 11.2 Sensitivity of MS detection techniques.

Figure 11.2 simply demonstrates the associated sensitivity and selectivity associated with MS and MS/MS under the different set ups that each can be performed. It is important to select a technique that delivers the right level of sensitivity and selectivity for the application without being overly complex. This is particularly true if the method concerned is likely to be transferred into a quality-control environment.

1. Scout optimal MS conditions (e.g. source, transmission, fragmentation, and detection) and optimal LCMS solvent and pH modifier for a pure impurity standard of appropriate concentration by flow injection analysis (the threshold of toxicological concern [TTC] level may be taken into account when preparing this solution).

2. Determine LOD/LOQ for a pure impurity standard of the target genotoxic analyte using the optimized set of LCMS conditions. Calculate required sample concentration, based upon this data, in order to meet target analyte levels.

3. Dissolve the sample in an LCMS compatible solvent system at the required sample concentration.

4. Develop appropriate HPLC separation based around the optimal eluent system previously described (0). Ideally, use fast, efficient chromatography of a column dimension that does not require pre-MS splitting of the eluent.

5. Finally, check the DL/QL for a dissolved standard spiked into the sample matrix, and also conduct recovery experiments, spiking the genotoxic impurity into the matrix at appropriate levels (50%–150% of the limit) and ensuring that a satisfactory recovery is achieved (see later validation section for details of typical validation criteria).

11.3.2.4 GC

Application   GC with direct injection and flame ionization detection (FID) is suitable for the analysis of a huge range of volatile and semi-volatile analytes. The advantages of the technique are the high efficiencies afforded by GC columns (>100,000 theoretical plates) that often result in excellent chromatographic resolution of the analyte from other components and the utility and robustness of FID detection. Where a volatile genotoxic impurity is present at a level of between 100 and 1000 ppm, and where there are no significant matrix interferences, GC is often the preferred technique.

Limitations   The primary limitation with direct injection GC as a tool for analysis of genotoxic impurities comes from matrix interferences. Since most DS molecules are nonvolatile and solutions need to be prepared at high concentrations, interference from the matrix is commonplace. It is not uncommon for DS molecules to undergo thermal degradation at the temperatures experienced within a GC instrument. Interference often occurs in the form of injection liner contamination. This can have a dramatic affect either activating the inlet liner, resulting in the complete retention of the analyte or even *in situ* generation of the analyte through degradation of the sample (API, intermediate).

Such affects can be minimized or even eliminated through techniques such as ALEX (automated liner exchange) and Dean switching to effect heart cutting, however such techniques are not as common place within the pharmaceutical industry as in other sectors, and their use is therefore likely to be restricted to nonroutine, specialist applications.

The flame ionization detector is not selective, and this may limit usage in materials where there are many organic impurities present at similar levels to that of the analyte being measured.

Experimental   Since the matrix will potentially be injected onto the column, it is important to establish the affect of repeated injections of matrix on the method at an early stage. Liquid/liquid extractions (refer Section 11.4.2.1) can be a very useful tool to accompany direct injection gas chromatographic analysis.

11.3.2.5   Static Headspace GC with Mass Spectrometery Detection
Application   The key area of application for static headspace GCMS is in the analysis of volatile analytes. The technique effectively extracts the analyte from the matrix and simultaneously concentrates it, improving sensitivity.

The use of this technique has found wide applicability in the analysis of volatile halides, halo alkenes, aldehydes, and sulphonate esters.

Limitations   The main limitation of static headspace GCMS is that as the volatility of the analytes decreases, extraction into the headspace is not as efficient, and sensitivity subsequently decreases. Injection repeatability of this technique can also be poor, but this can easily be compensated for by the use of an internal standard.

Dynamic headspace dramatically improves sensitivity for less volatile analytes; however, this technique is not widely used and thus its use is likely to be restricted to non-routine, specialist applications.

Experimental   The following sequence of tests can be used to quickly determine whether static headspace will work for a given application.

1. Identify a suitable solvent in which the analyte sample (API or intermediate) is soluble to the required level (typically >20 mg/mL). Solvents commonly used are DMSO, DMF, and water; mixtures of organic solvents and water are particularly useful. However, other solvents, including ionic liquids, may also employed.

2. Identify suitable headspace extraction and chromatographic parameters, this can be performed on an individual basis, but the application of "ready to use technology platforms" (refer section 5) can play a significant role in this area.

3. Run blank injection(s).

4. Run sample solution(s).

5. Run standard(s) at the appropriate limit, that is at the limit for the genotoxic impurity based on the appropriate TTC

6. Finally, check the DL/QL for a dissolved standard spiked into the sample matrix, and also conduct recovery experiments spiking the genotoxic impurity into the matrix at appropriate levels (50%–150% of the limit), and ensuring that a satisfactory recovery is achieved (see later validation section for details of typical validation criteria).

11.3.2.6 NMR

Application   To many people, the idea of using NMR for trace analysis, such as analysis of genotoxic impurities, would seem incongruous; the technique being dismissed as simply too insensitive for such analysis. Yet recent advances in NMR technology—the advent of high-strength systems 400–500 Mhz, combined with other improvements, such as cyroprobe technology (whereby cooling the sample in the instrument obtains an significant improvement in sensitivity), has made such analysis genuinely possible. In fact, as an inherently quantitative technique, method development can often be quick and easy. Moreover, it is applicable to a very wide range of genotoxic analytes.

In a 1H/19F NMR spectrum run under quantitative conditions, the strength of the resonance signal for protons/fluorines is directly proportional to the molar concentration of the compound. This is true for all nonexchangeable protons (this is not true though for exchangeable protons, for example OH and NH protons). By comparison of the areas of the substrate (known purity) with the signal from the genotoxic impurity, the levels of the genotoxic impurity can be calculated. This technique has proven to be very effective for genotoxic impurity analysis (see Chapter 13 where this is explored in more detail). The proton or fluorine signals in the NMR spectrum of a genotoxic impurity must however be well resolved from any substrate signals and possess the appropriate sensitivity in order for NMR to be applied successfully.

The sensitivity is dependant on a number of factors, such as:

1. Sample concentration (>100 mg/mL is generally required but the higher the better).

2. MW ratio of the genotoxic impurity to the substrate (API or intermediate).

3. Degree of resolution of genotoxic impurity signal selected from other resonances.

4. Spectral line width.

5. Number of proton or fluorine contributing to the signal.

6. Multiplicity of NMR signal (i.e. singlet will be twice as intense as a doublet).

Limitations   As with all analytical techniques, there are limitations to the use of NMR for GI analysis. If the spectra for instance is not "clean" in the area of the GI signal(s), then there is very little that can be done to rectify this.

Although a very general statement, NMR may not be sensitive enough to be able to, in some cases, really reach the very low limits (e.g. sub 10 ppm) that may sometimes be required.

Probably the biggest limitation of NMR though is the cost of equipment, which can be prohibitive or off-putting even to more well-funded organizations. But where this technology is available, it can provide a truly differentiating part of the arsenal for GI analysis.

It should be noted that as for all of the other techniques described in this document, the use of a reference material of the analyte is strongly recommended for high-quality quantitative data. There is a common misunderstanding that a reference material is not required when using NMR for GI analysis.

Experimental   The first stage in any such analysis is to obtain reference data for both the substrate and the genotoxic impurity. Using these spectra, the aim is then to try to identify a region in the two spectra where a resonance associated with the genotoxic impurity is likely to free from interference from any resonance associated with the substrate (typically the API). It is essential that the genotoxic impurity has a resonance in a region of the spectrum that is baseline resolved from anything other resonances to allow for it to be integrated and thus properly quantified.

The solubility of the substrate is also a key factor. In NMR, sensitivity increases linearly with concentration, but only to the square root of experimental time. Therefore, high concentrations (100 mg/mL) are advantageous, as long as this is not at the expense of spectrum quality (i.e. broader lines).

Expert knowledge, may, however, be required to optimize experimental conditions (relaxation times/pulse length/experiment time), and to ensure the right instrumentation is used. For lower detection limits, cryoprobe technology might be required, and selective excitation might be required to overcome dynamic range issues on some instruments. These specific techniques are explored in depth in Chapter 13.

Based on these factors, if NMR is considered a viable option, the next step is to confirm such an approach is feasible by performing some initial experimental work. An example of such an experiment is outlined below.

1. Perform spikes at a 500/1000 ppm of the genotoxic analyte into the sample to confirm these can be detected (using standard NMR conditions). If these spikes are successful, continue NMR development. If not, move to another technique.
2. Determine the level of genotoxic impurity present in your substrate and perform a series of low level spikes at or around the staged TTC level.
3. Confirm the substrate and genotoxic impurity are appropriately stable in your solvent of choice.

11.3.2.7   *Other Techniques*   Although the techniques described above are considered to be those that are most widely applicable to GI analysis, it is unrealistic to expect that those alone would deal with every single GI analysis given the number of different classes of GI and the wide variability seen within each class in terms of physicochemical properties.

The following section outlines other techniques that might be expected to play a lesser, but potentially important role, within this area.

For each of the techniques in this section, the potential area of application is briefly outlined, along with an assessment of the limitations of the technique concerned. These limitations are different for each technique; some relate to lack of widespread availability, for example dynamic headspace, others because a preferable alternative existed (such as ECD detection in GC), and others simply because they would be expected to have limited application.

Solid-Phase Microextraction (SPME)   SPME is a common technique for concentrating trace analytes, and is potentially useful for compounds where sensitivity is low due to poor headspace extraction. The fibers used are very delicate and require careful treatment to ensure that they remain useable for more than ca. 12–15 injections. As an adsorptive technique, there may also be issues with analyte carryover even with the bake-out processes typically built into the automation of the process. SPME is commercially available, although modification of standard GC instrumentation is often required.

Electron Capture Detector (ECD)   The ECD is a common detector used within the environmental field, used typically for the analysis of trace levels of pesticides. Based on its application in this area, it has built a reputation as being a very sensitive and selective technique. In GI analysis, it may have application for analysis of halogen containing and electron accepting classes of compounds, for example alkyl halides. However, sensitivity can vary greatly between compounds, and selectivity can also be problematic, since generally, any substance that accepts electrons can be detected. The ECD can also be susceptible (unstable) to environmental factors within a laboratory. If available, FID and Mass Spec are likely to be preferable approaches to detection.

Dynamic Headspace GC   Dynamic headspace is a technique with significant potential for application to analysis of semi-volatile compounds, where static headspace starts to reach its limitations. The technique involves purging the sample with gas (helium) while the headspace extraction takes place, a higher percentage of the analyte is thus transferred into the gas chromatograph, and the sensitivity can be improved by orders of magnitude when compared with static headspace.

Automatic Liner Exchange   Automatic liner exchange can be a useful capability to have when using GC where direct injection is required. In situations where the matrix is retained in the liner, automatically changing the liner between sample injections ensures that the analytical instrumentation remains free from contamination and matrix effects.

Heart Cutting/Dean Switching   Heart cutting using Dean switching technology has potential for use when direct GC injection is required, and where the matrix enters the analytical column. The Dean switching can be used to divert the matrix to "waste" and send only analyte to the detector, again ensuring that the instrumentation remains free from contamination and matrix effects.[5]

Capillary Electrophoresis Capillary electrophoresis (CE) is another potential option providing an orthogonal separative technique to chromatography (GC/LC). Thus, where no suitable separation can been achieved, chromatographically using LC, CE can be considered. It would also appear to be more robust to matix effects, and has been widely applied to the analysis of epoxides (see Chapter 10) in herbal products for this reason.

11.3.3 Sample Preparation

Sample preparation is one of the singularly most important, but still surprisingly undervalued aspects of GI analysis. In many pharmaceutical analyses, particularly those associated with the API, sample preparation is generally limited to dissolution in a chosen solvent at a specific concentration. Such an approach is often unsuitable for the analysis of a GI. This is due to matrix interference, compounded by analyte (GI) instability. Such challenges can be overcome by the appropriate preparation of the sample.

Another issue is solubility. For both chromatographic methods and NMR, high sample concentrations are often required (e.g. in excess of 100 mg/mL) to enable analyses of the low-level genotoxic impurity present in the sample. Achieving high solubilities can often be a significant challenge, and there is also the risk of the sample precipitating out of solution, especially if the sample solution needs to be cooled in order to control degradation.

At the outset of developing, a method it is recommended to consider sample preparation as an integral and vital part of the development process. Approaches to sample preparation are described below.

11.3.3.1 *Extractions*
As already described, the sample matrix can often have an adverse impact on the analysis of a GI. If the GI and matrix have diverse chemical properties, extraction can and should be considered. Many GIs of concern (e.g. alkylating agents) are small, neutral molecules that have high solubility in organic solvents, whereas the API may be ionizable, and thus have better solubility in water, particularly in the ionised form. Both classical liquid/liquid extractions as well as use of solid phase devices may be of use in such situations. To be able to accurately quantify the level of GI present standard addition should ideally be used and the recovery determined.

11.3.3.2 *Derivatization*
Derivatization is another long-established arm of analytical chemistry with a very important role to play in genotoxic impurity analysis.

Using derivatization to alter the chemical and/or physical properties of an analyte can often be the most effective and efficient way to optimize a method (when compared with attempts at adjusting instrumental and/or method parameters).

If the properties of the analyte are fundamentally responsible for problems in optimizing a method, then the best approach is often to seek to alter them via a derivatization. For many polar compounds with active and reactive functionalities, this can be the case. Unstable analytes in particular often require derivatization. As well as stabilizing the analyte, derivatization can be used to manipulate the physical properties of the analyte to aid analysis. Examples include increasing volatility to enable analysis by GC, increasing lipophilicity to improve retention in liquid chromatography, and introduction of a chromophore to allow UV detection.[6]

Many of the compounds, including alkyl sulfonates, mustards, halo alcohols, and boronic acids can all be successfully analyzed using simple and effective derivatization approaches (see Chapter 12).

One of the potential drawbacks of derivatization is that it involves a chemical reaction that may be difficult to control, a specific concern being as to whether or not it has gone to completion. For this reason, an internal standard is often employed in conjunction with derivatization, one that undergoes the exact same reaction as the analyte.

11.3.3.3 Use of Internal Standards for Trace Analysis Using Chromatographic Techniques
The use of internal standards for trace analysis offers a number of advantages that should be considered. The principle is to use a compound that by having similar chemical and physical properties to the analyte, will behave in an identical (or very similar) way. Any irregularities and idiosyncrasies associated with an analysis will be also be reflected by the internal standard. The main areas that the use of internal standards covers for are (1) improved repeatability of injection; (2) compensation for matrix effects; (3) identification of any issues during derivatization process; and (4) assurances that the result is genuine for analyses where no analyte is detected.

An ideal compound to use, as an internal standard, is a stable isotopically labeled version of the analyte, and many such compounds are available from commercial sources. In cases where these compounds are not available, homologues of the analyte may also be considered. One potential advantage of the use of a homologue is that it may not necessarily require the use of MS detection for selectivity purposes, as is the case for labeled materials. However, the downside of using a homologue is that it poses a great risk of inaccuracies through differing physicochemical properties, for example in terms of reaction rates (derivatization), etc.

The more complex the method, that is if it involves extraction or derivatization, the greater the value of the use of an internal reference standard. Similarly, techniques that have inherently poor repeatability, such as headspace GC, will also benefit from the use of such standards.

11.4 BUSINESS REQUIREMENTS

The advent of this strategy has meant in many instances, the analyst actually has a choice in terms of methodology they can look to employ, this being both between different chromatographic techniques and between chromatography and NMR. Thus when selecting the technique of choice, the analyst is able to take into consideration other factors beyond simply technical suitability to produce and use a method.

From an AZ perspective, an important factor was defined as being the stage of development of the project. In simplistic terms, stage of development can be split into three stages early, mid and late stage of development. Each of these from an analytical perspective has its own key requirements.

1. Early development: speed and efficiency are critical—how quickly can a result be obtained.

2. Mid-stage development: a transitional phase during which factors are often a trade-off between those defined for early and late stage development.

3. Late development: the robustness of the technique and its transferability become more critical factors.

Some techniques are quicker from the perspective of developing and running analyses than others, and since project attrition and likelihood of changes to synthetic routes are higher at the early stages of development, thus analyses that offer the potential for time savings in these areas would always be preferable. Therefore during the early stages of development the use of NMR and the generic "walk-up" methodology are strongly favored.

As a project approaches the later stages of development, the potential need to transfer methods into a QC environment becomes an important factor. At this stage, the robustness of the method becomes an important factor. Also critical in this assessment of suitability is the availability of a particular technique; this could, for instance, preclude the use of NMR.

Below is further guidance included within the AstraZeneca strategy to help understand the factors that may influence the technique and approaches chosen.

11.4.1.1 *Early Stage Project (Phase I)*   In the early phase of development, short clinical durations and the application of limits based on the staged TTC concept often mean that the limits associated with a genotoxic impurity are relatively high compared with limits associated with longer term use. This is an important factor to take into consideration when deciding on the most suitable analytical technique, as it allows less sensitive techniques such as HPLC-UV to be applied, often in the form of limit tests. This means that in most instances a rapid, fit for purpose approach can be employed. Therefore, method development and validation timings are the most important considerations. Based upon this, toolbox techniques that offer ready-to-use (generic) approaches may be considered in the first instance, ahead of ones which require significant amounts of development work.

In some instances, depending on the limit of detection required, it is even possible to simply apply the general impurities screen without further method development. In cases where there is no available methodology and where suitable equipment and expertise is available, NMR may well offer often an efficient starting point (See Table 11.1).

11.4.1.2 *Mid-Phase (Phase II)*   The "mid" phase of development is largely a transitional stage from an analytical method development perspective, often influenced by the specific requirements of the projects. Factors for consideration include:

TABLE 11.1 Relative Suitability of Techniques for Early-Stage Development Projects

	Fast method development	Minimum resources	Generic approaches
LC	••	•••	••
LCMS	••	••	••
GC	••	•••	••
GCMS	••	••	•••
NMR	•••	••	•••

•••, Most suitable; ••, suitable; •, potentially unsuitable.

TABLE 11.2 Relative Suitability of Techniques for Mid-Stage Development Projects

	Minimum resources	Long-term viability
LC	•••	•••
LCMS	••	••
GC	•••	•••
GCMS	••	••
NMR	••	•

•••, Most suitable; ••, suitable; •, potentially unsuitable.

1. *Appropriateness of existing methodology.* Redevelopment of the method may be required driven by a reduction in permissible limits for the genotoxic impurity in question, this itself then driving the need to develop methodology with a lower limit of detection.

2. *Likelihood of the method concerned being required as a long-term method of control.* If the method is likely to be retained and used on a long-term basis then it may be appropriate at this stage to look to finalize the method by developing a method that can be used long term, including transfer to other sites for use. Factors that themselves influence this decision include how fixed is the associated synthetic process and where in the synthetic process is the analysis conducted. For example, a method associated with an early stage in the process may simply be used for data collection purposes, whereas a method for analysis of a genotoxic impurity late in the synthesis has a much higher probability of being required on a long-term basis as part of a specification (see Table 11.2).

11.4.1.3 Late Phase and Commercial During the late phases of development, consideration of the robustness of the method and the ability to readily transfer it

TABLE 11.3   Relative Suitability of Techniques for Late-Stage
Development Projects

	Sample throughput	Long-term viability	Regulatory acceptability
LC	•••	•••	•••
LCMS	•••	••	•••
GC	••	•••	•••
GCMS	•••	••	•••
NMR	•••	•	••

•••, Most suitable; ••, suitable; •, potentially unsuitable.

into different laboratories becomes an increasingly important consideration. Equally sensitivity and selectivity may become more critical, as permissible limits for a genotoxic impurity are reduced due to the longer duration of clinical trials.

At this stage, the preferred approaches would always be simple and robust technologies that are accessible without the need for high levels of expertise, for example the simple chromatographic techniques (see Table 11.3).

As part of the strategy development within AZ, significant time and effort has been spent in looking to developing a thorough understanding of the technology side of genotoxic impurity analysis, looking to establish both current and future capabilities in terms of available technology across the organization. Linked to this, surveys were conducted to determine the type and frequency of genotoxic analysis. Through these activities, it has then been possible to identify areas where there would be a business benefit in developing generic technology platforms. Readily available "walk-up" systems that can be used for specific classes of genotoxic impurities, rather than having to develop individual methods. This has ultimately become a vital component of the strategy.

Based on this objective, AstraZeneca established a collaboration at the Research Institute of Chromatography to develop standard technology platforms for each of the main genotoxic impurity classes. This has ultimately delivered a series of standard methodologies for each specific compound class (see Table 11.4 for details of the techniques employed for specific analytes). Where appropriate, these methods have then been established on dedicated instruments, allowing analysts direct access to these methods on a "walk-up" basis. This has had a significant impact on the time taken to develop new methods as in many instances these "generic" methods have proved fit for purpose without the need for significant modification. This work is described in detail in Chapter 12.

At the onset of this work, a general target of 1 ppm for all analytes was set for the quantification limit, thus all of the methods utilize MS detection. However, where higher limits are applicable, other detectors, for example FID and UV would also be viable options.

Another facet of this work is that it has allowed a far greater insight in what technique (chromatographic) is most suited to the analysis of a particular genotoxic

TABLE 11.4 Standard Technology Platforms Developed for Specific Compound Classes

Compound class	Method/technique
Sulphonates	HS-GCMS-Deriv
Halides	HS-GCMS and SPME-GCMS
Haloalkenes	HS-GCMS & SPME-GCMS
Arylamines	LC-MS-Deriv
Mustards	SPME-GCMS
Aldehydes	LCMS-Deriv
Epoxides	HS-GCMS
Michael acceptors	HS-GCMS
Aziridines	LCMS-Deriv
Boronic acids	GCMS-Deriv
Hydrazines	LCMS-Deriv

impurity based on its class. This has allowed for a significant improvement in method development cycle times as even where the available generic method proves unsuitable; it provides a start point for the development of a specific method.

11.5 METHOD VALIDATION

Once an analytical method has been developed, it then needs to be validated in order to demonstrate its suitability for its intended purpose. Although analytical method validation is covered through ICH guidelines (ICH Q2A and Q2B), these guidelines do not specifically address validation of trace level methodologies. The criteria defined in the ICH guidelines that validation are performed against, for example specificity, precision, accuracy, are all vital aspects of the validation required for trace analysis; however the limits described within the ICH guidelines are not generally applicable to such methods. It is therefore necessary to adapt the existing guidelines in order that they can be applied to the validation of trace analytical methods for genotoxic impurity analysis. Such an approach is described below.

11.5.1 Assay versus Limit Test

In general, analytical methods are developed with the specific purpose of quantifying the level of an impurity. However, in the case of genotoxic impurities, the existence of a clear limit, as defined by the TTC (subject to factors including duration of exposure), allows for the potential use of limit tests to determine the suitability of an API /DP. Thus, when developing a method suitable for the analysis of GI, the analyst has the option to either develop a quantitative assay or to simply develop a limit test. As to which is the more appropriate, it becomes a matter of evaluating the specific purpose of the method. Certainly, a quantitative assay may prove more appropriate where there is a need to provide a clear absolute value of the level of a GI present. This is particularly true where used in support of process development and/or in conjunction with purging experiments. It can also be argued that since the acceptable limits as defined by the "staged" TTC change depending on dose/duration, a quantitative test is preferred. This is though somewhat mitigated against in the case of a limit test where the true LOQ of the method is significantly below both the limit defined by the TTC. The ideal scenario is where the true LOQ of the method is below the limit of the GI, which will be enforced at commercialization. Another key factor is project attrition. Is there value in developing a quantitative assay capable of ppm level detection limits if the GI of concern relates to a project that is yet to enter into early clinical trials? In many cases, the answer will be to apply a "fit for purpose" limit test during early stages of development.

11.5.2 Method Validation and Stage of Development

Another important aspect of validation that needs to be defined is how should validation relate to the different phases of development within projects. Within the AstraZeneca Strategy, the stages of development were defined quite simply as early and late stage.

11.5.2.1 Criteria for Validation at Early Stages
At this stage of development, the primary focus of validation was defined to be to demonstrate that the method is scientifically "fit for purpose". In order to achieve this, the following method parameters were defined as critical and thus requiring appropriate validation.

Specificity The method should be shown to be free from interferences from known components; this is often performed as part of the method development and should be a simple test appropriate to the technique being used.

Sensitivity The method should be demonstrated to be appropriately sensitive for the purposes required. It was recommended that as a minimum 50% of the staged TTC limit should be typically quantifiable.

Recovery The effect of the sample matrix on the analytical result should be demonstrated. Ideally, it should be shown to have no appreciable effect; however, if the effect is well understood and is consistent then a low or high recovery may be acceptable. Acceptance criteria are typically defined as 80%–120% recovery. In the case of a limit test this may be a single point calibration. However, even for a limit test, given the fact that limits will vary as a function of dose/duration, then further calibration points may be considered. This would typically take the form of a high/medium/low sample set. The lowest level being defined based on a worst-case (highest dose/longest) study duration scenario (or simply the lifetime TTC limit of 1.5 µg/day).

Stability The solutions should be demonstrated to be stable over the timeframe of the analysis.

11.5.2.2 Validation Criteria for Validation of Late-Stage Projects For late-stage method validation, the criteria described above are all required, but additionally precision and robustness parameters should also be considered. Again the key here, as with all validation, is to provide appropriate scientific justification of results provided by the analytical method in question.

Precision Precision (often also referred to as repeatability) should be demonstrated by the performance of multiple injections and an RSD established. Limits of between 10% and 20% (based on six injections) should be acceptable.

Robustness Where a method is required to demonstrate control over a GI on a long-term basis, that is is a specified impurity, it is highly likely that the method concerned will be transferred from an R&D environment into a QC environment. Ahead of such a transfer, it is appropriate to consider the robustness of the procedure concerned. Such testing is performed by subjecting the method concerned to a series of minor variations to key method parameters, for example flow rate/temperature/ mobile phase composition/detector parameters, etc.

Linearity Where the method concerned is a quantitative assay as opposed to a limit test then the linearity of the method needs to be demonstrated. This would typically as a minimum involve three data points with duplicate samples at each point.

11.6 SUMMARY

The analysis of GIs undoubtedly presents analytical chemists with a new and complex challenge, one involving a number of complicating factors, for example analyte reactivity/matrix interference. That the analysis of GIs at ppm levels is achievable is however beyond question, the question is now one as to how can this best be achieved. The goal is therefore to address this in a systematic manner that affords the analyst the best chance of achieving a suitable method in as short a space of time as possible, moving away from the empirical approaches so widely seen at the onset of the need to control GIs.

The preceding chapter describes the strategy that has been set up within AstraZeneca for this purpose. The strategy was very deliberately designed to be flexible and adaptable, and is aimed at maximizing the chances of quickly and efficiently developing a "fit for purpose" method that takes into consideration not just the nature of the GI, but also the business requirements at the time of the method conception. What is significant about the strategy is the use of NMR, as well as chromatographic techniques. This has made the development of methods truly a question of choice, allowing the technique selection to not only best fit analyte/ matrix properties, but also to fit the business needs.

What is clear is that the business needs, in terms of GI analysis, differ depending on a number of factors. These include permissible GI levels (based on duration of clinical studies) and therefore detection limits, limit tests versus quantitative assay, and also technical factors, such as method transferability. Each has different weightings depending on stage of development. We believe that the approach describe above has given us a genuine choice in relation to these factors, allowing us to appropriately weight all of the factors involved in such analysis to ensure that the method ultimately developed represents the right balance between short- and long-term factors, thus maximizing business efficiency while maintaining robust control over GIs.

Finally, another key factor in terms of the strategy is that because it is not reliant on a single technique, it should be possible for any organization to develop a similar approach irrespective of whether or not all of the techniques described are available to them.

ACKNOWLEDGMENTS

The author wishes to thank the team of people from AstraZeneca Global Pharmaceutical Development who developed the AstraZeneca guidance for Analysis of PGIs. Ingrid Lindberg, Janet Hammond, Carolyn Stevenson, Eivor Ornskov, Mark Harrison and Glyn Allsop. The author would also like to thank Dr Stephen Smith and Dr Adrian Clarke (AZ) for reviewing the manuscript.

REFERENCES

1. Elder DP, Teasdale A, Lipczynski AM. 2008. Control and analysis of alkyl esters of alkyl and aryl sulfonic acids in novel active pharmaceutical ingredients. *Journal of Pharmaceutical and Biomedical Analysis* 46:1–8.
2. Elder DP, Teasdale A, Lipczynski AM. 2008. Control and analysis of alkyl and benzyl halides and other reactive organohalides as potential genotoxic impurities in active pharmaceutical ingredients. *Journal of Pharmaceutical and Biomedical Analysis* 48:497–507.
3. David F, Vanhoenacker G, Sandra P, Jacq K, Baker A. 2010, December. *Method selection for trace analysis of genotoxic impurities in pharmaceuticals.* LCGC Article.
4. Sun M, Bai L, Terfloth GJ, Liu DQ, Kord AS. 2010. Matrix Deactivation: A general approach to improve stability of unstable and reactive pharmaceutical genotoxic impurities for trace analysis. *Journal of Pharmaceutical and Biomedical Analysis* 52:30–36.
5. David F, Jacq K, Sandra P, Baker A, Klee M. 2010. Analysis of potential genotoxic impurities in pharmaceuticals by two-dimensional gas chromatography with Deans switching and independent column temperature control using a low-thermal-mass oven module. AstraZeneca Internal Guidance for the Analysis of PGIs within Drug Substances and Chemical Intermediates. *Analytical and Bio-Analytical Chemistry* 396(3):1291–1300.
6. Vanhoenacker G, Dumont E, David F, Sandra P, Baker A. 2009. Determination of arylamines and aminopyridines in pharmaceutical products using in-situ derivatisation and liquid chromatography-mass spectrometry. *Journal of Chromatography A* 1216:3563–3570.

CHAPTER 12

STRATEGIC APPROACHES TO THE CHROMATOGRAPHIC ANALYSIS OF GENOTOXIC IMPURITIES

Frank David
Karine Jacq
Gerd Vanhoenacker
Pat Sandra

12.1   INTRODUCTION

Since the advent of the EMEA guideline relating to genotoxic impurities[1] it has become necessary to monitor and control such impurities to very low levels. This has led to the development of a series of analytical methods, which, in many cases, are "compound-specific" focused on a specific genotoxic analyte present in a specific product. In contrast to such specialized individual methods, the goal of our study was to develop a number of generic methods that could be applied to several impurities in a wide range of APIs. The major challenges faced in relation to this work were related to the extremely wide ranges of polarities and volatilities of the possible target analytes, in combination with a large range of matrices (APIs and intermediates) with different physicochemical characteristics (water soluble, ionic, polar, apolar, basic, acidic, etc.). Moreover, because of the low limits defined within the EMEA guideline, based on the threshold of toxicological concern (TTC) concept (1.5 µg/day for lifetime exposure),[2] such methods need to be able to quantify the potentially genotoxic impurities (PGIs) and genotoxic impurities (GIs) at trace level, sometimes around or below 1 ppm (1 µg/g), which is typically 500 times lower than for classical impurity analysis in pharmaceutical quality control (at 0.05% level).

Developing each method on an individual basis would be incredibly time and resource consuming for pharmaceutical companies. The project therefore aimed to develop a strategic approach, one based on knowledge of the physicochemical properties of the analyte/matrix, that would significantly improve both the effectiveness and timeliness of the method development process. Based on our research, a method

Genotoxic Impurities: Strategies for Identification and Control, Edited by Andrew Teasdale
Copyright © 2010 by John Wiley & Sons, Inc.

selection chart (decision tree) was constructed, which can be used to guide analysts through the selection of the most appropriate method to apply to a specific PGI/GI analysis.[3] Methods were developed either using gas chromatography (GC) or liquid chromatography (LC), both in combination with a single quadrupole mass spectrometer as a detector, since these techniques are commonly available in a routine QC environment. The same separation methods can, of course, also be applied using triple quadrupole instruments using multiple reaction monitoring (MRM), or using ion trap and time-of-flight mass spectrometers.

Next, for each class of PGI/GI, sample preparation was optimized. In each instance the ubiquity of the method was examined through evaluating it using a selection of APIs, with different physicochemical properties (polarity, functionalities, etc.). Attention was focused specifically on robust sample preparation methods that could be both automated and online coupled to GC or LC. The ultimate aim was to minimize method variability through minimizing manual sample handling and thus also reducing the reliance on the expertise of individual analysts.

The result of this research is the decision tree chart presented in Figure 12.1. Briefly, this chart starts from the question: Is the PGI/GI amenable to analysis by GC or not? If yes, the next question is whether the PGI/GI has sufficient vapor pressure to be present in the headspace phase of a concentrated solution of the API (in water, dimethylsulfoxide (DMSO), or other low volatile solvent). If yes, static headspace (SHS), solid-phase microextraction (SPME), or dynamic headspace (DHS) can be used. Since most APIs are not volatile, headspace methods can therefore be considered as "first-to-try," since the analytical system (GC inlet, column, detector) is not subsequently contaminated by the matrix. The choice between SHS, SPME, and DHS depends on the volatility of the analytes and the desired sensitivity. This is discussed in detail in the section relating to the analysis of alkyl- and aryl halides.

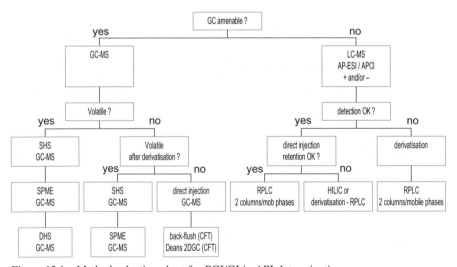

Figure 12.1 Method selection chart for PGI/GI in API determination.

In some cases, analytes do not have enough vapor pressure to allow them to be analyzed using headspace analysis. In such instances, *in situ* derivatization can be applied to generate a volatile derivative of the GI/PGI that can be then analyzed by SHS, SPME, or DHS. Examples of such approaches are described in detail in the later sections describing the analysis of sulfonates and N-mustards. If the analyte is GC amenable (stable and eluting from the GC column at moderate temperatures, for example <320°C), but not volatile enough for headspace techniques (even after derivatization), a direct injection of a concentrated API solution in GC can be used. Hereby, attention should be paid to the volatility and thermal stability of the analytes and the matrix (API). Since the matrix is also introduced, the API itself, other API impurities and/or API decomposition products (e.g. formed in the hot GC inlet), can interfere with the target PGIs/GIs or can influence the system performance (contamination). In this respect, state-of-the-art GC techniques such as backflushing and two-dimensional GC (2D-GC, GC-GC) can be very useful. Recently introduced tools based on capillary flow technology (CFT) such as splitters and microchannel column switching plates can be installed in GC instruments, making backflushing and 2D-GC accessible for routine analyses. The applicability of CFT is illustrated by the analysis of Michael acceptors and haloalcohols.

In our study, many of the classes of GTI/PGI studied were found amenable to GC, either directly or postderivatization. Because of the availability of robust and low-cost GC-MS systems, we recommend that the GC-MS option should be consideration as the first option. If the analytes are not amenable to GC, then LC-MS should be evaluated (Fig. 12.1, right path). In selecting LC-MS, first a selection of the ionization mode is needed. Both atmospheric pressure electrospray ionization (AP-ESI) and atmospheric pressure chemical ionization (APCI), either operating in the positive ion or negative ion detection mode, can be evaluated in terms of sensitivity and selectivity. Both modes are rather complementary. One mode can, for instance, result in a higher absolute response, but combined with lower selectivity and/or higher background, the overall result might be that the other ionization mode performs better for a given application. Flow injection of solutions of the PGI/GI and MS acquisition in alternating +/− scan mode and the use of a multimode ESI/APCI source can hereby be useful.

Once the ionization mode is selected, direct injection of a concentrated API solution, followed by reversed phase HPLC (RP-LC), is then the next step. Where the analyte is poorly retained, hydrophobic interaction liquid chromatography (HILIC) or precolumn derivatization (into more hydrophobic derivatives) can be used as alternative, as illustrated by the analysis of aziridines. Although MS is often considered as "universal" detection, some target analytes can give very low or nonselective response, in both ESI and APCI ionization modes. In these cases, derivatization to enhance detectability prior to LC-MS can be useful. Precolumn derivatization was used for aldehydes and hydrazines.

The details of the methods listed in the method selection chart and their application to different PGI/GI analytes and API matrices are described in the next sections. For each class of PGI/GI, a short method description is given, followed by typical operating conditions and a discussion on the results obtained.

12.2 INSTRUMENTATION

In our study, various systems were used. GC-MS methods were developed and validated on an Agilent 6890 or 7890 GC combined with a 5975 MSD (Agilent Technologies, Wilmington, DE, USA). A typical GC configuration for PGI/GI analysis is presented in Figure 12.2.

The GC was equipped with a split/splitless inlet and/or a programmed vaporizing inlet (CIS 4 PTV, Gerstel GmbH, Mulheim, Germany). Injection was performed using a multipurpose sampler (MPS2, Gerstel), which allows liquid injection, SHS, and SPME. A dual rail configuration, as shown in Figure 12.2, allows automated sequences of sample preparation steps, such as dilution, reagent and internal standard (IS) addition, and derivatization. This is followed by liquid, headspace, or SPME injection. This is possible, since two arms are available that can carry different liquid or gas syringes (or SPME syringe). Different vial trays (2 mL, 20 mL vials, reagents, rinse solvents) and thermostated agitators can also be installed. The system could

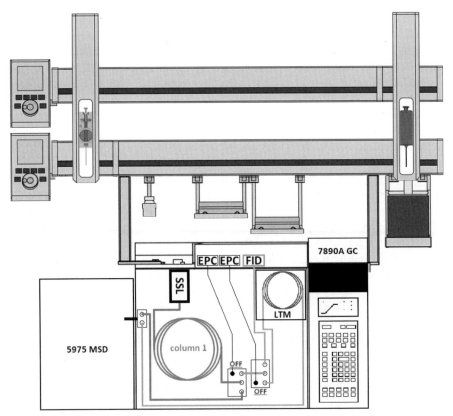

Figure 12.2 Typical GC-MS configuration. System includes dual rail sampler for liquid and headspace injection, split/splitless (SSL) inlet, Deans switch, and low thermal mass (LTM) oven.

also be equipped with thermal desorption (TDU), dynamic headspace (DHS) (Gerstel) and capillary flow technology options. The flow from the GC column can be directed to the MSD or to a second column, situated in a separate low thermal mass oven (LTM, Agilent Technologies) for further separation of heart-cut fractions. Carrier gas flows through the columns, and restrictors were controlled by electronic pressure control (EPC) modules.

LC-MS methods were developed on an Agilent 1100 or 1200 LC combined with a 1100 Series Quadrupole MSD (version SL) equipped with an electrospray ionization (ESI) or atmospheric pressure chemical ionization (APCI) source (Agilent Technologies, Walbronn, Germany). A typical LC-MS configuration is shown in Figure 12.3.

The HPLC system consisted of a binary pump (with solvent selection valve), an automated liquid sampler, a thermostated column oven equipped with a column switching valve, and a diode array detector (optional). In the six-port/two position valve two columns were installed allowing unattended column selection. Automated sample introduction can either be done using a standard liquid sampler (autosampler 1) or a XYZ robot (MPS 3, Gerstel) allowing more flexibility in sample preparation options, such as dilution, shaking, reagent and IS addition, etc. (autosampler 2).

The MSD was used in SIM mode either using positive or negative ion detection. During the elution of the API, the LC column effluent could be diverted to waste, not to contaminate the ionization chamber.

These instrumental configurations are only listed as a guideline. Equivalent systems can also be applied.

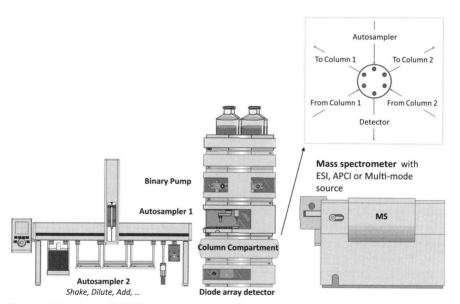

Figure 12.3 Typical HPLC-MS configuration. System includes autosampler (Agilent ALS or Gerstel MPS3), binary pump, thermostated column compartment with column selection valve, DAD detector, and MSD.

The analytes studied are representative of each class with structural alert functionalities.[4] All are commercially available from Sigma-Aldrich. Commercially available APIs were used as "matrix" for method development and validation. These covered different physicochemical properties, and included promethazine (base, apolar), carbamazepine (neutral, intermediate polarity), ampicillin (polar, zwitter-ions), Vitamin C (acid, polar), penicillin V (polar, acidic), ephedrine (basic, medium polar), asperin (acid, intermediate polar), bromhexine (base, medium polar), guai-fenesin (neutral, polar), and doxylamine (basic, medium polar).

12.3 ALKYL HALIDES AND ARYL HALIDES

12.3.1 Method Description

Alkyl halides are used as alkylating agents in synthesis. Analytical methods for this class of PGIs/GIs were recently reviewed by Elder et al.[5] and include both GC and LC methods. A typical list of possible target analytes is given in Table 12.1. Most of these target analytes are stable, amenable to GC, and are also volatile enough to allow headspace analysis.

Classical static headspace (SHS) analysis in combination with GC and MS detection was therefore initially evaluated in this study.

SHS is often available in pharmaceutical QC labs, since the same methodology is used for residual solvent analysis. While residual solvents are normally analyzed using flame ionization detection (FID), the selection of mass spectrometric detection operating in selected ion monitoring (SIM) mode results in enhanced selectivity and sensitivity needed for trace analysis. Therefore, static headspace—GC-MS analysis is a good starting point for method development.

For less volatile compounds, a headspace enrichment method, such as solid-phase microextraction (SPME) can be evaluated. Halogenated alcohols, however, are not volatile enough to be analyzed by headspace techniques. These more polar analytes are analyzed by direct injection—GC-MS after derivatization, as described in Section 12.8.

12.3.2 Analytical Conditions

12.3.2.1 Sample Preparation The following sample/standard preparations were made in order to evaluate method suitability. The API (50 mg) was dissolved in 2 mL DMSO/water (1:1) in a 20 mL headspace vial. The solvent(s) can be adapted according to API solubility (first dissolved in 1 mL DMSO, then add 1 mL water or vice versa; alternatively, other high boiling solvents can be used, e.g. dimethyl acetamide [DMAC]).

For calibration, a set of target compounds was prepared in methanol (at a concentration of 50 ng/µL). Aliquots (0.5–10 µL) of this solution were spiked in the API solution. Resulting spiked concentrations are in the order of 0.5–10 ppm (µg/g API). Also an internal standard, such as fluorobenzene or 3-fluorotoluene (or a deuterated analyte) can be added. Such internal standards are utilized where there is a need to enhance the precision of the analysis.

TABLE 12.1 Typical Alkyl and Aryl Halides Analytes

Peak	Analytes	RT (min)	Ion Quant	Ion Qual	LOD ppm SHS	LOD ppm SPME
1	chloromethane	4.21	50	52	0.42	ND
2	vinyl chloride	4.49	62	64	0.65	ND
3	bromomethane	5.04	94	96	0.31	1.05
4	vinyl bromide	5.62	106	108	0.09	0.10
5	1-chloropropane	6.30	63	42, 78	0.11	0.61
6	iodomethane	6.71	142	127	0.13	0.01
7	2-chloropropane	7.23	63	42, 78	0.08	0.07
8	E-1,2-dichloroethene	7.65	61	96	0.02	0.03
9	2-bromopropane	8.13	43	122, 124	0.06	0.57
10	Z-1,2-dichloroethene	8.66	61	96	0.03	0.03
11	2-chloroacrylonitrile	9.04	87	52	0.08	0.01
12	1-chloro-2-methylpropene	9.11	55	90	0.02	0.04
13	1-bromopropane	9.24	122	43, 124	0.11	0.19
14	2-iodopropane	10.56	127	70	0.64	0.68
15	1-bromo-2-methylpropene	11.34	55	134	0.17	0.03
16	1-iodopropane	11.75	127	43, 170	0.13	0.13
17	E-1,2-dibromoethene	12.38	186	105	0.11	0.01
18	Z-1,2-dibromoethene	13.21	186	105	0.12	0.01
19	2-iodoethanol	14.20	172	127	ND	<1
20	3-bromo-2-methylacrylonitrile (cis)	15.11	66	145	0.29	0.02
21	3-bromo-2-methylacrylonitrile (trans)	16.45	66	145	2.24	0.20
22	4-fluorobenzyl chloride	19.04	109	144	0.25	0.01
23	benzyl chloride	19.04	91	126	0.38	0.01
24	4-fluorobenzyl bromide	20.83	109	83	2.50	0.27
25	benzyl bromide	20.86	91	170	ND	2.70
26	4-methylbenzyl chloride	21.28	105	140	1.83	0.02
27	4-methylbenzyl bromide	22.98	105	184	ND	3.70
28	4-chlorobutylether	26.11	91	55	1.15	0.01

ND, not detected.

12.3.2.2 GC-MS Parameters

SHS was performed at 80°C during 15 min. One milliliter headspace was injected in split mode (split ratio 1/10, inlet temperature: 250°C).

Headspace SPME (HS-SPME) was performed using a 75 µm/85 µm Carboxen/PDMS fiber at 80°C equilibration and extraction temperature during 20 min.

GC-MS conditions were identical for SHS-GC-MS and SPME-GC-MS:

Column: 60 m × 0.25 mm i.d. × 1.4 µm D_f DB-VRX (Agilent Technologies)
Carrier gas: Helium, constant flow (1.5 mL/min)
Oven: 40°C—2 min—10°C/min—250°C—4 min
Detection: MS in simultaneous SIM/SCAN mode

Scan range: 29–350 m/z
Selected ions (SIM): see Table 12.1
Solvent delay: 3.5 min

12.3.3 Results

A typical chromatogram (SIM trace) obtained for an API (promethazine) spiked with 28 analytes (Table 12.1) at 5 ppm (5 µg/g API) level is shown in Figure 12.4.

From the chromatogram, it is clear that most analytes are well detected. Good linearity ($r^2 > 0.99$) was obtained in a range from 0.5 to 10 ppm (µg/g API). Repeatability was better than 10% RSD at 5 ppm level, except for chloromethane (RSD ≈ 20%). The limit of detection was below 0.5 ppm for most analytes, as shown in Table 12.1. It is clear from these results that very volatile analytes, such as vinyl-chloride can be analyzed with excellent sensitivity using these SHS-GC-MS conditions. It can also be observed that the relative response of the late eluting, less volatile compounds drops significantly, as can be expected from their lower vapor pressure. 4-methylbenzylbromide (analyte 27) could not be detected at this level and also a more polar analyte, such as iodoethanol (analyte 19), was not detected with the SHS-GC-MS method. Also, other haloalcohols, such as 2-chloroethanol, 2-bromoethanol, and 2-(2-chloroethoxy) ethanol were tested, but these more polar analytes could also not be detected by SHS-GC-MS.

Based on these results, however, it is clear that the SHS-GC-MS procedure described can be utilized as a general screening method applicable to the analysis of a wide range of alkyl and aryl halides.

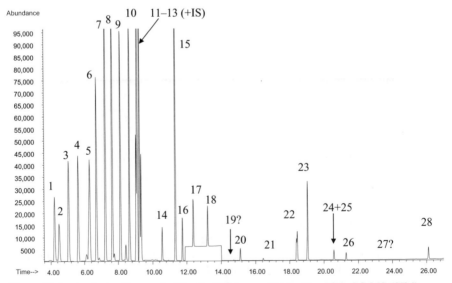

Figure 12.4   Analysis of organohalides in API (promethazine) by SHS-GC-MS (SIM). Sample spiked at 5 µg/g API. SHS at 80°C. Analytes: see Table 12.1.

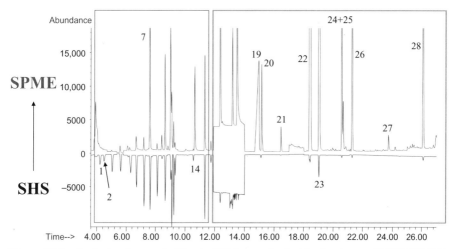

Figure 12.5   Analysis of organohalides in API (promethazine) by headspace-SPME-GC-MS (SIM) (top) and SHS-GC-MS (SIM) (bottom, inversed). Sample spiked at 0.5 µg/g. SPME at 80°C. Analytes: see Table 12.1.

In order to increase the sensitivity for some analytes, HS-SPME was also evaluated. A Carboxen/PDMS fiber was used, since this fiber is recommended for the analysis of volatile organic compounds (VOCs). The SIM chromatograms for the analysis of promethazine, spiked at 0.5 ppm level, obtained by respectively SPME and SHS are compared in Figure 12.5. The LODs for the 28 analytes obtained by SPME are compared with SHS in Table 12.1. It is clear that the late eluting analytes, with favorable PDMS-air partitioning coefficients ($K_{PDMS/air}$), are concentrated in the fiber and enriched, resulting in very low detection limits. This is obvious for the analytes eluting after 12 min (peaks 16–28). As shown in Table 12.1, the gain in sensitivity can be as high as a factor 10 (as illustrated by, for instance, dibromoethenes, 4-fluorobenzylchloride and 4-chlorobutylether). 4-methylbenzylbromide (peak 27), not detected by SHS-GC-MS, can now be detected. Also, iodoethanol (peak 19) could be detected, but repeatability was not good and another method is therefore recommended (see Section 12.8). From these result, it is clear that SPME is complementary to SHS and for analytes typically eluting after toluene on an apolar column (log $K_{PDMS/air}$ > 3), SPME leads to higher sensitivity. It should, however, be noted that for the very volatile analytes (e.g. chloromethane [1], vinylchloride [2]), SHS is superior to SPME, since no enrichment on the fiber is obtained for these analytes.

Another option to increase sensitivity is the use of dynamic headspace (DHS). In this case, the headspace of the sample, placed in, for instance, a 20 mL vial, is purged with a controlled flow of inert gas (usually carrier gas). The gas is sent though a trap containing an adsorbent, such as Tenax® (a porous polymer resin based on 2.6-diphenylene oxide; Scientific Instrument Services, Inc., Ringoes, NJ) or charcoal. The trapped compounds can subsequently be desorbed using dedicated thermal desorption equipment.[6] Typically, a gain in sensitivity in the order of a factor 10–50 can be obtained versus static headspace.

It can be concluded that for the analysis of most alkylhalides, static headspace followed by GC-MS operated in SIM mode can be employed and this should be start point when looking to determine a suitable method. It is though recommended that SPME-GC-MS be employed for volatile analytes with log $K_{PDMS/air} > 3$, to enhance sensitivity.

12.4 SULFONATES

12.4.1 Method Description

Sulfonate esters, including the methyl, ethyl, and isopropyl esters of methanesulfonic acid (mesylates), benzenesulfonic acid (besylates), and toluylsulfonic esters (tosylates), are probably the best-known class of GIs. These esters can be formed potentially from the reaction of volatile alcohols (used as solvent) and sulphonic acids (used as the salt counterion). The formation reaction is given in Figure 12.6A. The most important sulfonate and sulfate esters are listed in Table 12.2.

The analysis of sulfonate esters is not straightforward. Indeed, a recent review conducted by Elder et al.,[7] described a variety of different approaches. Sulfonate esters cannot be analyzed directly by headspace techniques, since the vapor pressure is too low. Moreover, direct injection in GC or HPLC is difficult and prone to artifacts, such as possible formation of the GIs by decomposition of the API salts (e.g. in the GC inlet = false positives), hydrolysis of the sulfonates (e.g. in aqueous media), and/or API interference. An elegant method was described by

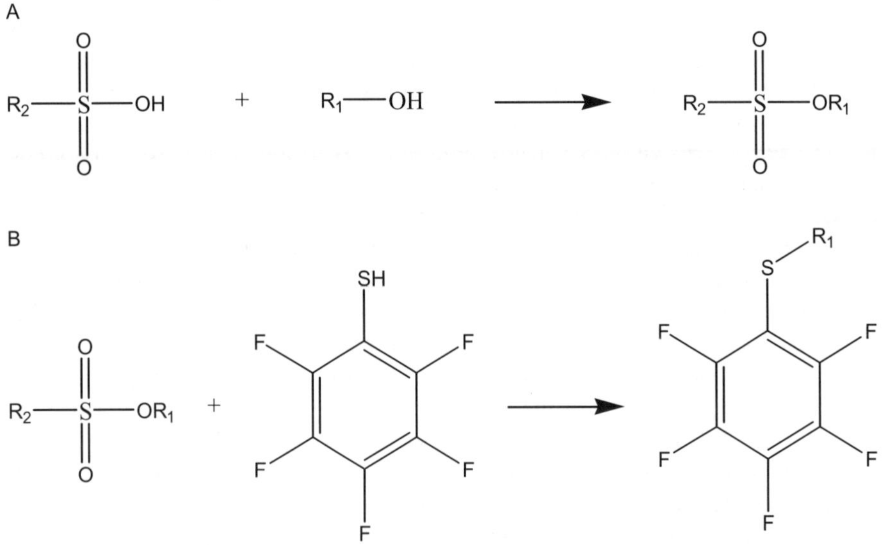

Figure 12.6   Sulfonate ester formation reaction (A) and sulfonate ester derivatization reaction (B).

TABLE 12.2 Sulfonate and Sulfate Ester Target Compounds

Name	Abbreviation	R_1	R_2	Synthesis	
				Alcohol	Acid
Dimethyl sulfate	DMS	CH_3	OCH_3	Methanol	Sulfuric acid
Diethyl sulfate	DES	C_2H_5	OC_2H_5	Ethanol	Sulfuric acid
Diisopropyl sulfate	DIS	C_3H_7	OC_3H_7	Isopropanol	Sulfuric acid
Methyl methane sulfonate	MMS	CH_3	CH_3	Methanol	Methane sulfonic acid
Ethyl methane sulfonate	EMS	C_2H_5	CH_3	Ethanol	Methane sulfonic acid
Isopropyl methane sulfonate	IMS	C_3H_7	CH_3	Isopropanol	Methane sulfonic acid
Methyl benzene sulfonate	MBS	CH_3	C_6H_5	Methanol	Benzene sulfonic acid
Ethyl benzene sulfonate	EBS	C_2H_5	C_6H_5	Ethanol	Benzene sulfonic acid
Isopropyl benzene sulfonate	IBS	C_3H_7	C_6H_5	Isopropanol	Benzene sulfonic acid
Methyl p-toluene sulfonate	MpTS	CH_3	C_7H_8	Methanol	p. Toluene sulfonic acid
Ethyl p-toluene sulfonate	EpTS	C_2H_5	C_7H_8	Ethanol	p. Toluene sulfonic acid
Isopropyl p-toluene sulfonate	IpTS	C_3H_7	C_7H_8	Isopropanol	p. Toluene sulfonic acid

Alzaga et al.[8] using *in situ* derivatization—SHS-GC-MS. In this method, the sulfonates are derivatized (and thereby also stabilized) by reaction with pentafluorothiophenol (Fig. 12.6b). The methyl, ethyl, or isopropyl derivatives are stable and volatile, and can be analyzed by SHS-GC-MS. Isotope-labeled analytes, prepared in-house from deuterated alcohols reacting with sulphonic acids or sulfonyl chlorides, are used as internal standards. This method was completely automated on a dual rail autosampler (Gerstel), and could also be applied to study sulfonate ester formation kinetics.[9]

It should be noted that using this methodology, differentiation between sulfonates is only made based on differences in the R_1 group (Fig. 12.6). This means that no differentiation can be made between ethyl methanesulfonate (EMS), ethyl benzenesulfonate (EBS), and ethyl para-toluenesulfonate, since all three result in the same reaction product (ethyl-PFTP). Differentiation can only be made between the different mesylates: methyl methanesulfonate (MMS), EMS, and isopropyl methanesulfonate (IMS). In pharmaceutical QC, this is sufficient, since in most cases, it is known if mesylates, besylates, tosylates, or sulphates are potentially formed.

The suitability of the Alzaga method was examined in detail, and the outcome of this evaluation is described below.

If confirmation analysis is required or speciation is needed, additional GC-MS or LC-MS analysis can be used. In this case, direct injection can be used; however, precautions need to be taken to avoid/control analyte and/or API degradation. An example of this approach is described below, demonstrating the use of programmed temperature vaporizing (PTV) injection in combination with GC-MS.

12.4.2 Analytical Conditions

12.4.2.1 Sample Preparation
The following sample/standard preparations were made in order to evaluate method suitability.

The API (50 mg) was dissolved in 4 mL of a dimethylacetamide/water or DMSO/water mixture (1:1, v/v) in a 20 mL HS vial. (DMAC gives a lower background than DMSO if sulfates should be monitored, DMSO gives slightly higher sensitivity).

An internal standard was added (typically 10 μL of a 5 ng/μL solution, see below). For spiking experiments, the sulfonate esters are also added from an acetone solution. One hundred microliters of the derivatization solution, containing 6.4 mg/mL pentafluorothiophenol in 1 M NaOH, was added through the septum of the vial. Derivatization was performed for 15 min at 105°C ("headspace equilibration time and temperature").

Synthesis of deuterated internal standards:

A deuterated internal standard were synthesized for each analyte from the corresponding acid and deuterated alcohol (see Table 12.2).

For each IS, 100 μL deuterated alcohol (e.g. d6-ethanol) and 0.188 mmol acid (e.g. methane sulfonic acid) were mixed in 5 mL reagent tubes, heated for 2 h at 100°C, then cooled down at room temperature and diluted in 5 mL acetone. These solutions were stored at 4°C (stock solution). The exact concentration and purity of these solutions were measured using GC-FID and GC-MS against a nondeuterated standard.

12.4.2.2 GC-MS Parameters
SHS: 15 min equilibration, 105°C
Injection: 1 mL, 1/10 split ratio, 250°C
Column: 60 m × 0.25 mm i.d. × 1.4 μm D_f DB-VRX (Agilent)
Carrier gas: Helium, constant flow (2.4 mL/min)
Oven: 60°C—1 min—10°C/min—200°C—30°C/min—250°C—1.33 min
Detection: MS in SIM mode
Selected ions (SIM):
10.50–13.27 min: 199, 200, 214, 217
13.28–14.00 min: 200, 201, 228, 233
14.00–18.00 min: 200, 201, 242, 249
Dwell times: 100 ms
Solvent delay: 10.5 min
Quantification was performed using ions:
214 for methylthiopentafluorobenzene (methyl-PFTP)

217 for deuterated methylthiopentafluorobenzene (methyl-PFTP-d₃)
228 for ethylthiopentafluorobenzene (ethyl-PFTP)
233 for deuterated ethylthiopentafluorobenzene (ethyl-PFTP-d₅)
242 for isopropylthiopentafluorobenzene (isopropyl-PFTP)
249 for deuterated isopropylthiopentafluorobenzene (isopropyl-PFTP-d₇)

12.4.3 Results

An example of a chromatogram obtained by the derivatization—SHS-GC-MS method for the analysis of ampicillin spiked at 1 ppm level with methyl methanesulfonate (MMS) and ethyl methanesulfonate (EMS), is shown in Figure 12.7. Detection was performed in SIM mode at m/z 214 (MMS derivative), 217 (d3-MMS derivative), 228 (EMS derivative), and 233 (d5-EMS derivative). The target analytes and their respective internal standards were easily detected.

The method was validated (Table 12.3). The linearity, measured in a concentration range from 0.2 to 10 ppm (adding 10, 25, 50, 100, 250, and 500 ng/50 mg API) was excellent. The LODs (S/N = 3) were below 0.5 ppm, except for IMS (isopropyl-PFTP derivative) which showed a slightly lower sensitivity (LOD = 3 ppm). RSDs were measured at 1 ppm level (at 5 ppm for IMS) and were below 10%.

The full automation of the method and the resulting repeatability allowed us to use this method to be applied for kinetic studies on the formation of sulphonate esters from alcohol/acid mixtures under different reaction conditions (pH, temperature, water content).[9]

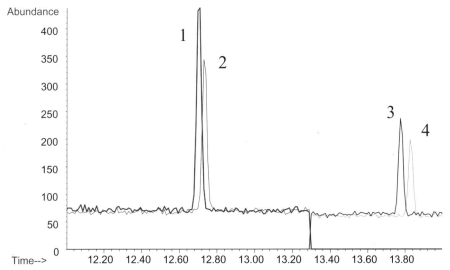

Figure 12.7   Analysis of sulphonate esters in API (ampicillin) by derivatisation—SHS-GC-MS (SIM). Sample spiked at 1 µg/g. Derivatisation with pentafluorothiophenol. Analytes: 1. d3-MMS, 2. MMS, 3. d5-EMS, 4. EMS.

TABLE 12.3 Validation Results for Sulfonate Ester Analysis by Derivatization-SHS-GC-MS

Type	Analyte	LOD	Linearity	RSD (%)
		ppm (50 mg API)	r^2 (0.2–10 ppm)	(@ 1 ppm)
Tosylates	*MpTS*	0.08	0.998	3
	EpTS	0.11	0.999	7
Besylates	*MBS*	0.06	0.998	3
Mesylates	*MMS*	0.11	0.998	6
	EMS	0.26	0.999	9
	IMS	3.2	0.999	9
Sulfates	*DMS*	0.04	0.999	9
	DES	0.08	0.999	8

12.4.4 Confirmation Analysis by ALEX-GC-MS

As described above, the generic SHS-GC-MS does not allow differentiation between mesylates, besylates, and tosylates as the derivatization reaction simply results in formation of methyl, ethyl, or isopropyl derivatives of pentafluorothiophenol.

Should it be necessary to discriminate between such species then, depending on the API and the possible sulfonate, either GC or LC methods can be selected.[7]

An example of an approach using GC-MS is described below. In this case, direct liquid injection of a concentrated API solution was done in a GC-MS system equipped with a programmed temperature vaporizing (PTV) inlet and an ALEX system (Automated Liner EXchange). This system allows automated liner exchange after a single or a few injections, avoiding cross-contamination and reducing contamination of the analytical column and detector. The PTV exchangeable liner was filled with polydimethylsiloxane (PDMS) particles that retain the API and avoids the introduction of the drug product in the GC. As an illustration, a 50 mg/mL solution of promethazine (API) was spiked with 0.5 μg (10 ppm) sulfonates (EMS, IMS, and EpTS) in chloroform. From this solution, 1 μL was injected in splitless mode. The PTV injector was heated from 20 to 220°C at 12°C/s. Separation was done on a 30 m × 0.25 mm ID × 0.25 μm HP-5MS column using a temperature program from 40°C (1 min) at 8°C/min to 280°C (2 min). Carrier gas was helium at a constant flow of 1.6 mL/min. MS detection was done in scan/SIM mode.

The chromatogram is shown in Figure 12.8A. EMS, IMS, and EpTS are clearly detected. The relatively low end temperature of the PTV (220°C) avoided the introduction of the bulk of the API, while the target analytes are quantitatively transferred in the column. As an illustration, the obtained mass spectra for EMS and EpTS are given in Figure 12.8B and C, respectively.

Using this method, the presence of sulfonates can be confirmed and differentiation can be made between mesylates (EMS) and tosylates (EpTS).

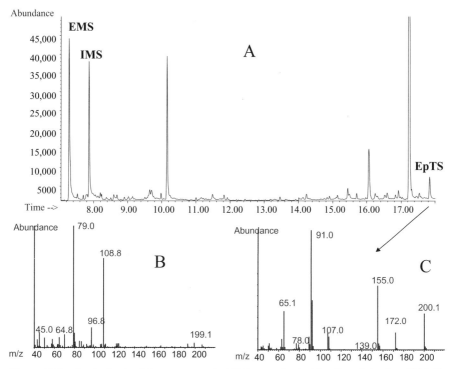

Figure 12.8   Analysis of sulphonate esters in API (promethazine) by direct injection-GC-MS (scan) using an automated liner exchange system. (A) TIC chromatogram, (B) mass spectrum of EMS, C. mass spectrum of EpTS.

12.5   S- AND N-MUSTARDS

12.5.1   Method Description

Mustards are β-halogenated dialkylsulfides (S-mustards) or β-halogenated amines (N-mustards). These compounds are used as alkylating reagents in chemical synthesis. Typical representatives of this class of PGIs/GIs are given in Table 12.4.

Some of these analytes, such as 2-chloroethyl methyl sulfide and 2-chloroethyl ethyl sulfide, are volatile and can be analyzed by static headspace GC-MS using the method described for halides (Section 12.3).

N-mustards (or "mustard-like" analytes), with a primary or secondary amine functionality, on the other hand, do not have sufficient vapor pressure to be analyzed by headspace techniques. For these analytes, a method based on derivatization followed by SHS or SPME was developed. A derivatization reaction that can be performed in situ in aqueous media was selected. The same method could also be applied in nonaqueous solvent systems.

Successful analysis of the target N-mustard analytes could be achieved by in situ derivatization using ethylchloroformate. This derivatizsation is also used for the

TABLE 12.4 Selected S- and N-Mustard Target Analytes

		CAS $n°$	RT	Target Ion	Qualifiers
2,2,2-trifluoroethylamine[a]	CF₃EtNH₂	870-24-6	11.05	144	106, 126
2-chloroethyl methyl sulfide	ClEtSMe	542-81-4	12.10	61	110, 112
2-chloroethyl ethyl sulfide	ClEtSEt	693-07-2	13.50	75	124, 126
2-chloroethylamine[a]	ClEtNH₂	821-48-7	17.27	102	63
3-chloropropylamine (IS)[a]	ClPropNH₂	5535-49-9	19.71	102	165
bis-(2-chloroethyl)amine[a]	Bis ClEtNH	753-90-2	22.42	164	56, 92
2-chloroethyl phenyl sulfide	ClEtSPhe	6276-54-6	22.28	123	172, 174

[a] As derivatives.

RT, retention time (minutes).

GC analysis of amino acids. Primary amine groups (–NH₂) are derivatized into carbamates (-NH-CO-OEt). The resulting compounds are more volatile and can be enriched on an SPME fiber.

12.5.2 Analytical Conditions

12.5.2.1 Sample Preparation The following sample/standard preparations were made in order to evaluate method suitability.

The API (100 mg) was dissolved in 2 mL of a solvent mixture containing water/ethanol/pyridine (2:1:1, v/v). Depending on the API solubility, the order of solvent addition can be changed. Next, 50 µL ethylchloroformate was added, and the derivatization performed at room temperature over a 15 min period in an ultrasonic bath. The derivatized samples were analyzed by SPME-GC-MS.

An internal standard (for instance: 3-chloropropylamine, in the form of a hydrochloride salt) can also be incorporated into the method to improve precision.

12.5.2.2 GC-MS Conditions
SPME: PDMS fiber (100 µm), 2 min incubation and 10 min extraction time at 80°C
Injection: split/splitless inlet in split (1/10) mode, 250°C
Column: 60 m × 0.25 mm i.d. × 1.4 µm D_f DB-VRX (Agilent Technologies)
Carrier gas: Helium, constant pressure (235.9 kPa)
Oven: 50°C—1 min—10°C/min—250°C (4 min); run time: 20 min
Detection: MS in simultaneous SIM/SCAN mode
Scan range: 29–350 m/z
Selected ions (SIM): see Table 12.4
Solvent delay: 3.5 min

12.5.3 Results

As described above, the S-mustards 2-chloroethyl methyl sulfide and 2-chloroethyl ethyl sulfide can be analyzed using static headspace—GC-MS (SHS at 80°C, 10 min equilibration). Using the GC conditions described above, these analytes elute in a

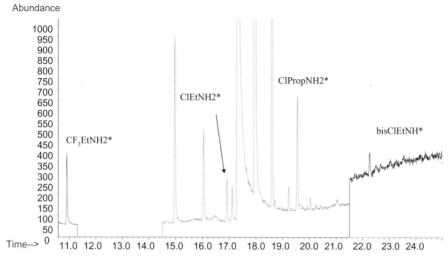

Figure 12.9 Analysis of N-mustards in API (doxylamine) by derivatization—SPME-GC-MS. Sample spiked at 0.5 µg/g. Derivatization with ethylchloroformate. Analytes: acyl-derivatives of trifluoro-ethylamine (CF$_3$EtNH$_2$), 2-chloroethylamine (Cl-EtNH$_2$), 3-chloropropylamine (IS) and bis(2-chloroethyl)amine (bisClEtNH$_2$).

time window between 11.3 and 14.5 min. The LOD was lower than 1 ppm for a 50 mg API in 2 mL solvent solution.

The N-mustards were derivatized using ethylchloroformate. The chromatogram (EIC of SIM) obtained for an API sample (doxylamine) spiked at 0.5 ppm level is shown in Figure 12.9. The derivatives of trifluoro-ethylamine (CF$_3$EtNH$_2$) (ion 144), 2-chloroethylamine (Cl-EtNH$_2$) (ion 102), 3-chloropropylamine (IS) (ion 102), and bis(2-chloroethyl)amine (bisClEtNH) (ion 164) were all detected. The linearity was tested in the range from 0.5 to 10 ppm, and the correlation coefficients were in the order of 0.995–0.999. The RSDs measured for APIs spiked at 1 ppm level were in the order of 13%–15%. The LODs, measured using the lowest spike level and corresponding to a signal-to-noise of 3 were 0.2 ppm for trifluoroethylamine (as derivative) and 2-chloroethylamine (as derivative), 0.1 ppm for 3-chloropropylamine (IS, as derivative), 0.4 ppm for 2-chloroethyl phenyl sulfide, and 0.5 ppm for bis(2-chloroethyl)amine (as derivative). The response for this later compound is lower. In order to obtain higher sensitivity for this analyte, derivatization followed by direct injection can be considered, as could the employment of alternative detection techniques, for example triple quadrupole MS.

12.6 MICHAEL REACTION ACCEPTORS

12.6.1 Method Description

Michael reactive acceptors are reagents that have an α,β-unsaturation next to an electron withdrawing functionality (such as a carbonyl or nitrile). The selected target analytes studied are listed in Table 12.5.

TABLE 12.5   Selected Michael Reaction Acceptor Target Analytes

Peak nr	Analyte	CAS no.	RT (min)	Target ion	Qualifiers Q1
1	Acrylonitrile	107-13-1	6.19	53	52
2	Methacrolein	78-85-3	6.99	70	39, 41
3	Methyl acrylate	96-33-3	7.85	55	85
4	2-Chloroacrylonitrile	920-37-6	7.96	52	87
5	Crotononitrile (Z)	4786-20-3	8.70	67	39, 41
6	Ethyl acrylate	140-88-5	9.73	55	99
7	cis-2-Pentenenitrile	25899-50-7	10.75	54	81
8	4-Methyl-3-pentene-2-one	141-79-7	12.25	83	55, 98
9	Methyl tiglate	6622-76-0	13.57	83	55, 114
10	2-Cyclohexen-1-one	930-68-7	15.20 7.44 (*)	68	96
11	Methyl-3-aminocrotonate	14205-39-1	15.80 8.83 (*)	84	42, 115
12	3-Ethoxy-2-cyclohexenone	5323-87-5	20.24 13.13 (*)	68	140
13	Cinnamonitrile	1885-38-7	20.25 13.07 (*)	129	102

Retention times (RTs) refer to the SHS method, except (*): retention time measured with direct GC-MS method (20 m × 0.18 mm ID × 1 µm DB-VRX column).

An initial evaluation was performed using static headspace—GC-MS. This approach was successful for a number of the volatile analytes studied; however, several of the less volatile analytes simply were not detected by SHS-GC-MS. In order to analyze these, direct liquid injection was required. A major drawback of direct injection is that it introduces a concentrated API solution directly into the GC-MS system. This can lead to contamination of the system. To avoid this, backflushing or Deans switching was applied. The principle of backflushing and its application to the analysis of nonvolatile Michael reaction acceptors are described in this section. The application of Deans switching is discussed in detail in Section 12.9.

12.6.2   Analytical Conditions

12.6.2.1   Sample Preparation   The following sample/standard preparations were made in order to evaluate method suitability.

For SHS analysis, the API (50 mg) was dissolved in 2 mL of a solvent mixture containing water/DMSO (1:1, v/v) in a 20 mL headspace vial. Depending on the API solubility, the order of solvent addition can be changed. The target analytes were dissolved in acetone for spiking in the API solution. Typically, 5 µL of a 10 ng/µL solution was added to obtain a 1 ppm spike level in the API.

For the nonvolatile analytes, a 50 mg/mL solution was made in dichloromethane. Also, pyridine could be used as solvent. Injection of 1 µL in splitless mode corresponds to the introduction of 50 µg API and a 1 ppm PGI/GI level corresponds to the injection of 50 pg PGI/GI on column.

12.6.2.2 SHS-GC-MS Parameters
Static headspace was performed at 80°C during 15 min. One millimeter headspace was injected in split mode (split ratio 1/10) in a PTV inlet with a Tenax TA packed liner.

PTV inlet temperature program: 20°C (0.1 min)—720°C/min—250°C, CO_2 cooling
GC-MS conditions:
Column: 60 m × 0.25 mm i.d. × 1.4 µm D_f DB-VRX (Agilent Technologies)
Carrier gas: Helium, constant pressure (200 kPa, with QuickSwap at 28 kPa)
Oven: 60°C (0.5 min)—8°C/min—100°C (3 min)—30°C/min—250°C (7.5 min)
Detection: MS in simultaneous SIM/SCAN mode
Scan range: 29–350 m/z
Selected ions (SIM): see Table 12.5, dwell times: 100 ms
Solvent delay: 3.5 min

12.6.2.3 Direction Injection GC-MS Conditions
Injection was performed in a PTV inlet with an empty, baffled liner. 1 µL was injected in splitless mode.

PTV inlet temperature program: 60°C (0.1 min)—720°C/min—250°C
GC-MS conditions:
Column: 20 m × 0.18 mm i.d. × 1 µm D_f DB-VRX (Agilent Technologies)
Carrier gas: Helium, constant flow 1.0 mL/min (with QuickSwap at 28 kPa)
Oven: 60°C (1 min)—10°C/min—250°C (10 min)
Detection: MS in simultaneous SIM/SCAN mode
Scan range: 45–350 m/z
Selected ions (SIM): see Table 12.5, dwell times: 100 ms
Solvent delay: 5 min
Postrun backflush at 20 min:
MS is switched off
Inlet pressure: 1 kPa
Pressure at the QuickSwap connector: 300 kPa
Backflush time: 10 min

12.6.3 Results

12.6.3.1 SHS with PTV
Static headspace was first used in combination with a classical split/splitless inlet. For the selected analytes, better results were obtained using a PTV inlet at 20°C (and using a Tenax packed liner). This resulted in peak focusing before introduction in the column. Good peak shapes were obtained for the volatile analytes.

The SHS-GC-MS analysis is illustrated by the analysis of a promethazine sample spiked with 1 ppm of the target analytes. The obtained chromatograms (extracted ion chromatograms from SIM acquisition mode) are shown in Figure 12.10. Analytes 1–9 in Table 12.5 can easily be detected. The last four analytes (2-cyclohexen-1-one, methyl-3-aminocrotonate, 3-ethoxy-2-cyclohexenone and cinnamonitrile) are not volatile enough and cannot be detected (although they elute

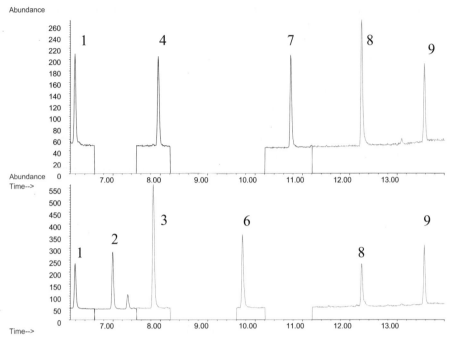

Figure 12.10 Analysis of Michael reaction acceptors in promethazine spiked at 1 ppm level by SHS-GC-MS (SIM). Peaks and extracted ions: see Tables 12.5 and 12.6.

from the column using the conditions listed above, as tested by liquid injection—retention times: see Table 12.5).

For the volatile analytes, the method was validated and excellent linearity ($r^2 > 0.99$ in the range from 0.2 to 5 ppm), repeatability (RSD < 5% at 1 ppm), and sensitivity (LOD < 0.1 ppm) were obtained as summarized in Table 12.6.

12.6.3.2 Direct Injection The target analytes 10–13 in Tables 12.5 and 12.6 were not volatile enough to allow headspace analysis to be performed successfully. For these compounds, direct injection of a concentrated (5%) solution of the API was used. In this case, the API and/or its impurities and degradation compounds are also present in the GC column. To eliminate these, column backflushing was used. To do this, the pressure at the outlet of the capillary column should be controlled. This can be achieved using a QuickSwap connector installed on the MS transfer line.

The principle of column backflush is illustrated in Figure 12.11. In normal GC mode, a high pressure on the inlet and a low pressure at the QuickSwap results in a forward capillary column flow rate of 1–2 mL/min. Typically, the outlet pressure is set at 4 psi (=28 kPa), which results, in combination with a 17 cm × 110 μm capillary in the transfer line at 260°C, with a flow rate of about 2 mL/min to the MS.

After elution of the analytes of interest (target PGI/GI), the inlet pressure is decreased (to a minimum, just enough to flush the inlet), and the pressure at the

TABLE 12.6 Validation Results for Michael Reaction Acceptor Analysis by SHS-GC-MS and Direct Injection GC-MS

Peak no.	Analyte	Method	RSD (%)	R^2	LOD
1	Acrylonitrile	SHS	3.6	0.999	0.02
2	Methacrolein	SHS	2.9	0.997	0.02
3	Methyl acrylate	SHS	1.4	0.996	0.02
4	2-Chloroacrylonitrile	SHS	3.9	0.994	0.02
5	Crotononitrile (Z)	SHS	3.4	0.994	0.04
6	Ethyl acrylate	SHS	3.4	0.996	0.02
7	cis-2-Pentenenitrile	SHS	3.7	0.999	0.02
8	4-Methyl-3-pentene-2-one	SHS	2.5	0.994	0.05
9	Methyl tiglate	SHS	3.2	0.993	0.05
10	2-Cyclohexen-1-one	Direct	7.6	0.995	0.02
11	Methyl-3-aminocrotonate	Direct	3.7	0.974	0.30
12	3-Ethoxy-2-cyclohexenone	Direct	8.2	0.999	0.30
	3-Ethoxy-2-cyclohexenone	*Direct—2D*	*1.5*	*nm*	*0.05*
13	Cinnamonitrile	Direct	12.5	0.997	0.03
	Cinnamonitrile	*Direct—2D*	*1.6*	*nm*	*0.01*

Direct: direct liquid injection of 5% solution, GC-MS and backflush.

Direct—2D: direct liquid injection of 5% solution, two-dimensional GC-MS (see Section 12.8).

nm, not measured; SHS, static headspace GC-MS method.

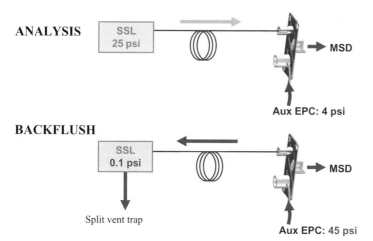

Figure 12.11   Principle of capillary column backflush.

outlet (transfer line) is raised. The MS is switched off (too high flow). In this way, outlet pressure is higher than inlet pressure, and capillary column flow is reversed. Higher molecular weight analytes (such as the API) are backflushed and exit via the split vent. Backflush times need to be optimized according to final GC oven temperature and column choice.[10]

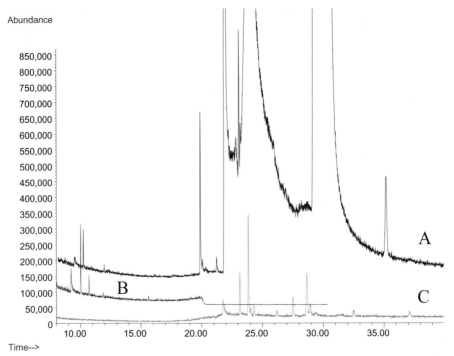

Figure 12.12   Analysis of carbamazepine using backflush. (A) No backflush,
(B) Backflush at 20 min, C. Blank run after backflush.

A direct injection GC-MS method was applied for the less volatile Michael reaction acceptors. A sample of carbamazepine spiked at 1 ppm level with the four analytes (compounds 10–13, Table 12.5) was analyzed. The chromatogram obtained in scan mode without backflush is shown in Figure 12.12A. The analytes could not be detected (present at 50 pg level), but the peaks for carbamazepine and its degradation compound (iminostilbene) overload the chromatogram. Next, the same analysis was performed with a backflush initiated at 20 min (Fig. 12.12B). A blank run (solvent injection) was performed afterwards. API (carbamazepine) and iminostilbene were completely removed; only some minor peaks (solvent impurities) were detected (Fig. 12.12C).

The extracted ion chromatograms from the SIM acquisition are shown in Figure 12.13. The target analytes (2-cyclohexen-1-one, methyl-3-aminocrotonate, 3-ethoxy-2-cyclohexenone, and cinnamonitrile) can easily be detected. The method was validated, and the results are included in Table 12.6. RSDs at 1 ppm level were between 5% and 15%, and LODs lower than 0.5 ppm.

Target analytes 12 and 13 were also analyzed by using two-dimensional heart-cutting GC-MS.[11] Details on the analytical method are included in Section 12.8. The validation results obtained by 2D-GC-MS are included in Table 12.6, and show that

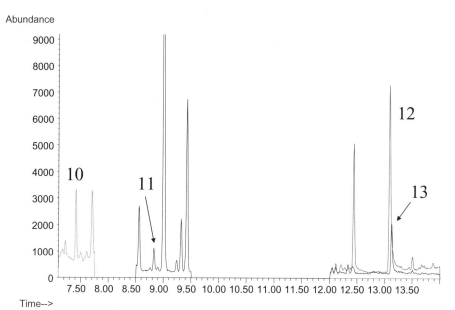

Figure 12.13   Analysis of Michael reaction acceptors in carbamazepine spiked at 5 ppm by direct injection-GC-MS (SIM), using backflush. Peaks and extracted ions: see Tables 12.5 and 12.6.

repeatability, measured on a carbamazepine sample spiked at 1 ppm level, was better than 2% ($n = 6$), and that the LOD was lower than 0.1 ppm. This enhanced sensitivity observed is mainly due to the removal of background (matrix) interference by the two-dimensional approach. Moreover, the 2D-GC approach also resulted in complete separation of 3-ethoxy-2-cyclohexenone and cinnamonitrile (co-eluting in Fig. 12.13).[11]

12.7   EPOXIDES

12.7.1   Method Description

For the analysis of epoxides, the same approach was used as for the Michael reaction acceptors. First, static headspace—GC-MS was applied. For the analytes that could not be detected, direct injection—GC-MS in combination with backflush or Deans switch 2D-GC was applied.

In Table 12.7, a selection of 17 epoxide target analytes is described. All these analytes were analyzed by liquid injection and by SHS-GC-MS using the conditions listed below. If the analytes could not be detected with the SHS method (at levels below 10 ppm), they were analyzed by a direct liquid injection method, as described in Sections 12.6 and 12.8.

TABLE 12.7 Selected Epoxide Target Analytes

Name	CAS n	RT (min)	Ions	Method
2-methyloxirane = propylene oxide	75-56-9	6.19	43, 58	SHS
1,2-epoxybutane = ethyloxirane	106-88-7	7.87	71, 41, 57	SHS
2,3-epoxy-2-methylbutane	5076-19-7	8.44	58, 41, 43	SHS
2-propyloxirane = 1,2-epoxypentane	1003-14-1	10.03	71, 41	SHS
2-oxiranylmethanol = glycidol	556-52-5	10.23	44, 43	**Direct**
epichlorohydrin	106-89-8	10.44	57, 27	SHS
glycidyl isopropyl ether	4016-14-2	13.42	43, 59	SHS
methyl 2-methylglycidate	58653-97-7	13.52	43, 57, 84	SHS
cyclohexene oxide	286-20-4	13.96	83, 41, 54	SHS
exo-2,3-epoxynorbornane	3146-39-2	15.68	81, 39, 54	SHS
glycidyl acrylate	106-90-1	15.92	55, 27	SHS
2-(4-fluorophenyl)oxirane	18511-62-1	17.33	137, 119	SHS
styrene oxide	96-09-3	17.37	119, 91	SHS
1-phenylpropylene oxide (S,S)	4518-66-5	17.97	90, 105, 133	SHS
(2,3-epoxypropyl)benzene	4436-24-2	18.52	91, 134, 105	SHS
ethyl 3-methyl-3-phenylglycidate I	77-83-8	21.62	132, 104, 205	**Direct**
ethyl 3-methyl-3-phenylglycidate II	77-83-8	23.05	132, 104, 205	**Direct**
2-(4-nitrophenyl)oxirane (R)	78038-43-4	23.40	89, 118, 148	**Direct**

12.7.2 Analytical Conditions

Sample preparation was identical to the methods described in Sections 12.6 and 12.8. For SHS, 50 mg API is dissolved in 2 mL DMSO/water (1/1).

12.7.2.1 SHS-GC-MS Parameters
Static headspace was performed at 80°C during 15 min. One milliliter headspace was injected in split mode (split ratio 1/10) in a PTV inlet with a Tenax TA packed liner.

PTV inlet temperature program: 50°C (0.1 min)—720°C/min—250°C, CO_2 cooling
GC-MS conditions:
Column: 60 m × 0.25 mm i.d. × 1.4 μm D_f DB-VRX (Agilent Technologies)
Carrier gas: Helium, 1.2 mL/min constant flow (with QuickSwap at 28 kPa)
Oven: 50°C (0.1 min)—8°C/min—150°C—25°C/min—250°C (7.5 min)
Detection: MS in simultaneous SIM/SCAN mode
Scan range: 27–350 m/z
Selected ions (SIM): see Table 12.7, dwell times: 100 ms
Solvent delay: 3.5 min

12.7.3 Results

The target analytes listed in Table 12.7 were all analyzed by liquid injection first, using the GC-MS conditions described above. All analytes are GC amenable and the retention times are included in the table.

Next, SHS-GC-MS was applied. As for the Michael reaction acceptors, better peak shape and sensitivity was obtained using a PTV inlet for the SHS injection. The optimum initial PTV temperature was 50°C.

Most of the analytes could be detected at LODs below 1 ppm. These analytes are marked with SHS in the method column. Using SHS-GC-MS, three compounds were not detected: glycidol, ethyl-3-methyl-3-phenylglycidate (both isomers), and 2-(4-nitrophenyl)oxirane. The last two higher molecular weight compounds do not elute. Glycidol, on the other hand, elutes relatively early, but the presence of the hydroxyl-function makes this analyte less volatile for headspace analysis and more difficult to analyze by GC. For these analytes, a method based on direct injection was used. For glycidol, derivatization was also performed, using the same method conditions as applied for haloalcohols.[11]

12.8 HALOALCOHOLS

12.8.1 Method Description

During the method development for alkyl halides (Section 12.4), it was observed that some polar halogenated compounds, such as 2-iodoethanol, could not be extracted from an API solution using headspace techniques, and/or that poor peak shape and low repeatability/linearity were obtained (see compound 19, Figs. 12.4 and 12.5). Other haloalcohols were also tested, but SHS-GC-MS or SPME-GC-MS methods could not be successfully applied. Furthermore, no suitable in situ derivatization method could be developed that could be successfully combined with headspace analysis (SHS or HS-SPME).

Haloalcohols are generally amenable to analysis by GC, and therefore direct analysis by GC could be considered. For trace-level analysis, however, better data in terms of repeatability, sensitivity, and robustness are obtained if the hydroxyl-function is derivatized. This is easily done by silylation (formation of trimethylsilyl-ethers), but silylation reactions are normally performed in nonaqueous media, and removal of residual reagent (or derivatisation by-products) can be difficult. Silylation followed by direct liquid injection and GC-MS analysis was found to work well for different haloalcohols, but since the derivatized analytes are quite volatile, interferences from the residual reagent and derivatization by-products was observed. Moreover, in contrast to HS techniques, a complex mixture is introduced in the analytical system containing derivatized analytes, excess reagent, reaction by-products, and (derivatized) API. All this (plus more abundant impurities and/or degradation compounds of the API) can interfere with PGI/GI determination, and, moreover, contaminate the analytical system (GC column, MS detector). For this reason, heart-cutting two-dimensional GC was evaluated as an alternative.[11] The analytical set-up for this approach is shown in Figure 12.14.

A concentrated solution of the API was injected (in split/splitless inlet) on an apolar first dimension column (column 1). Inlet pressure was set at 170 kPa, and outlet pressure at the CFT Deans switch device was 120 kPa. This results in a flow of about 1 mL/min through column 1. The flow from the additional electronic

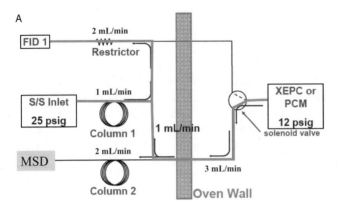

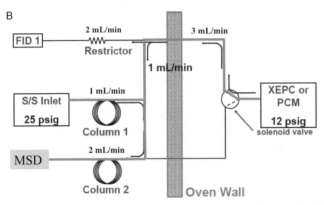

Figure 12.14   Deans switch 2D-GC-MS set-up for the analysis of GI/PGI in API by direct injection. (A) column 1 effluent diverted to monitor FID; (B) heart-cut fraction to column 2.

pressure module connected to the Deans switch device (XEPC or PCM) was 3 mL/min. A three-way valve, located outside the oven (and not in contact with the sample), diverts this flow to the lower part of the CFT device, to column 2 (2 mL/min), and adds 1 mL/min to the exit flow of column 1 (Fig. 12.14A). In this mode, the early eluting fraction containing the solvent and excess derivatization reagent was sent to a monitor FID detector (combined flow = 2 mL/min), no effluent of column 1 enters column 2.

Immediately prior to the elution of the fraction containing the PGI/GI analytes, the three-way valve was switched. The flow from the Deans switch EPC was diverted to the top of the Deans switch device, and the fraction of interest was heart-cut to the second dimension column (Fig. 12.14B). In the heart-cut mode, no effluent of column 1 was sent to the FID detector; instead, the fraction of interest was quantitatively transferred to column 2 (held in a separate low thermal mass column oven).

After the heart-cut, the remaining fraction eluting from the first column was again diverted to the monitor FID (mode: Fig. 12.14A) or can be backflushed. The target analytes within the heart cut fraction were then further separated on the second dimension column from other potentially interfering impurities and detected by MS (scan/SIM mode). In this way, the main analytes (API, derivatisation reagents, solvent, etc) are not introduced in the second column, avoiding overloading and contamination of this column and of the MS source. The use of the separate low thermal mass oven enables an independent temperature control of the second dimension column, and consequently more flexibility in method optimization.

The heart-cutting was applied to several haloalcohol analytes (2-chloroethanol, 2-bromoethanol, 2-iodoethanol, 4-chloro-1-butanol, 2-(2-chloroethoxy)ethanol, and 11-bromo-1-undecanol), and to glycidol, an epoxide that could not be analyzed by the methods described in Section 12.7. The same method can also be applied for less volatile epoxides and Michael reaction acceptors.[11]

12.8.2 Analytical Conditions

12.8.2.1 Sample Preparation The following sample/standard preparations were made in order to evaluate method suitability.

Carbamazepine was dissolved in dry pyridine at 50 mg/mL. From this solution, 100 μL (=5 mg carbamazepine) was placed in a 2 mL vial and spiked with 5 μL of a 1 ng/μL PGI/GI test mixture (=5 ng PGI, corresponding to 1 ppm). Then, 100 μL Bis (Trimethylsilyl) trifluoroacetamide (BSTFA) was added. The vial was heated at 70°C for 30 min. After cooling, 500 μL dichloromethane and 500 μL water were added. The mixture was vortexed, and injection (1 μL in splitless mode) was performed from the lower organic layer. This sample preparation could be fully automated on an MPS2 autosampler.

12.8.2.2 2D-GC-MS Parameters The analysis was performed on a GC-MS equipped with a split/splitless inlet, an FID, a capillary flow technology Deans switch, a LTM oven, and a MSD detector, using the following parameters:

Injection: 1 μL in splitless mode, 250°C
Column 1: 30 m × 0.25 mm i.d. × 0.25 μm D_f HP-5MS (in GC oven)
Column 2: 30 m × 0.25 mm i.d. × 0.25 μm D_f DB-17 (in LTM oven)
Carrier gas: Helium, 170 kPa at inlet (1 mL/min for column 1 at 50°C)—
    120 kPa at Deans switch (2 mL/min for column 2 at 50°C)
GC oven temperature: 50°C (1 min)—20°C/min—300°C (20 min)
LTM oven temperature: 50°C (11 min)—10°C/min—140°C (4 min)—25°C/
    min—300°C (3.1 min)
Monitor detector: FID, 300°C, 30 mL/min H_2, 400 L/min air
Main detection: MS in simultaneous SIM/SCAN mode
Scan range: 45–350 m/z
Selected ions (SIM) (100 ms dwell times), see Table 12.8

12.8.3 Results

The application of Deans switching is illustrated by the analysis of the silylated derivatives of two haloalcohols (bromoethanol, iodoethanol) and an epoxide (glycidol,

TABLE 12.8 Figures of Merit for 2D-GC-MS Analysis of Haloalcohols and Glycidol

Haloalcohols[a]	Ion	r^{2b}	RSD (%)			LOD[c]
			1 ppm	5 ppm	10 ppm	ppm
glycidol	59, 101	0.999	5.4	4.8	7.0	0.34
2-chloroethanol	93, 137, 73	0.998	7.5	8.2	9.1	0.15
2-bromoethanol	137, 139, 181, 183	0.999	2.5	3.1	3.0	0.17
2-iodoethanol	185, 229	1.000	1.2	2.6	3.2	0.06
4-chloro-1-butanol	93, 123, 165	1.000	2.2	2.4	2.8	0.10
2-(2-chloroethoxy)ethanol	73, 93, 137, 181	0.998	9.8	7.1	1.5	0.16
11-bromo-1-undecanol	97, 169, 83, 75	0.999	13.0	10.6	8.2	0.38

[a] As TMS-derivatives.

[b] r^2 from 6 replicates at 1, 5, and 10 ppm.

[c] LOD in ppm calculated for S/N = 3.

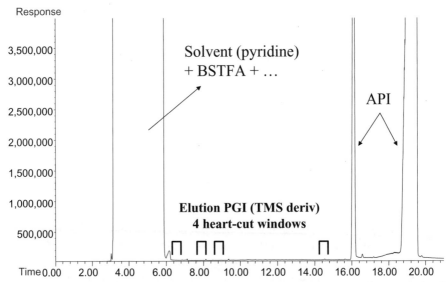

Figure 12.15   FID monitor detector trace from first dimension separation of the analysis of haloalcohols and glycidol in API (carbamazepine) by 2D-GC-MS.

2,3-epoxy-1-propanol) in carbamazepine. The first dimension separation was done on an apolar HP-5MS column (in GC oven). The profile obtained on a monitor FID detector after this first dimension is shown in Figure 12.15.

The PGIs cannot be detected (present at 50 pg), while solvent, residual silylating agent and API (also derivatized) overload this column. The target analytes eluting between 8 and 14 min were heart-cut using small heart-cut windows around the peak elution times (typically retention time +/− 0.1 min). The retention times of

Abundance

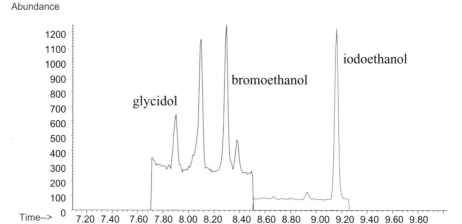

Figure 12.16 Extracted ion chromatogram from second dimension GC-MS analysis of haloalcohols and glycidol in API (carbamazepine) by 2D-GC-MS.

the target analytes were monitored from a scouting run without heart-cutting through injection of a high-concentrated solution of the analytes in question.

The fractions are further analyzed on the second dimension column. The chromatogram in Figure 12.16 (extracted ion chromatogram from SIM acquisition) shows the detection of 2-bromo-ethanol, 2-iodo-ethanol and glycidol as their silylated derivatives, free from interferences.

The method was validated,[11] and the results are summarized in Table 12.8. The linearity was very good ($r^2 > 0.99$) in the range from 1–10 ppm, the RSDs are below 10%, except for the late eluting bromo-undecanol (RSD: 10–15%). The LODs were below 0.5 ppm, which is also better than obtained by direct liquid injection and one-dimensional GC-MS. The 2D-GC approach is thus very useful for problem cases where no headspace extraction is possible.

12.9   AZIRIDINES

12.9.1   Method Description

Initial attempts to apply GC were unsuccessful. Problems encountered included peak tailing, often compounded by a generally low response. Thus, the focus was therefore moved to the development of suitable LC-MS methodology. Initially, electrospray ionization, operating in the selected ion monitoring (SIM) mode, was examined.

It is, of course, possible to develop a specific method through the application of selective sample preparation methods based on (micro-) liquid–liquid extraction or solid phase extraction. However, the purpose of our work was to develop a standardized approach to such analysis, and hence it was necessary to avoid such specific, individual approaches. Thus, direct injection was employed. As with GC,

TABLE 12.9 Selected Aziridine Target Analytes

Peak	Name	CAS Nr	MW	LC mode	SIM ion
1	1-(2-cyanoethyl)aziridine	1072-66-8	96	HILIC	97.2
2	1-isobutyrylaziridine	20286-12-8	113	HILIC	114.2
3	Cis-2,3-diphenyl-1-propylaziridine	314062-46-9	237	RPLC	238.1
4	2-aziridin-1-yl-1-(4-nitrophenyl)-ethanol	21719-28-8	208	RPLC	209.1

the introduction of a concentrated solution of API into an LC system can be hugely problematic, causing both interference and ion suppression. It was quickly established that it is not possible to develop a single HPLC method that is applicable to all analyses. We therefore developed in parallel a number of HPLC methods based on two columns, each with (minimum) two mobile phase combinations, resulting in 4 methods that can be applied in an automated sequence during method selection/ optimization. The instrument diagram is shown in Figure 12.3. In this way, scouting runs can be made to select the optimal column/phase combination for a given set of PGIs/GIs in a given API. Either, two reversed phase HPLC columns (e.g. C18 + phenyl) or a RP-LC and hydrophobic interaction liquid chromatography (HILIC) method can be combined. HILIC is very complementary to RP-LC, especially for more polar analytes that elute after the (less polar) API.

The RP-LC/HILIC approach was applied for the analysis of four aziridines. The selected test analytes are shown in Table 12.9.

12.9.2 Analytical Conditions

12.9.2.1 Sample Preparation The following sample/standard preparations were made in order to evaluate method suitability.

A 100 mg/mL solution was prepared in either acetonitrile (HILIC) or water/ acetonitrile 90/10 (v/v, RPLC). The mixture was placed in an ultrasonic bath for 5 min to complete extraction and dissolution. Some samples were not completely dissolved, but the selected aziridines were easily solubilized and extracted. The sample was centrifuged and/or filtered if necessary.

Spiked sample solutions can be prepared from a standard solution of the aziridines. To obtain a 1 ppm spiked sample, 100 ng (10 μL of 10 ng/μL solution) was added to the sample at a concentration of 100 mg/mL.

12.9.2.2 HPLC-MS Parameters
RPLC Method
Column: Altima HP C18 column, 15 cm × 3 mm ID × 3 μm, (Grace, Lokeren, Belgium)
Column temperature: 30°C
Injection: 50 μL
Mobile phase A: 0.1% ammonium acetate + 0.1% acetic acid in water

Mobile phase B: acetonitrile.
RPLC gradient: 10% B to 100% B at 10 min (5 min hold)
Flow rate: 0.5 mL/min.
MSD: ESI, positive ion detection mode, SIM acquisition
RPLC method: 350°C drying gas, 12 L/min, 40 psig pressure, cap V: 3.6 kV
SIM ions: see Table 12.9.

HILIC Method
Column: Prevail Silica HILIC column, 15 cm × 4.6 mm ID × 3 μm, (Grace),
Column temperature: 20°C
Injection: 50 μL
Mobile phase A: 0.1% ammonium acetate + 0.1% acetic acid in water
Mobile phase B: acetonitrile.
HILIC gradient: 100% B (2 min hold) to 50% B at 15 min (1 min hold)
Flow rate: 1 mL/min
MSD: ESI, positive ion detection mode, SIM acquisition
HILIC method: 320°C drying gas, 12 L/min, 45 psig pressure, cap V: 2.8 kV
SIM ions: see Table 12.9.

Note that for both methods, the same solvents (A and B) are used. This allows automatic switching between methods in a sequence if a column selection valve is installed (Fig. 12.3).

For the analytes listed in Table 12.9 and the tested APIs, these conditions resulted in sufficient selectivity. It might be needed to adapt the gradients for other analytes and matrices.

12.9.3 Results

The chromatograms (EIC from SIM) for a Vitamin C sample, dissolved at 100 mg/ mL in acetonitrile/water (9/1), and spiked at 1 ppm level with the 4 analytes, are presented in Figure 12.17. Test compounds 1 (1-(2-cyanoethyl) aziridine) and 2 (1-isobutyrylaziridine), were not retained on RP-LC, and thus were instead analyzed using the orthogonal HILIC method. Excellent peak shapes were obtained.

Test analytes 3 (Cis-2,3-diphenyl-1-propylaziridine) and 4 (2-aziridin-1-yl-1 (4-nitrophenyl)-ethanol), on the other hand, showed more retention in RP-LC. No interferences from the API or other impurities (present a higher level) were observed.

For all analytes, excellent signal-to-noise ratios were obtained using either approach. LODs were well below 0.1 ppm. Only compound 4 (2-aziridin-1-yl-1(4-nitrophenyl)-ethanol) showed a lower response. Peak broadening (using the RPLC method) was also observed for this analyte; this is probably due to the acid/base characteristics of this analyte.

The RPLC and HILIC methods were subsequently validated. The linearity was good ($r^2 > 0.99$) in the range from 0.1 to 20 ppm for the RPLC method, and $r^2 > 0.97$ in the range from 0.1 to 2 ppm for the HILIC method. At higher concentrations, deviation was observed for the HILIC method, probably due to detector saturation. Sample dilution or reduced injection volume could be used here, since sensitivity is high.

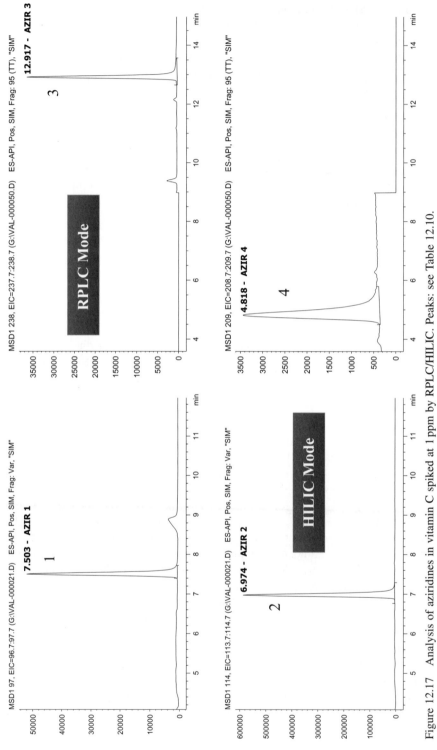

Figure 12.17 Analysis of aziridines in vitamin C spiked at 1 ppm by RPLC/HILIC. Peaks: see Table 12.10.

12.10   ARYLAMINES AND AMINOPYRIDINES

12.10.1   Method Description

A similar approach to that applied to aziridines was also applied to the analysis of arylamines and aminopyridines.[12] The list of selected target analytes is shown in Table 12.10.

In this case, direct analysis of these target analytes was done using reversed-phase LC methods. For the analytes with low retention in RPLC (mostly those with primary amine functions and no alkyl group), precolumn derivatization was used. The primary amine function was reacted with hexylchloroformate to form a $-NH-CO-O-C_6H_{13}$ derivative. This improves detectability (M + 128 = higher mass ion) and retention in RPLC due to the hydrophobicity of the hexyl group.

A set of methods was developed that allows the analysis of different aryl-amines and aminopyridines in different APIs at less than 1 ppm level. Two columns (C18 and phenyl) were used, and for each column, four gradients (combinations of solvents A1/B1, A1/B2, A2/B1, and A2/B2) could be applied to optimize the selectivity of the separation between API and the PGIs/GIs. A concentrated solution of the API was injected, and detection was performed using a single quadrupole mass spectrometer in the selected ion monitoring (SIM) mode. Each sample was analyzed with and without derivatization.

12.10.2   Analytical Conditions

12.10.2.1   Sample Preparation   The following sample/standard preparations were made in order to evaluate method suitability.

TABLE 12.10   Selected Target Analytes for Arylamine and Aminopyridine Analysis

Peak	Analyte	CAS No	Retention[a]	MW	MW der[b]
1	1-phenylpiperazine	92-54-6	Yes	162	290
2	N,N-dimethyl-m-toluidine	121-72-2	Yes	135	—
3	5-amino-2-Chloropyridine	5350-93-6	Yes	128	256
4	4-aminopyridine	504-24-5	No	94	222
5	4-amino-2-methylpyridine	18437-58-6	No	108	236
6	3-aminobenzonitrile	2237-30-1	Yes	118	246
7	2-aminophenol	95-55-6	No	109	237
8	5-amino-2-methylpyridine	3430-14-6	No	108	236
9	4-methyl acetanilide	103-89-9	Yes	149	—
10	3-aminopyridine	462-08-8	No	94	222
11	5-fluoro-2-methyl aniline	367-29-3	Yes	125	253
12	N-ethyl anthranilic acid	89-50-0	Yes	165	293
13	5-aminoindole	5192-03-0	No	132	260
14	Aniline	62-53-3	No	93	221

[a] Retention under standard RPLC conditions: yes = well retained (retention factor k > 3).

[b] MW after hexylchloroformate derivatization.

The API was prepared at 100 mg/mL concentration in acetonitrile. Internal standard and spiking solutions (for instance 10 μL of 10 ng/μL PGI/GI) were added to this sample. The injected concentration of the PGI/GI corresponds to 0.1 ng/μL.

Solubilization was accelerated by using ultrasonic treatment during 5 min. An aliquot of this sample was filtered and analyzed directly (=nonderivatiszed PGI/GI method).

From the same solution, 1 mL was added to 9 mL borate solution (15 mM sodium tetraborate, adjusted to pH 9.5 with sodium hydroxide 1N) in a 20 mL vial. Next, 0.5 mL hexachloroformate solution (2% in acetonitrile) was added. Reaction was performed at room temperature during 30 min. Finally, 0.2 mL of phosphoric acid solution (85%) was added to stop the reaction and neutralize the mixture. This mixture was analyzed for the derivatised PGIs/GIs.

12.10.2.2 HPLC-MS Parameters

Column A: Zorbax Eclipse Plus C18, 150 mm L × 3.0 mm ID, 3.5 μm particle size (Agilent Technologies)

Column B: Zorbax Eclipse XDB Phenyl, 150 mm L × 3.0 mm ID, 3.5 μm particle size (Agilent Technologies)

Column temperature: 30°C

Injection volume: 5 μL (underivatized sample)—50 μL (derivatized sample)

Mobile phase: A1 = 0.05% v/v formic acid in water, B1 = acetonitrile

(A2: 10 mM ammonium formate in water, B2: methanol)

Gradient 1: from 5% B1 to 100% B1 at 10 min (4 min hold)

(other gradients: see text and Vanhoenacker et al.[12])

Flow: 0.5 mL/min

MSD: ESI, positive ion detection mode, SIM acquisition

Nitrogen drying gas: 350°C, 12 L/min,

Nebulizer pressure: 35 psig

Capillary voltage: 4 kV

SIM ions: see Table 12.11

The difference in injection volume takes into account the dilution during the derivatization step. For the nonderivatized and derivatized sample, the same quantity of API is injected.

12.10.3 Results

The chromatograms (extracted ion chromatograms) obtained for a nonderivatized and derivatized sample of ephedrine spiked at 1 ppm level with the target analytes are shown in Figures 12.18 and 12.19, respectively. The peak identification, retention times and measured ions (SIM) are listed in Table 12.11. The 7 target analytes that have sufficient retention using standard RPLC conditions (C18 column, gradient 1) are well detected. The seven target analytes that initially showed low retention in RPLC, are better retained, and easily detected in the API after derivatization. Some analytes (such as target analyte 3, 5-amino-2-chloropyridine) can be detected in both analyses.

TABLE 12.11   Retention Times, Selected SIM Ions, and Recovery for Arylamines and Aminopyridines in Ephedrine

Peak	Analyte	Nonderivatized			Derivatized		
		RT (min)	Ion	Rec[a]	RT (min)	Ion	Rec[a]
1	1-phenylpiperazine	5.54	163	51.4			
2	N,N-dimethyl-m-toluidine	5.85	136	90.9			
3	5-amino-2-chloropyridine	6.15	129	80.4	*11.25*	*257*	
4	4-aminopyridine				7.02	223	94.2
5	4-amino-2-methylpyridine				7.19	237	67.2
6	3-aminobenzonitrile	7.29	119	81.4			
7	2-aminophenol				7.34	238	94.1
8	5-amino-2-methylpyridine				7.34	237	93.1
9	4-methyl acetanilide	7.77	150	76.5			
10	3-aminopyridine				7.88	223	34.1
11	5-fluoro-2-methyl aniline	8.39	126	78.9			
12	N-ethyl anthranilic acid	8.80	166	86.7			
13	5-aminoindole				10.80	261	65.1
14	Aniline				11.61	222	99.4

[a] Recovery (accuracy) measured as response relative to external standard.

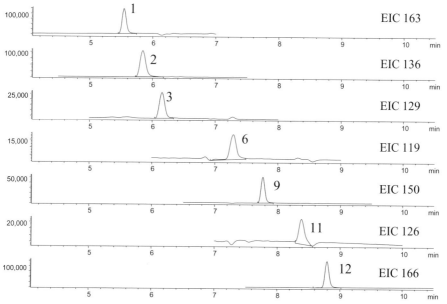

Figure 12.18   Analysis of nonderivatized arylamines and aminopyridines in ephedrine spiked at 1 ppm by RPLC-MS. Peaks: see Table 12.12.

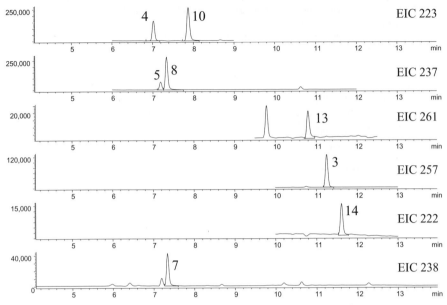

Figure 12.19 Analysis of derivatized arylamines and aminopyridines in ephedrine spiked at 1 ppm by RPLC-MS. Peaks: see Table 12.12.

The responses for the compounds were compared with the responses for the injection of the same concentration of target analytes in a 0.1 ng/μL standard solution without API (same injected amount of PGI/GI), and the obtained recoveries (%, =[area target analyte in API/area in standard solution] × 100) are also given in Table 12.11.

For the analysis of the nonderivatized samples, good recoveries (between 75% and 100%) were obtained using the standard reversed phase (column A) conditions for all of the analytes except for 1-phenylpiperazine (51%). For this analyte, the analysis on column B (phenyl phase) resulted in better recovery.[12]

For the analysis of the derivatized samples, recoveries were between 65% and 100%, except for 3-aminopyridine. Also for this analyte, better recovery was obtained using the phenyl column.[12]

These lower recoveries are often due to ion suppression by co-eluting API or other impurities (at higher concentration). This was clearly observed for the analysis of 5-aminoindole (analyte 13) in bromhexine API. The extracted ion chromatogram (ion 261) of a bromhexine sample spiked at 1 ppm level, derivatized and analyzed using method A (C18 column, gradient 1 using A1/B1 solvents), is shown in Figure 12.20A. The target analyte elutes at 10.8 min, but is hardly visible in the chromatogram. By changing the gradient to solvents A1/B2 (methanol instead of acetonitrile, 10% B2 to 100% in 10 min, 4 min hold), the chromatogram shown in Figure 12.20B

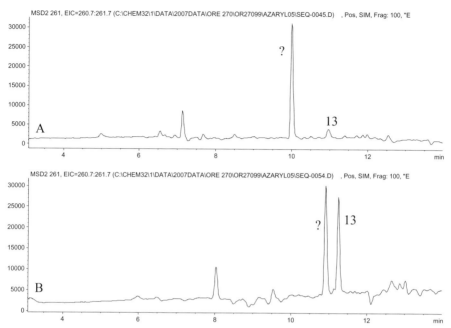

Figure 12.20 Analysis of derivatized arylamines and aminopyridines in bromhexine spiked at 1 ppm by RPLC-MS. Analysis using default method (formic acid in water + acetonitrile gradient). Analysis using modified method (formic acid in water + methanol gradient).

was obtained. The target analyte now elutes at 11.5 min and can clearly be detected. This example illustrates that selectivity tuning can be necessary with some combinations of PGIs/GIs and APIs. It should also be noted, as illustrated by the presence of another significant peak of an unknown impurity detected both in Figure 12.20A and B, that detection by single quadrupole MS in SIM mode has limited selectivity. This unknown compound also elutes in the same elution window and gives the same mass ion. Where such matrix interference occurs, the use of MS/MS (by triple quadrupole MS systems, for instance) may be required in order to achieve the required sensitivity.

12.11 HYDRAZINES

12.11.1 Method Description

A similar approach as described for the arylamines was applied for the analysis of hydrazines. These analytes, having a free primary amine function, were also analyzed after derivatization using hexylchloroformate, resulting in N-acyl derivatives

TABLE 12.12 Selected Hydrazine Target Analytes

Peak Nr	Name (CAS)	CAS	MW$_{original}$	MW$_{derivative}$
1	1-Methylhydrazine	60-34-4	46	174
2	Acetohydrazide	1068-57-1	74	202
3	2-Hydrazinoethanol	109-84-2	76	204
4	Phenylhydrazine	100-63-0	108	236

showing higher retention in RP-LC and better detectability by MS. The selected target analytes are listed in Table 12.12.

12.11.2 Analytical Conditions

12.11.2.1 Sample Preparation The following sample/standard preparations were made in order to evaluate method suitability.

APIs (Vitamin C, Penicillin V) were dissolved at 100 mg/mL in acetonitrile and spiked with 1-methylhydrazine, acetohydrazide, 2-hydroxyethanol, and phenylhydrazine at 1 ppm level. To the sample, 7 mL borate buffer (15 mM sodium tetraborate, pH 9.5 in 10% acetonitrile) was added, followed by 0.5 mL hexylchloroformate solution (2% in acetonitrile). After reaction during 15 min at room temperature, the reaction was stopped by adding 0.5 mL phosphoric acid (17% in water) and injection was performed.

12.11.2.2 HPLC-MS Parameters

Column: Zorbax Eclipse Plus C18, 150 mm L × 3.0 mm ID, 3.5 μm particle size (Agilent Technologies)
Column temperature: 35°C
Injection volume: 50 μL
Mobile phase: A1 = 0.05% formic acid, B1 = acetonitrile
Gradient: from 15% B1 to 100% B1 at 19 min
Flow: 0.5 mL/min
MSD: ESI, positive ion detection mode, SIM acquisition
Nitrogen drying gas: 340°C, 12 L/min
Nebulizer pressure: 35 psig
Capillary voltage: 4 kV
SIM ions: M + 1 ions at m/e 175, 203, 205, and 237 were monitored.
Alternative methods were also validated for additional selectivity and separation between API and PGI/GI. These methods included:
Column B: Zorbax Eclipse XDB Phenyl, 150 mm L × 3.0 mm ID, 3.5 μm particle size (Agilent Technologies)
Mobile phase A2: 10 mM ammonium acetate
Mobile phase B2: methanol

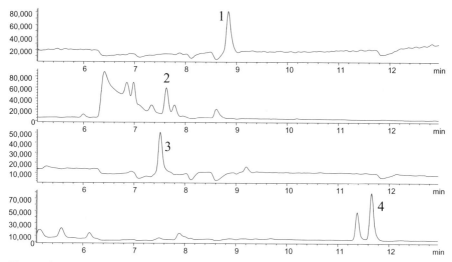

Figure 12.21   Analysis of hydrazines in vitamin C spiked at 1 ppm level by derivatisation—RPLC. Analytes: see Table 12.13.

12.11.3   Results

The chromatogram (EICs from SIM) obtained for the analysis of a Vitamin C sample spiked at 1 ppm level with the four selected analytes is shown in Figure 12.21.

All four analytes were detected at the 1ppm level. Analyte 2 (acetohydrazine) was not fully resolved from other impurities. In such circumstances, further confirmatory analysis employing for example MS/MS may be appropriate. Alternatively, the method may be revised. This can be achieved using a HPLC configuration equipped with two columns and four solvents, as illustrated in Figure 12.3, through an automated sequence.

The repeatability of this derivatization method was better than 10% RSD, and the derivatization was linear ($r^2 > 0.99$) in a range from 0.25 to 5 ppm.

Another example is shown in Figure 12.22. A Penicillin V sample, also spiked at 1 ppm level, was analyzed by the default method (C18 column, formic acid/acetonitrile). The extracted ion chromatogram for phenylhydrazine (analyte 4) is shown in Figure 12.22A.

The peak just elutes after another peak detected at m/e 237 and is largely suppressed (recovery <10%). The same sample was reinjected using the Phenyl column and an ammonium formate (A2)/acetonitrile (B1) gradient (10% B1 to 100% B1 at 19 min). The EIC at 237 is shown in Figure 12.22B. The analyte elutes at 10.75 min, while the interference is shifted to a longer retention time. Phenylhydrazine can be detected and recovery was >90%.

This example again shows how selectivity can be effectively and quickly modified using the instrument set-up described in Figure 12.3.

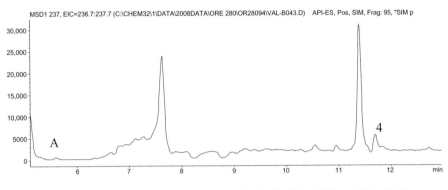

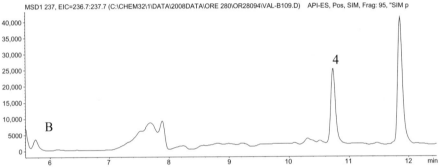

Figure 12.22 Analysis of phenylhydrazine in penicillin V spiked at 1 ppm level by derivatisation—RPLC. (A) Analysis using default method (C18 column, formic acid in water + acetonitrile gradient). (B) Analysis using modified method (Phenyl column, ammonium formate + acetonitrile gradient).

12.12 ALDEHYDES AND KETONES

12.12.1 Method Description

Aldehydes and ketones can be analyzed either by GC or with LC. Method selection is thus based on ease-of-use of the method, robustness, and possible automation. Generally, for aldehydes and ketones this issue is not one of the separation itself but the difficulty of detection. Formaldehyde, for instance, elutes very fast in GC-MS, and no specific ions are present for sensitive and selective detection. In LC-MS, detection is also difficult, especially for low MW aldehydes/ketones. Therefore, derivatization of aldehydes and ketones is often applied to enhance detectability, both in GC and LC.

In our study, precolumn derivatization using 2,4-dinitrophenylhydrazine (DNPH) was applied for analytes with carbonyl functionality. This method allowed the analysis of relatively volatile analytes (e.g. C1-C10 aldehydes) and less volatile analytes (e.g. 4-hydroxybenzaldehyde) using the same method. Isotopically labeled aldehydes were used as internal standards (IS1, IS2 and IS3) to improve the repeatability and accuracy of the method.

TABLE 12.13 Selected Aldehyde Target Analytes

Peak	Name (CAS)	CAS No.	$MW_{original}$	$MW_{derivative}$
1	Formaldehyde	50-00-0	30	210
2	Propionaldehyde	123-38-6	58	238
3	Hexanal	66-25-1	100	280
4	Nonanal	124-19-1	142	322
5	4-Hydroxybenzaldehyde	123-08-0	122	302
6	4-Cyanobenzaldehyde	105-07-7	131	311
7	2,3-Dimethylbenzaldehyde	5779-93-1	134	314
8	3,4-Dimethylbenzaldehyde	5973-71-7	134	314
9	4-Hydroxy-3-methylbenzaldehyde	15174-69-3	136	316
IS1	Formaldehyde-13C,d2		33	213
IS2	Propionaldehyde-2,2-d2		60	240
IS3	4-Hydroxybenzaldehyde-2,3,5,6-d4		126	306

The selected target analytes and some commercially available internal standards are listed in Table 12.13.

12.12.2 Analytical Conditions

12.12.2.1 Sample Preparation
The following sample/standard preparations were made in order to evaluate method suitability.

The sample was dissolved in a mixture of methanol/acetonitrile/water (2/1/1) at 50 mg/mL.

Derivatization was automated in the Agilent 1100/1200 series ALS. Internal standard was added at 0.5 ppm level. From the sample solution, 4 µL was drawn in the sampler, followed by 1 µL DNPH solution (500 mg 2,4-dinitrophenylhydrazine is dissolved in 10 mL methanol, 1 mL conc. sulfuric acid is added and the solution is diluted to 50 mL with methanol, resulting concentration: 1%).

12.12.2.2 HPLC-MS Parameters
Column: Zorbax Stablebond Phenyl column, 150 mm L × 3.0 mm ID, 3.5 µm particle size (Agilent Technologies)
Column temperature: 40°C
Injection volume: 5 µL (with injector program)
Draw 4 µL sample
Add 1 µL DNPH reagent
Mix
Wait 4 min
Mix
Inject
Mobile phase: A = 10 mM ammonium acetate in water, B = acetonitrile
Gradient: from 36% B to 100% B at 12.5 min, 3.5 min hold
Flow: 0.65 mL/min

MSD: ESI, negative ion detection mode, SIM acquisition
Nitrogen drying gas: 330°C, 11 L/min,
Nebulizer pressure: 50 psig
Capillary voltage: 3.5 kV
SIM ions: M-1 ions were monitored (Table 12.13)

12.12.3 Results

Figures 12.23 and 12.24 show the analysis of a 0.1 ng/μL standard solution of, respectively, the aliphatic and aromatic selected aldehyde analytes. This concentration corresponds to 2 ppm relative to the API (50 mg sample). All compounds, including the internal standards, are easily detected. The most volatile aldehyde (formaldehyde) can also be detected at this level without API interference. The retention times for the analytes are given in Table 12.14.

The method was validated using several API. Aliphatic aldehydes were assayed using IS1 and IS2, aromatic aldehydes using IS3.

In general, good linearity ($r^2 > 0.99$) was observed in a concentration range from 0.5 to 10 ppm. Repeatability (RSD) was better than 10% at 1 ppm level. The recoveries for the analytes (accuracy) were determined in Vitamin C and ephedrine (spiked at 1 ppm) versus a standard solution, and are listed in Table 12.14. In most cases, recoveries were between 80% and 120%, except for 4-hydroxy-3-methylbenzaldehyde in Vitamin C. In this case, significant ion suppression was observed, thus revision of the method conditions would be required to successfully analyze the analyte in question.

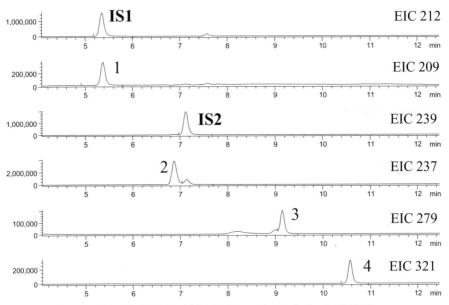

Figure 12.23 Analysis of aliphatic aldehydes in standard solution by DNPH derivatisation—RPLC. Analytes: see Table 12.14.

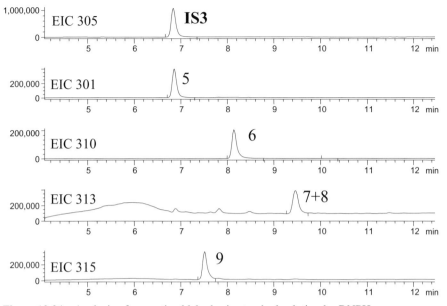

Figure 12.24   Analysis of aromatic aldehydes in standard solution by DNPH derivatisation—RPLC. Analytes: see Table 12.14.

TABLE 12.14   Retention Times, SIM Ions, and Recovery for Aldehydes Spiked in Vitamin C and Ephedrine

Peak	Name (CAS)	RT (min)	Ion	Recovery % (Vit C)	Recovery % (ephedrine)
1	Formaldehyde	5.37	209	a	110
2	Propionaldehyde	7.14	237	83	96
3	Hexanal	9.14	279	98	102
4	Nonanal	10.57	321	105	101
5	4-Hydroxybenzaldehyde	6.86	301	106	98
6	4-Cyanobenzaldehyde	8.14	310	121	108
7	2,3-Dimethylbenzaldehyde	9.46	313	124	103
8	3,4-Dimethylbenzaldehyde	9.46	313	(co-elutes with 7)	
9	4-OH-3-methylbenzaldehyde	7.51	315	18	97
IS1	d2,C13-Formaldehyde	5.35	212	—	—
IS2	d2-Propionaldehyde	7.12	239	—	—
IS3	d4-Hydroxybenzaldehyde	6.84	305	—	—

[a] Trace of formaldehyde was present in the vitamin C sample at the 10 ppm level. Hence no recovery value was calculated.

12.13 CONCLUSIONS

Through the studies described, it has been possible to develop a systematic approach applicable to the analysis of GIs that is based on the physicochemical properties of the class of GI concerned. This eliminates the need to develop individual compound-specific methods, resulting not only in a less empirical approach to method development, but also one that considerably reduces the time/effort spent on such activities. This strategy is outlined graphically in the chart shown in Figure 12.1.

In terms of the techniques employed, GC was used in preference, combined with, where possible, static headspace. This work has shown that such an approach can be used for the most volatile organohalides. Where such an approach was unsuccessful, techniques such as SPME and DHS were used to extend the headspace extraction to less volatile analytes, and also offer very high sensitivities. For non-volatile analytes, such as sulphonate esters and N-mustards, derivatization-SHS or derivatization-SPME were employed.

In some instances where headspace techniques could not be used, for example for haloalcohols, derivatization (silylation) followed by direct injection was employed. This was combined with heart-cutting 2D-GC to avoid analyte interference and MS source contamination.

Nonvolatile compounds were analyzed by LC-MS. An automated selectable column approach, using two reversed phase LC or a RP-LC/HILIC approach was used for aziridines, arylamines, and aminopyridines. Precolumn derivatization was successfully employed for analytes poorly retained by RP-LC. Derivatization was also found to be a useful to increase detectability in MS, as demonstrated by the analysis of aldehydes and hydrazines.

In conclusion, it has been possible to demonstrate that the analysis of GIs can be addressed systematically through the deployment of a small number of generic methods that not only dramatically reduce the time spent in method development, but also provide robust procedures that can be readily established within laboratories and where required transferred between facilities.

ACKNOWLEDGMENTS

The authors would like thank all the individuals and technical groups within AstraZeneca who contributed to the set up and running of this project, in particular Hans Jurgen Federsel and the members of Global Process R&D External Sciences Leadership Group.

REFERENCES

1. European Medicines Evaluation Agency, Committee for Medicinal Products for Human Use. 2006. *Guideline on the Limits of Genotoxic Impurities*. CPMP/SWP/5199/02, London, June 28, 2006. Available at http://www.emea.europa.eu/pdfs/human/swp/519902en.pdf (accessed September 20, 2010).

2. Muller L, Mauthe RJ, Riley CM, et al. 2006. A rationale for determining, testing and controlling specific impurities in Pharmaceuticals that possess potential for genotoxicity. *Regul. Toxicol. Pharmacol.* 44:198–211.

3. David F, Jacq K, Vanhoenacker G, Sandra P, et al. 2009. Method selection for trace analysis of genotoxic impurities in pharmaceuticals. *LC.GC Europe* 22(12):552.

4. Serafimova R, Fuart Gatnik M, Worth A. 2010. Review of QSAR Models and Software Tools for Predicting Genotoxicity and Carcinogenicity. JRC Scientific and Technical Reports, EUR 24427 EN —2010. Available at http://ecb.jrc.ec.europa.eu/DOCUMENTS/QSAR/EUR_24427_EN.pdf.

5. Elder DP, Lipczynski AM, Teasdale A. 2008. Control and analysis of alkyl and benzyl halides and other related organohalides as potential genotoxic impurities in active pharmaceutical ingredients (API). *J.Pharm. Biomed. Anal.* 48:497–507.

6. *DHS Brochure Gerstel GmbH.* Available at http://www.gerstel.com/en/dynamic-headspace.htm (accessed September 20, 2010).

7. Elder DP, Teasdale A, Lipczynski AM. 2008. Control and analysis of alkyl esters of alkyl and aryl sulfonic acids in novel pharmaceutical ingredients. *J. Pharm Biomed. Anal.* 46:1–8.

8. Alzaga R, Ryan RW, Taylor/Worth K, et al. 2007. A generic approach for the determination of residues of alkylating agents in active pharmaceutical ingredients by *in situ* derivatization-headspace-gas chromatography-mass spectrometry. *J. Pharm. Biomed. Anal.* 45:472–479.

9. Jacq K, Delaney E, Teasdale A, et al. 2008. Development and validation of an automated static headspace gas chromotography-mass spectrometry (SHS-GC-MS) method for monitoring the formation of ethyl methane sulfonate from ethanol and methane sulphonic acid. *J. Pharm. Biomed. Anal.* 48:1339–1344.

10. Klee MS. 2009. Optimizing capillary column backflush to improve cycle time and reduce column contamination. *J. Sep. Sci.* 32:88–98.

11. David F, Jacq K, Sandra P, et al. 2010. Analysis of potential genotoxic impurities in pharmaceuticals by two-dimensional gas chromatography with Deans switching and independent column temperature control using a low-thermal-mass oven module. *Anal. Bioanal. Chem.* 396:1291–1300.

12. Vanhoenacker G, Dumont E, David F, et al. 2009. Determination of arylamines and aminopyridines in pharmaceutical products using in-situ derivatization and liquid chromatography-mass spectrometry. *J. Chromatographr. A.* 1216:3563–3570.

CHAPTER 13

ANALYSIS OF GENOTOXIC IMPURITIES BY NUCLEAR MAGNETIC RESONANCE SPECTROSCOPY

Andrew Phillips

13.1 INTRODUCTION TO NMR

NMR is a familiar technique in the sphere of structure elucidation. In combination with mass spectrometry, the information present in an NMR spectrum can allow the full determination of unknown structures. Less well known is that NMR is increasingly playing a key role within the pharmaceutical industry for quantitative analysis.

NMR is an inherently insensitive technique, and therefore not the natural choice for trace analysis. However, if sufficient sensitivity can be achieved through the correct experimental setup or the development of new technology, NMR becomes a natural choice for GI analysis because of its structural specificity and quantitative nature.

The aim of this chapter is to describe the theory required to understand the advantages and challenges of GI analysis by NMR and present a number of salient examples.

For a more general background to NMR, the book *High-Resolution NMR Techniques in Organic Chemistry* by T.D.W. Claridge provides an excellent introduction.[1] A wealth of other useful background information can be found in books by leading NMR experts.[2–5]

13.2 WHY IS NMR AN INSENSITIVE TECHNIQUE?

13.2.1 Nuclear Spin

The nuclei of some atoms have an intrinsic property called nuclear spin angular momentum, which is characterized by the quantum number, I. This quantum number

Genotoxic Impurities: Strategies for Identification and Control, Edited by Andrew Teasdale
Copyright © 2010 by John Wiley & Sons, Inc.

takes half-integer values. Nuclei with $I = 0$ are NMR silent, such as carbon-12. Nuclei with $I > 1/2$ are NMR active, but often display "exotic" NMR properties, which result in effects such as very broad lines. Therefore, nuclei that are suitable for trace analysis have $I = 1/2$, for example ^{1}H and ^{19}F.

For a spin 1/2 nucleus, there are two possible quantum states, denoted α and β, that in a magnetic field have different energies. The energy difference, ΔE, increases with increasing magnetic field strength:

$$\Delta E = h\nu = \frac{h\gamma B_0}{2\pi}$$

where ν is the Larmor frequency in s^{-1}, γ is the gyromagnetic ratio in $rad\,s^{-1}T^{-1}$, and B_0 is the magnetic field the nucleus experiences in T.

13.2.2 Boltzmann Distribution

What is crucial here is that for a collection of similar nuclei, the total signal depends on the population difference between the α and β states—this is given by the Boltzmann distribution:

$$\frac{N_\alpha}{N_\beta} = e^{\Delta E/k_B T}$$

where $N_{\alpha,\beta}$ are the number of nuclei in that state, k_B is the Boltzmann constant, and T the temperature.

At the field strengths that are used in NMR at room temperature, this corresponds to a very small population difference—about 1 part in 10,000 for protons. This explains why NMR is such an insensitive technique.

The sensitivity depends on the nuclei used, both because of the different gyromagnetic ratio and the natural abundance. Table 13.1 lists selected spin-1/2 nuclei and shows very clearly that the relative sensitivity of ^{1}H and ^{19}F is significantly higher than other spin-1/2 nuclei and hence these are the only nuclei that are suitable for trace analysis.

TABLE 13.1 Sensitivity of Common Spin-1/2 Nuclei

Nuclei	Natural abundance (%)	Gyromagnetic ratio/$10^6 rad\,s^{-1}T^{-1}$	NMR frequency ν/MHz	Relative sensitivity
^{1}H	99.98	267.5	400.0	1.0
^{13}C	1.11	67.3	100.6	1.76×10^{-4}
^{15}N	0.37	−27.1	40.5	3.85×10^{-6}
^{19}F	100.00	251.8	376.3	0.83
^{29}Si	4.7	−53.2	79.5	3.69×10^{-4}
^{31}P	100.00	108.4	161.9	6.63×10^{-2}

Frequencies are for a 400 MHz (9.4 T magnet).

13.3 HOW COULD NMR BE USED FOR TRACE ANALYSIS?

To understand how NMR could be used for trace analysis, it is first important to explain a little about how an NMR spectrum is generated.

13.3.1 Generating an NMR Spectrum

The easiest way to understand how an NMR spectrum is generated is to think of the population difference between two spin states giving rise to a bulk magnetization vector, M_0, which behaves according to classical mechanics. This means, if perturbed, the vector will precess like a gyroscope around any applied field.

For example, if a radiofrequency (RF) pulse of the correct frequency is applied, it will cause the magnetization to precess. A correct choice of amplitude and length for this pulse results in rotation onto the x–y plane. The vector then precesses around the static field at a specific frequency, referred to as the Larmor frequency, causing an induced voltage in the RF coil surrounding the NMR sample. Over time, the system will return to equilibrium resulting in a decay of this voltage—this is termed relaxation.

Traditionally, this signal is called the free induction decay (FID), an amplitude time signal. Fourier transformation converts this into an amplitude frequency signal—with a peak appearing at the Larmor frequency. The whole process is illustrated in Figure 13.1.

Two features of acquiring a spectrum that become important when thinking about GI analysis are, first, the ability to change how the RF pulse is applied (see Section 13.4.8.1), and, second, understanding the relaxation in the system to ensure the experiments are quantitative (see Section 13.3.5).

13.3.2 Chemical Shift

If all ^1H nuclei had the same Larmor frequency, NMR would not be a very useful technique. However, the beauty of NMR is that the local chemical environment alters the exact magnetic field a particular nucleus experiences. As these differences are tiny, it is conventional to express frequency in terms of a chemical shift, δ, in parts per million (ppm) defined as:

$$\delta = \frac{v - v_{ref}}{v_0}$$

where v is the frequency of the nucleus in question compared with a reference, v_{ref}, and v_0 is the operating frequency of the NMR instrument. Table 13.2 lists some examples—for more detailed information, see *Spectroscopic Methods in Organic Chemistry* by Dudley Williams and Ian Fleming.[6]

In favorable circumstances, it is this chemical shift difference between atoms than can give resolution between a substrate and a potential genotoxic impurity.

For example, it can be seen that a common structural alert, an aldehyde functionality, has a distinct chemical shift in comparison with most other functional groups. It is, therefore, very likely when trying to detect an aldehyde proton in the presence of a substrate that it will be resolved.

There is also a dependence on the NMR solvent used (any solvent can be used for NMR as long as it is deuterated). It is conceivable that even if no resolution

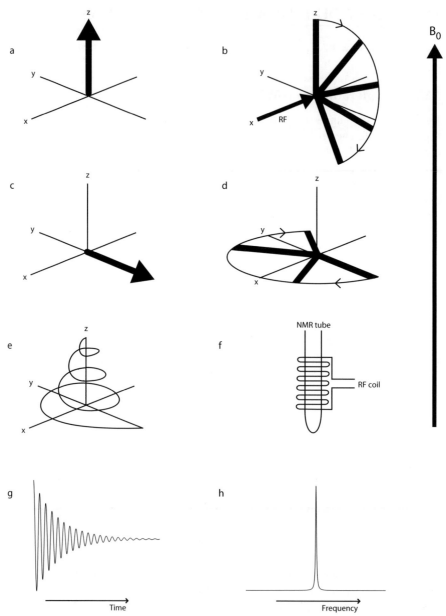

Figure 13.1 Diagrammatic representation of how a NMR spectrum is generated. (a) The bulk magnetization vector, $\mathbf{M_0}$, at equilibrium. (b) Precession due to the applied RF pulse. (c) After a RF pulse has been applied for the correct length to time to rotate the magnetization by 90°. (d) Precession at the Larmor frequency around the static field, B_0. (e) Relaxation of magnetization back to equilibrium. (f) The RF coil that detects the precessing magnetization which results in panel (g) the Free Induction Decay. Finally Fourier Transformation gives a spectrum shown in panel (h).

TABLE 13.2   Example ^1H and ^{13}C Chemical Shifts

Functional group	Range of ^1H chemical shifts (ppm)	Range of ^{13}C chemical shifts (ppm)
	9.5–10.0	180–220
	6.5–9.0	100–160
	4.5–6.5	100–140
O**CH₂**CH₂CH₃	3.5–4.0	55–70
OCH₂**CH₂**CH₃	1.0–2.0	10–50
OCH₂CH₂**CH₃**	0.5–1.0	0–40

between two atoms is seen in one solvent the choice of a different solvent may achieve sufficient resolution.

The chemical shift of atoms near a possible protonation site will also change depending on the protonation state. This effect can be utilized to achieve resolution between nuclei that may not be resolved originally. For example, in compounds (1) and (2), the two protons A and B have approximately the same chemical shift in deuterated dimethyl sulfoxide (d_6-DMSO), and hence are not resolved from each other. The addition of a base deprotonates the NH_2 group, causing a change in the chemical shift of H_B. H_B is now resolved from H_A.

13.3.3   Scalar Coupling

The chemical shift of a given nucleus is not only affected by the local chemical environment, but the exact frequency also depends on the spin-state of other nearby nuclei. For example, if you consider two nearby protons A and B, as in Figure 13.2. The frequency of proton A is different depending on whether proton B is in spin-state α or β. The result of this is that the signal from proton A appears as a doublet. The effect, called scalar coupling, continues for all nearby protons, often resulting in a complex multiplet structure.

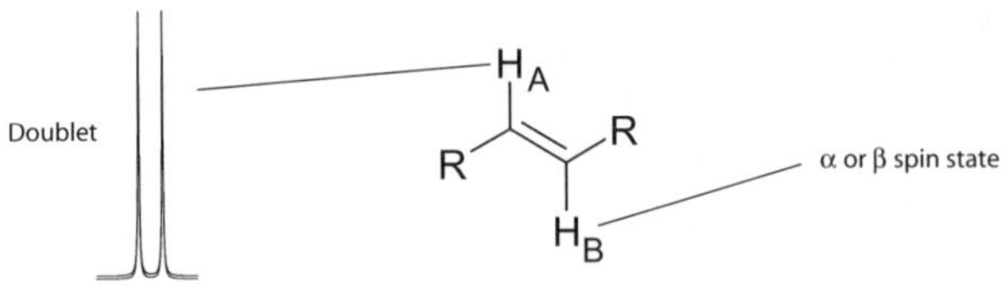

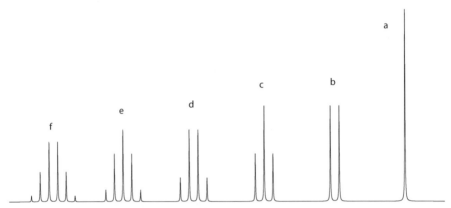

Figure 13.2   The different spin-states of H_B causes the signal from H_A to split into a doublet.

Figure 13.3   The effect of coupling on a single nucleus (a) not coupled, coupled to (b) 1, (c) 2, (d) 3, (e) 4, and (f) 5 other equivalent nuclei. As the degree of coupling increases the peak intensity is reduced, leading to less sensitivity and the width of the peak increases leading to an increase in the likelihood of peak overlap.

Scalar coupling is extremely useful for structure elucidation, because it contains a wealth of molecular connectivity information. However, the coupling can cause a problem for trace analysis, as it not only reduces sensitivity, but can also result in less resolution between signals as shown in Figure 13.3.

13.3.4   The Quantitative Nature of NMR

Despite the chemical shift and the scalar coupling dramatically changing the nature of the NMR spectrum, neither affects the total intensity that arises from each nucleus. This means that the intensity, as long as relaxation is taken into account, is a direct reflection of the total number of nuclei present. This is the basis of assay measurement. It is possible to calculate the purity of a substrate by the addition of a known purity standard and the measurement of the integral ratio between the purity standard and the substrate in question, using the formula:

$$\text{Assay } \%w/w = \frac{I_s \times MW_s \times P_p \times N_p \times W_p}{I_p \times MW_p \times N_s \times W_s}$$

where $I_{p,s}$ are the respective integrals of the internal purity standard (p) and substrate (s), $MW_{p,s}$ are the molecular weights, $N_{p,s}$ are the number of protons in the signals integrated, $W_{p,s}$ the weights added, and P_p the percentage purity of the standard.

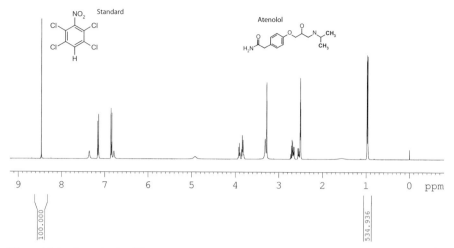

Figure 13.4   Quantitative ^{1}H spectra of atenolol (12.36 mg, molecular weight 266.3 gmol^{-1}) in d$_6$-DMSO recorded at 400 MHz. 13.50 mg TCNB (purity 99.8%, molecular weight 260.9 gmol^{-1}) has been added as internal standard.

In Figure 13.4, integration of the internal purity standard, tetrachloronitroben-zene (TCNB) relative to the 6 protons from the two CH$_3$ groups in atenolol enables an assay value for atenolol of 99.2% to be calculated.

In the same way, the ratio between a substrate and a residual solvent or a trace level impurity can be used to calculate the amount present. The following equation can be used to calculate the % w/w of any impurity relative to the main component:

$$\mathrm{Imp}\ \%w/w = 100 \times \frac{I_i \times MW_i \times P_s \times N_s}{I_s \times MW_s \times N_i}$$

where $I_{i,s}$ are the respective integrals of the impurity (*i*), and substrate (*s*), $MW_{i,s}$ are the molecular weights, $N_{i,s}$ the number of protons in the signals integrated, and P_s the purity. For trace impurities, it is more convenient to convert to parts per million (do not confuse with the NMR chemical shift):

$$\mathrm{Imp}\ (\mathrm{ppm}) = \mathrm{Imp}\ \%w/w * 10000$$

Many examples of quantitative NMR applied to pharmaceutical analysis can be found in Wawer et al.[7]

13.3.5   Relaxation

In NMR, there are two important relaxation phenomena, termed longitudinal and transverse relaxation.

Longitudinal relaxation can be understood as the exponential recovery of magnetization along the *z*-axis (M_z) following a RF pulse as shown in Figure 13.1e. Mathematically, this is given at a time *t* as:

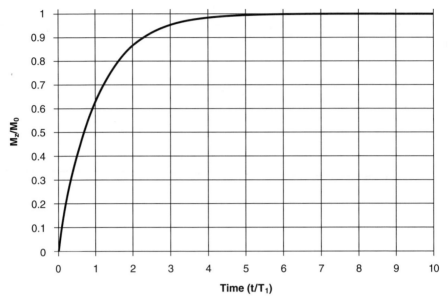

Figure 13.5   The return to equilibrium magnetization is governed by the relaxation time T_1 and is greater than 99% complete after a period of $5 \times T_1$.

$$M_z = M_0\left(1 - e^{-t/T_1}\right)$$

where T_1 is the time constant in seconds.

Figure 13.5 shows this decay, and as can be seen after $3 \times T_1$, 95% of magnetization has returned to z, while after $5 \times T_1$, 99.3% has.

For small- to medium-sized organic molecules, proton T_1 values range from 0.4 to 10 s. Generally, the smaller the molecule, the longer the T_1, and it must be remembered that different nuclei in a molecule will have different T_1 values. Measurement of T_1 values can be done using the inversion recovery sequence—see Claridge[1] for practical details.

Therefore, what is important for any quantitative NMR experiment is to ensure that following a 90° pulse, sufficient time ($5 \times T_1$) is left to allow full relaxation before the experiment is repeated (for signal averaging). Otherwise, the differential relaxation across the spectrum will result in the integrals not being a direct reflection of the number of that nuclei present in the sample.

It should be noted that a fully quantitative spectrum is obtained at the expensive of sensitivity—see Section 13.4.5 for more details.

Transverse relaxation can be described as the "fanning out" of magnetization in the x–y plane. The time constant, T_2, for this relaxation, manifests itself in the linewidth of signals. However, there is also a contribution to the linewidth from magnetic field inhomogeneity ($T_{2(\Delta B_0)}$). Traditionally, a combined time constant T_2^*, which is related to the actual observed linewidth, is defined as:

$$\frac{1}{T_2^*} = \frac{1}{T_2} + \frac{1}{T_{2(\Delta B_0)}}$$

In small- to medium-sized organic molecules in normal low-viscosity NMR solvents the greatest contribution to the linewidth comes from this inhomogeneity term. In terms of quantification, because in general T_2 is similar to, but never bigger than T_1, it is not significant when ensuring experiments are quantitative.

13.3.6 Summary

In summary, there a number of reasons why NMR could be a great tool for GI analysis:

- Chemical shift differences and the ability to manipulate them to give resolution between substrates and GIs.
- The NMR spectrum is quantitative. As long as the correct precautions are taken, it is possible to directly calculate impurity levels without need for any calibration.
- Sample preparation is straightforward, and often little method development is required. More often than not, whether resolution can be achieved can be determined using reference data for each of the components, and so the substrate simply needs to be dissolved in the NMR solvent, and the sample is ready for analysis.

As a result of these factors, NMR can be considered as a true orthogonal technique to LC/GC for GI analysis. However, this is of little value unless we can overcome the sensitivity issues. This is the topic of the next section.

13.4 WHAT CAN BE DONE TO MAXIMIZE SENSITIVITY?

We have already discussed the inherent insensitivity of NMR. This section explores the different factors that determine the sensitivity of a given experiment.

The signal-to-noise ratio (S/N) of a given signal depends on many factors, and for our purposes can conveniently be represented by:

$$\frac{S}{N} \propto P \cdot C \cdot MW_i^{-1} \cdot NS^{1/2} \cdot A \cdot \gamma^{5/2} \cdot N \cdot T_2^*$$

where P is a "performance factor" for the NMR system used, C is the substrate concentration, N is the number of atoms contributing to a signal, T_2^* is the apparent transverse relaxation time constant, NS is the number of scans, A is the natural abundance of the nuclei, γ is the gyromagnetic ratio, and MW_i is the molecular weight ratio of the GI. Additionally, the sensitivity is also affected by signal multiplicity, as was illustrated in Figure 13.3.

Each of these factors will be considered in turn along with the impact of signal resolution.

13.4.1 System Performance

The performance factor, P, of a given NMR system depends on a number of features primarily the magnetic field strength, B_0, and the probe performance for a given nuclei.

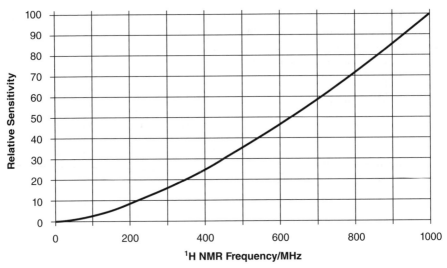

Figure 13.6 Relative sensitivity of the NMR experiment as a function of magnetic field strength.

13.4.1.1 *Field Strength* In terms of field strength:

$$\frac{S}{N} \propto B_0^{3/2}$$

This means increasing the field strength does give a significant sensitivity enhancement (e.g. going from 400 to 600 MHz gives a theoretical increase of ×1.8) (Fig. 13.6). However, as field strength increases, magnet costs also increase dramatically.

13.4.2 Probe Performance

Probe performance depends on a number of factors:

13.4.2.1 *Probe Design* Most NMR probes are designed to allow RF pulses to be applied to two or more nuclei at different frequencies at the same time. This allows the acquisition of a wide range of different experiments. For example, acquisition of one nuclei while the other is being decoupled (such as the common ^{13}C experiment with ^{1}H decoupling) or advanced two-dimensional experiments.

These experiments are achieved by the presence of two or more separate coils surrounding the sample (Fig. 13.7). The ability of the coil to detect an NMR signal depends on many factors, such as choice of material and geometry. However, one generally accepted factor is the "filling factor," or how "close" the coil is to the sample.

The traditional design places the coil for the less sensitive nuclei (referred to as the X channel) nearest the sample. With the correct electronic setup (and dependant on the exact probe design), this coil is able to observe all nuclei except for proton: that is ^{13}C, ^{15}N, ^{31}P, and ^{19}F. Proton observation is then performed with the ^{1}H coil outside this X coil.

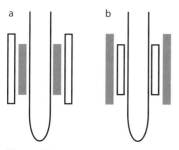

Figure 13.7   Probe design. (a) Traditional and (b) inverse probe designs. The ^{1}H coil is shown in white and the X coil in gray.

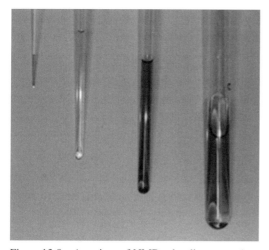

Figure 13.8   A variety of NMR tube diameters: 1 mm, 3 mm, 5 mm, and 10 mm.

In comparison, the so-called inverse design places the proton coil nearer the sample. Clearly, to optimize sensitivity for the nuclei used for GI analysis, it is important to select a probe that is optimized: that is a traditional design for ^{19}F and an inverse design for ^{1}H.

13.4.1.2   Probe Diameter   The second important factor when choosing an appropriate probe is the sample size. Probes are available that will allow the use of NMR tubes with an outside diameter of between 1 and 10 mm (or larger) as shown in Figure 13.8. Clearly, the larger the tube size, the larger the active volume within the coil.

There are two ways to understand the sensitivity these different probe sizes allow. One way is to consider a fixed mass of material that is dissolved in an appropriate amount of NMR solvent. This method is of crucial importance when looking at mass limited samples, for example if an impurity has actually been isolated using chromatography, and, let us say, 50 μg of material is available. In this case, dissolving the material in a small amount of solvent and using a probe designed for a smaller NMR tube results in better mass sensitivity.

TABLE 13.3 Concentration Sensitivity of Some Example Probe Designs at Different Field Strengths

Field	Probe type	0.1% ethyl benzene sensitivity
400	Traditional 5 mm	220:1
500	Traditional 5 mm	330:1
500	Inverse 5 mm	900:1
600	Inverse cryogenic probe	6000:1

However, in the case of GI analysis, we are not usually sample limited. Generally, a large amount of substrate is available, and to maximize sensitivity, we need to maximize the total amount of material within the coil (i.e. by increasing the concentration). Therefore, what is relevant is the concentration sensitivity of the probe. The best way to measure this is to consider the signal to noise obtained from the classic measure of instrument sensitivity—0.1% ethyl benzene in $CDCl_3$. In this case, the sensitivity will be proportional to the amount of material actually within the coil and hence the sample volume. This, of course, means the larger the probe diameter the better the concentration sensitivity. Table 13.3 lists the concentration sensitivity of a number of probe designs at different field strengths—the importance of correct probe design is clear.

13.4.2.2 Cryogenically Cooled Probes Table 13.3 makes reference to cryogenic probes that give significantly enhanced sensitivity, but what are these?

In a "normal" probe, the RF coils are at room temperature. However, it is possible to represent the noise generated by the electronic hardware by the equation:

$$\frac{S}{N} \propto \frac{1}{\sqrt{T_C R_C + T_a(R_C + R_s) + T_S R_S}}$$

where T_C and R_C represent the temperature and resistance of the coil, T_S the sample temperature, R_S the resistance generated in the coil by the sample, and T_a the effective noise temperature of the preamplifier.[8] Although complex, this equation simply means that a decrease in temperature of the coil results in increased signal to noise.

Despite the engineering challenges of having a RF coil at a very low temperature while keeping the sample at room temperature, cryogenic probes that cool the RF coils and preamplifier down to 25 K have recently been developed.

As can be seen in Table 13.3, these type of probes result in at least a fourfold increase in sensitivity (the additional increase seen arises from the increase in field strength). A cryoprobe installation is shown in Figure 13.9.

13.4.3 Substrate Concentration

As has already been stated, NMR reflects the actual number of nuclei within a sample. This means that the sensitivity linearly increases with concentration.

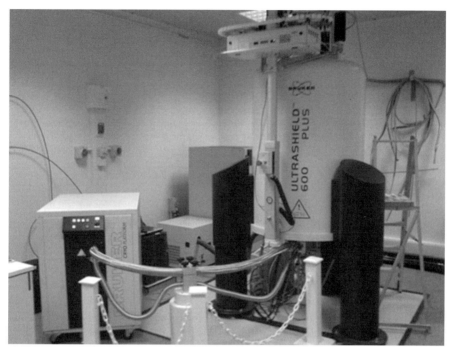

Figure 13.9   A cryoprobe installation on a 600 MHz magnet. The unit on the left generates cold helium gas, which is transferred into the probe by the top connecting pipe. The bottom connecting pipe provides the vacuum which isolates the sample from the cold coils.

Increasing sample concentration is therefore probably the easiest and cheapest option to obtain sufficient sensitivity. In GI analysis, the aim is to detect and measure the impurity relative to the substrate. Hence, if you need to detect at 1 ppm in your substrate if you only dissolve 1 mg in 1 mL of solvent, the NMR needs to be capable of detecting 1 ng of GI. In contrast, if you dissolve 100 mg in 1 mL of solvent, the NMR only needs to be capable of detecting 100 ng of GI. Therefore, the concentration that can be achieved in solution will have a direct correlation with the levels of detection that are likely to be achieved.

Generally, the higher concentration the better, that is there is no limit as long as the material stays in solution for the period of the experiment, does not cause stability problems or cause significant spectral broadening due to the high viscosity of the solution.

So can NMR detect at these levels? Focusing on two amounts, 100 ng (1 ppm at 100 mg/mL) and 2 µg (20 ppm at 100 mg/mL), and using the signal-to-noise ratios in Table 13.3, it is possible to estimate levels of detection. This assumes a molecule weight identical to ethyl benzene.

As can be seen in Table 13.4, it is conceivable that even on a "normal" probe 20 ppm could be detected, whereas 1 ppm might be difficult unless circumstances are favorable. However, on a cryoprobe system, it appears theoretically possible to

TABLE 13.4 Theoretical Signal-to-Noise Ratios

Signal to noise of 0.1% (1 mg) ethyl benzene in 1 scan	Signal to noise in 1 h of acquisition	Signal to noise of 1 ppm	Signal to noise of 20 ppm
220:1	5903:1	0.6:1	12:1
900:1	24120:1	2.4:1	48:1
6000:1	160800:1	16:1	320:1

Signal to noise in 1 h calculated assuming it is possible to pulse every 5 s, corresponding to 720 scans in 1 h and hence a 26.8 times increase in S/N ratio. Signal to noise ratio at 1/20 ppm calculated assuming peak shape, molecular weight, and multiplicity is identical to ethyl benzene.

detect even 1 ppm. At this point, it should be stated that this is a theoretical calculation—practically, there are problems that will discussed in Section 13.4.8.

13.4.4 Molecular Weight Ratio

Sensitivity is proportional to the molecular weight of the GI. Table 13.4 estimated whether there was enough sensitivity in an NMR experiment, assuming that the molecular weight was identical to ethyl benzene. A ppm level is calculated on a weight to weight basis, so for example, 1 ppm at 100 mg/mL always corresponds to 100 ng. If this GI had a molecular weight 10 times that of ethyl benzene in the 100 ng, there are 10 times less the number of a particular proton, and hence the sensitivity will be 10 times less.

Therefore, it will always be easy to detect small MW GIs by NMR in comparison with GIs that are perhaps analogues of bigger MW drug substances.

13.4.5 Acquisition Time and Signal Averaging

As noise is random, it adds more slowly than signal leading to a square-root relationship between signal-to-noise and the number of times the experiment is repeated, NS. As can be seen in Figure 13.10, this means to double the signal-to-noise ratio from 0.5 to 1 takes four times the number of scans (25 versus 100 scans)—and hence four times the time. This means that although running the sample of interest for more time to increase the signal-to-noise has great benefit, it only goes so far. For example, if you need to run the sample for 12 h to detect say 10 ppm—to get the same signal-to-noise on 5 ppm would take $12 \times 4 = 2$ days—very quickly, the time required can become very long. It is therefore much more beneficial to optimize the system in terms of correct probe/instrument selection and sample concentration rather than relying on simply running the sample for longer and longer. In addition, the issue of dynamic range means there comes a point when running the sample for longer will make no difference anyway.

The other time optimization factor that we can change is of course how long is left between each scans to allow for complete relaxation. As had already been said, if we wish our experiment to be totally quantitative, we must leave $5 \times T_1$.

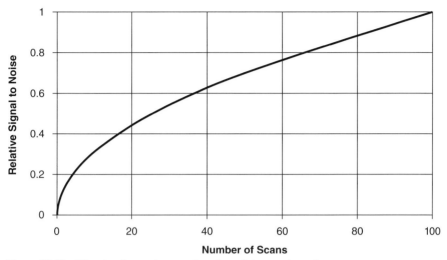

Figure 13.10 The signal-to-noise as a function of the number of scans.

Therefore, based on our approximate measurements of the T_1 values for both the substrate peaks of interest and our GI, we have a minimum repetition time between scans. This of course can have a dramatic impact on the sensitivity we will be able to obtain. For example, consider two systems: in system (a), the longest relaxing species has a T_1 of 500 ms. Therefore, our repetition between scans is 2.5 s. Therefore, in 1 h of acquisition, we are able to acquire 1440 scans. In system (b), the longest relaxing species has a T_1 of 4 s (not unreasonable for a small GI molecule). Therefore, the repetition times between scans is 20 s, and so in 1 h, we are able to acquire only 180 scans (eight times less scans than in system a). Taking into account the square root factor, this corresponds to 2.8 times less signal-to-noise in system (b) than system (a) in the same time.

However, there is something we can do when all other factors, such as concentration or choice of instrument, etc., have been exhausted. Although leaving $5 \times T_1$ gives quantitative spectra, it essentially *wastes time*—if pulses were applied more quickly, more sensitivity could be achieved in the same time but at the expense of quantitation.

In fact, there is also for a given repetition time, T_R, and a given T_1, a pulse angle (i.e. not a 90° pulse) that optimizes sensitivity. This is called the Ernst angle, α, which over time maximizes the signal intensity.[3]

$$\cos \alpha = \exp\left(-\frac{T_R}{T_1}\right)$$

The strategy to maximize the sensitivity is to have a repetition time as fast as possible, and then optimize the pulse angle based on this time and the relaxation time of the GI. How short T_R can be is governed by T_2^*, and hence how long the FID takes to decay. If the FID is truncated, this leads to unwanted artifacts. It is also important to optimize the pulse angle based on the GI relaxation time, as of course, this is the signal for which the maximum sensitivity is required.

The amplitude of each signal, ε is given by:

$$\varepsilon = \frac{1 - \exp\left(-\dfrac{T_R}{T_1}\right)}{1 - \exp\left(-\dfrac{T_R}{T_1}\right)\cos\alpha}\sin\alpha$$

and hence for a given pulse angle and T_R, it is possible to calculate the signal intensity expected from each signal of interest in the spectrum (with different T_1 values), and hence the expected error in any quantitative measurement. Of course, this error is only a guide, and so if this approach is used, a calibration curve must be generated.

For example, in a particular GI problem, when ^{19}F NMR was used, it was shown that at a concentration of 400 mg/mL substrate, it was possible to detect the impurity down to the required level of 8 ppm. A sample spiked with 1000 ppm was used to measure T_1 values. As relaxation times depend on the sample conditions, it is important to measure them in as representative sample as possible. In this case, while it was possible that the relaxation time of the GI was different when present at 8 or 1000 ppm, it was clearly not feasible to perform the measurement on a 8 ppm sample. It was, however, very important to measure the GI relaxation time in the presence of the substrate.

In this case, using the inversion recovery experiment the T_1 of the substrate was estimated at 0.6 s and the GI at 1.0 s. Therefore, to ensure the experiment was quantitative, 5 s was left between scans. Using this repetition time, however, it was shown that 17 h would be required to achieve the required signal-to-noise ratio at 8 ppm—this was deemed too long. It was therefore decided to optimize the experiment time at the expense of quantification. Looking at the FID (see Fig. 13.11), it was possible to reduce the repetition time down to 1.3 s—therefore using the GI relaxation time, the optimum pulse angle of 74° was used. In addition, by calculating the amplitude expected from the substrate and GI signals, it was shown that the expected error in quantification is about 16% (as the GI is relaxing more slowly than the substrate, its intensity will be less than if the experiment was quantitative).

It is also possible to calculate the theoretical sensitivity enhancement. As can be seen in Figure 13.12, at the Ernst angle for a single scan a repetition time of 1.3 s results in only 75% of the signal. However, in a fixed time, it is possible to acquire nearly four times as many scans, taking into account the square root factor giving a final enhancement of 1.5 times. This equates to a 2.2 times reduction in time. This is borne out experimentally, as using this setup, it was possible with sufficient sensitivity down to detect to 8 ppm with an acquisition time of approximately 6 h as shown in Figure 13.11.

13.4.6 Number of Protons and Linewidth

NMR signals in a spectrum have areas that are proportional to the number of nuclei, N, present. However, each signal is not of equal height. Theoretically, NMR lines have a Lorentzian lineshape given by the following equation:

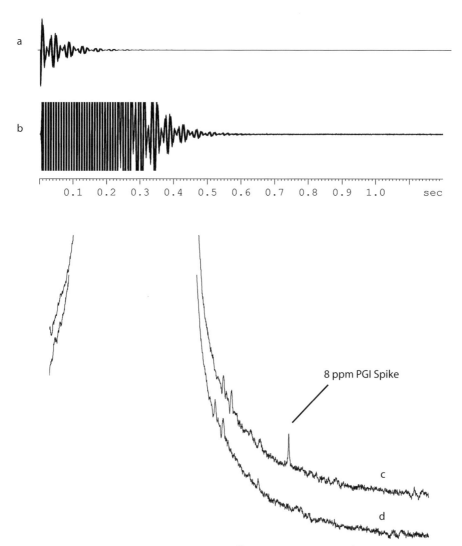

Figure 13.11   400 mg/mL substrate (a) FID of ^{19}F NMR spectrum with ^{1}H decoupling
(b) Same FID expanded vertically. As can be seen, 1.3 s is more than enough time to allow
the any signal to disappear. (c and d) Fourier transformed spectrum, showing region where
GI appears with and without 8 ppm spike. Signal from substrate is on the left disappearing
upwards. Data was acquired as per the text with a 74° pulse angle and 1.3 s repetition time in 6 h.

$$S(\omega) = \frac{R}{R^2 + (\omega - \Omega)^2}$$

where $S(\omega)$ is the signal height at a frequency ω of a peak centred at Ω. R is defined
as $1/T_2^*$. From this equation, it is easy to see (by setting $\omega = \Omega$) that the peak height
is $1/R = T_2^*$, hence sensitivity is directly proportional to the relaxation time, T_2^*.

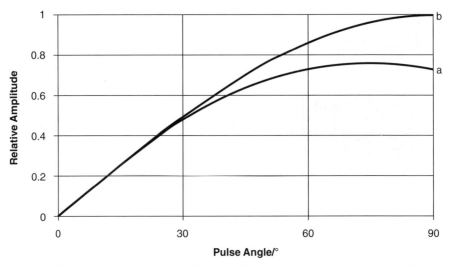

Figure 13.12 Relative amplitude as a function of pulse angle for a fixed relaxation time of 1 s and (a) repetition time of 1.3 s, (b) 5 s (quantitative conditions). Although the maximum amplitude is less when the repetition time is only 1.3's in a fixed time, more scans will have been acquired leading to 1.5 times enhancement in sensitivity.

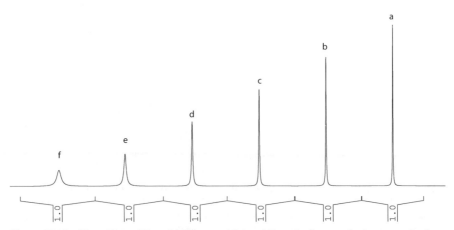

Figure 13.13 The effect of linewidth on sensitivity. All peaks from a single proton (a–f) have the same intensity but increasing linewidth. This leads to a reduction in sensitivity.

Figure 13.13 shows the effect of increasing linewidth on the intensity and sensitivity of signals. Therefore, in terms of GI analysis, the linewidth of any GI signal will have a direct impact on the levels of detection that are achievable. This needs to be remembered when optimizing experiments in terms of concentration, solvent choice, and temperature, all of which can have an effect on linewidth.

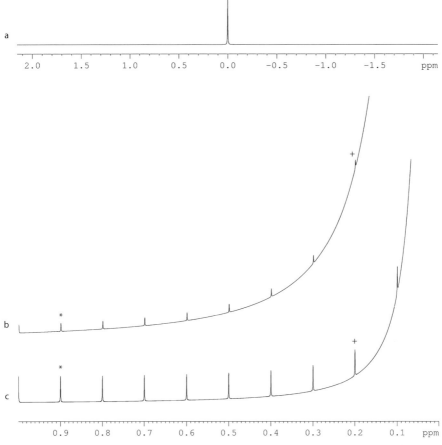

Figure 13.14   (a) Simulated spectra (with no noise) of a substrate peak at 0 ppm with a series of GI signals at 0.1 ppm intervals from 1 ppm down to 0 ppm at (b) 1 ppm and (c) 20 ppm with respect to the substrate signal. Signals at a chemical shift of 0.9 ppm (marked by *) are easily detected in both cases, but at a chemical shift of 0.2 ppm (marked by +), the 1 ppm GI signal is virtually obscured by the tail of the huge substrate signal.

13.4.7 Resolution

We have now addressed all the terms in the original equation at the start of Section 13.4, leaving just the resolution between signals to consider. In this context, the line-width of substrate signals and the frequency difference between a GI signal and substrate will directly influence the sensitivity that can be achieved. This is because NMR Lorentzian lines have long tails that at part per million levels can easily obscure very small signals. This is clearly seen in Figure 13.14 as, for example, a peak present at a level of 1 ppm with a chemical shift difference of 0.9 ppm from the substrate signal is easily detected and resolved, whereas a peak with a chemical shift difference of 0.2 ppm is only just detected and certainly could not be integrated. However, at a level of 20 ppm, a peak with a chemical shift difference of 0.2 ppm is easily detected.

13.4.8   Dynamic Range

So far all the discussion has been around the theoretical ability of NMR to detect the very low mass amounts of GIs that are present in solution. It has been argued that although a large number of factors have an impact, NMR does possess enough sensitivity to make such analysis a practical reality. However, what we have yet to consider is the impact of the substrate—does the fact that you are trying to detect a peak that could be a 1 million times smaller than most peaks in the NMR spectrum cause a problem? To answer this question, we have to consider whether the NMR instrumentation has sufficient dynamic range to detect these small signals.

When the FID is detected, it is digitized by an analogue to digital converter (ADC). The performance of this ADC determines both the frequency and amplitude range that can be detected. Traditionally, ADCs have 16 bits, one is reserved for the sign of the signal leaving a dynamic range of $2^{15} - 1 = 32767$ to represent the values.

Assuming the receiver gain of the instrument is adjusted in such a way that it exactly fills the ADC (with a value of 32767), the smallest signal that can be detected has a value of 1; anything smaller than this will not be detected in a single scan. Therefore, if we are looking at ppm levels, this dynamic range can prevent detection of the small signals even if the sensitivity is theoretically high enough.

The situation is improved by the fact that in reality, smaller signals will be detected, as they can "ride" on the noise and with signal averaging will gradually sum to give signals. Additionally, the most recent ADCs available in spectrometers have up to 22 bits. This corresponds to $2^{21} - 1 = 2097151$, which is clearly significantly more favorable.

Figure 13.15 shows the dramatic difference between an older instrument with a 16-bit digitizer and a new instrument with a 22-bit digitizer when detecting very small signals in the presence of a very large water peak. Spectra (b) and (d) show little difference (approximately 10,000 difference in intensity between the water signal and the impurity signal, whereas there is a huge difference in the sensitivity between (c) and (e) when the intensity difference is nearer 100,000.

An additional problem, that of distortion, can be encountered particularly with the more sensitive cryoprobe systems. If the largest peak in the system is so large that it cannot fit into the ADC range, even after adjustment of the receiver gain, this results in severe distortion of the spectra, as can be seen in Figure 13.16.

Cryoprobes are traditionally used for mass limited samples and are not designed to look at high concentration samples. The use of a 16-bit digitizer for samples at 100 mg/mL or higher concentration will almost certainly cause this distortion, which will prevent any GI detection.

13.4.8.1   Selective Excitation   These dynamic range and receiver overload problems are very common in the field of biological NMR when looking at proteins dissolved in water. There is a very intense water signal and then a large number of very small signals from the protein. To overcome this, there is a large number of so-called "solvent suppression" strategies that remove the water signal from the spectra, hence allowing an increase in receiver gain and so detection of the protein signals.[9–11]

Figure 13.17 shows an example of a spectrum acquired with water suppression.

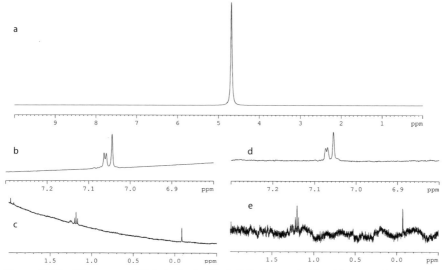

Figure 13.15 ^{1}H spectra of H_2O (spiked with 5 % D_2O for a lock) with impurities present. (a) Full expansion, (b and c) acquired on a new generation spectrometer 400 MHz spectrometer with 22 bit ADC, and (d and e) acquired on an older 400 MHz spectrometer with 16-bit ADC. In both cases, the sample and all experimental conditions were identical. In spectra (b and d) the intensity difference between the impurity and the water signal is approximately 10,000, whereas in (c and e) it is nearer 100,000.

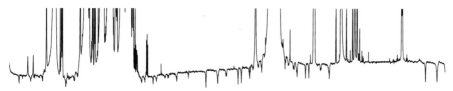

Figure 13.16   Example of the distortion caused by receiver overload. The form of the distortion can vary significantly depending on the sample concentration and the instrumentation used.

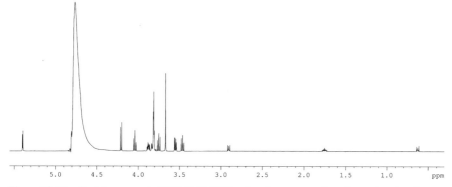

Figure 13.17   2 mM sucrose in 90% H_2O. Without water suppression, the water signal would be huge, but using simple presaturation, the size of the water signal is reduced, allowing the detection of the sucrose signals.

Unfortunately, this approach is not useful for GI analysis, because the substrate is not a single signal but a large number of very intense peaks, and there are no suppression sequences that can suppress more than two or three peaks at once.

The solution is therefore to take the opposite approach—instead of trying to suppress the large signals, the experiment is performed in such a way as to only "excite" the small GI signal using selective pulses.

A normal 90° pulse often described as a hard pulse can take 10 μs (t_{90}) to rotate the magnetization from the z-axis onto the x-y plane. This rotation can be translated into a frequency:

$$\frac{\omega_1}{2\pi} = \frac{1}{4t_{90}}$$

If t_{90} is 10 μs then $\omega_1 = 157 \times 10^3$ rad s^{-1}. In addition, one can choose at which chemical shift or frequency in the spectrum to apply the pulse. The distance between a peak and this chosen frequency is referred to as the spectral offset, Ω.

The general condition is that if $\omega_1 \gg |\Omega|$, then the full spectrum will receive a complete 90° pulse. For example, in a proton spectrum, peaks appear between 0 and 10 ppm, so if the RF pulse is applied at 5 ppm, the maximum offset, Ω, is $5 \times 400 = 2000$ Hz (or 13×10^3 rad s^{-1}) at a field strength of 400 MHz. It is clear then that ω_1 is significantly larger than any possible offset, hence all peaks will be excited.

If you significantly reduce the power of the RF pulse, and so increase the length of time it takes to rotate the magnetization, the width of excitation will decrease. Figure 13.18 shows the excitation profile for a 10 μs, 100 μs, and 10 ms

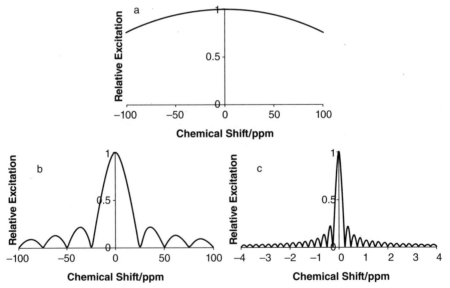

Figure 13.18 Excitation profiles for rectangular 90° pulses of (a) 10 μs, (b) 100 μs, and (c) 10 ms duration. Both a 10 μs and a 100 μs easily excite the full spectral width of a proton spectrum (maximum 10–15 ppm), whereas a 10 ms pulse will only excite a very small region around where the pulse is applied.

90° pulse. If a 10 ms pulse was applied, only a small region of the spectrum would be excited. This is termed a selective or soft pulse.

Using this selective pulse, a region where a GI peak is known to appear can be excited fully while the more intense regions are not, removing the problem that the intense peaks cause.

The wiggly nature of the excitation profile, as illustrated in Figure 13.18, can cause a problem, as some peak significantly far away from the central excitation region are still excited to a small degree. Given that these could be the very intense signals, they could still be large enough to cause a problem.

13.4.8.2   *Shaped Pulses*   It is possible to describe the normal RF pulse, whether applied in a *hard* or *soft* manner as a rectangular pulse, that is the RF is turned on for a given period and then turned off. Mathematically, is it possible to calculate the shape of the excitation profile by Fourier transformation of the shape of the RF pulse. The Fourier transform of a rectangle is a sinc function—hence the wiggly nature. However, the Fourier transform of a Gaussian shape is another Gaussian shape. If the RF power is therefore turned on and off in a Gaussian profile, the resulting excitation will be much flatter outside the main region.[12]

This principle can be extended much further to a whole a range of different shapes that have different properties, and that can be used in a wide range of applications. This is beyond the scope of this chapter; however, further details can be found in references[1,13,14]. For the case studies described in this chapter, the Gaussian pulse has been applied and has proved to be more than adequate.

Figure 13.19a shows how this is applied in practice on a cryoprobe system— by excitation of a small peak present in this case at approximately 4.8 ppm. Although the intense signals appear, their intensity is significantly reduced, removing receiver distortion and allowing a dramatic increase in the instrument receiver gain. The result is being able to fully utilize the theoretical sensitivity of the instrument.

From our experience, this type of experiment is beneficial over a normal pulse on a cryoprobe system or normal probe systems with older type ADCs. For normal probe systems with new higher dynamic range ADCs, no benefit is seen.

13.4.8.3   *Quantification Using Selective Pulses*   The selection of only the GI signal removes the reference to integrate against; so how can one of the big advantages of NMR, quantification, be utilized?

The easy solution is to make use of the flexibility of shaped pulses. By modulating the amplitude and phase of the pulse, it is possible to cause two regions of the spectrum to be excited. How this is achieved is beyond the scope here— see Freeman[13] for more details.

However, in practical terms, by exciting the GI and then choosing a second signal present in the spectrum at an intermediate level, that is not as low as the GI but not as intense as the substrate signals, it is possible to obtain an accurate ratio of the two signals.

Then, a normal *companion* proton spectrum is acquired, in which the intermediate signal can be integrated relative to the substrate. This allows a ratio between the substrate and GI to be obtained.

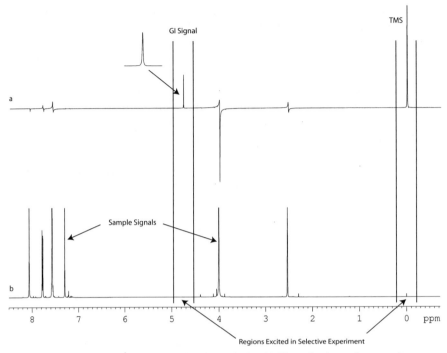

Figure 13.19   Using selective pulses for GI analysis. (a) The selective pulse experiment integrated in combination with (b) a normal companion proton.

The only challenge here is to make sure relaxation conditions are the same in the two experiments, and ensure there is no distortion due to receiver overload in the companion proton experiment. This is easily achieved by significantly reducing the pulse angle of the hard pulse. The whole process is summarized in Figure 13.19.

It is possible to choose any signal present at an intermediate level to excite with the GI, but in our experience, tetramethylsilane (TMS), the chemical shift reference, is an ideal choice, as it is always resolved and present at an appropriate level.

13.4.8.4   *Excitation Sculpting*   Although selective-pulse acquire experiments dramatically reduce the intensity of the strong signals (as shown in Fig. 13.19), they still appear as dispersive (positive and negative components) signals. These dispersive signals have long tails, and if there is not sufficient resolution between the GI signal and other signals, these tails can prevent accurate integration. As per any quantitative method, integration on a flat baseline is crucial for accurate results.

The solution to this is the use of a slightly more complicated NMR pulse sequence—called excitation sculpting[15,16]—which actively removes unselected signals. This pulse sequence comes in two varieties, incorporating either a single- or double-gradient echo.

The only disadvantage of these sequences is a slight loss in the signal-to-noise ratio, and therefore their application should be limited to cases when intense signals are causing a problem.

The difference between spectra obtained from the simple experiment and the excitation sculpting experiment can clearly be seen by comparison of Figure 13.26a and Figure 13.21c.

13.4.9 Limit Tests

NMR is an inherently quantitative technique, and so it is possible to calculate levels without calibration. However, in many GI problems, all that is required is a limit test, that is is the GI present at a level of concern (typically the TTC) or not?

This type of test can easily be performed by NMR—by simple comparison of spectra with and without a spike at the appropriate level. In many cases, for extra certainty, once a spectra has been run to detect a GI, spiking into the sample and then rerunning can confirm that nothing else in the sample is preventing detection.

13.4.10 Summary

In this section, we have discussed the many factors which determine the sensitivity of the NMR experiment—and highlighted that perhaps the most important for trace analysis is obtaining sufficient solubility.

In addition, the difficulties of using high sensitivity probes have been highlighted and a solution proposed by the use of selective pulses.

We are now in a position to consider some real examples to highlight how useful NMR can be in this area.

13.5 CASE STUDIES

As has been shown, if sufficient solubility can be achieved, NMR does have enough sensitivity to detect at ppm levels. The following examples highlight the use of ^1H NMR using normal systems, cryoprobe systems coupled with selective excitation, and the use of ^{19}F NMR.

13.5.1 Case Study 1: An Aldehyde Functionalized GI

During early Phase I development of compound (4), a synthetic intermediate functionalized with an aldehyde group (3) was identified as a GI. A fit-for-purpose method was therefore required to detect and if present, quantify this impurity down to about 50 ppm.

By a simple comparison of the API structure (4) and the aldehyde (3), it was immediately obvious that the proton signal from the aldehyde would be likely to appear in a totally unoccupied region of the API NMR spectrum.

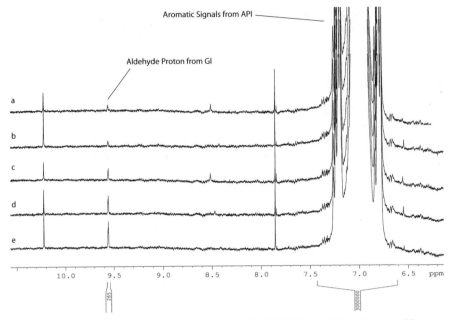

Figure 13.20   Proton spectra of 100 mg API(4) in d_6-DMSO (a and b) duplicates with no spike. Spiked with (c) 50 ppm aldehyde GI, (d) 100 ppm, (e) 150 ppm. Spectra run at 400 MHz at 300 K over 3 h of acquisition.

A solubility of 100 mg/mL of the API was easy achieved in d_6-DMSO. To this solution, a 500 ppm spike of the aldehyde impurity was added. This sample was run under normal proton conditions, ensuring the spectrum was quantitative. As this 500 ppm spike was clearly resolved, a further series of two duplicates of a "blank" sample, along with 50/100/150 ppm spikes, were successfully performed again under normal proton conditions on a 400 MHz instrument. Figure 13.20 summarizes the results of these experiments. They clearly demonstrate that low levels of the impurity are present in the API.

As a comparison, the same samples were run on a 600 MHz instrument with a cryoprobe using a simple selective experiment with companion proton (Fig. 13.21). There is a signal-to-noise increase, along with a dramatic decrease in experiment time (3 h to 10 min).

Simple integration of the aldehyde signal relative to a drug signal allowed quantification of the levels present as shown in Table 13.5. Excellent recoveries were also observed.

If lower detection limits were required it would have been possible to acquire data for longer. It is estimated that in 3 h a level of detection <5 ppm could have been achieved.

All the work required for this project was performed in less than one day and provided all the answers that were required at that time.

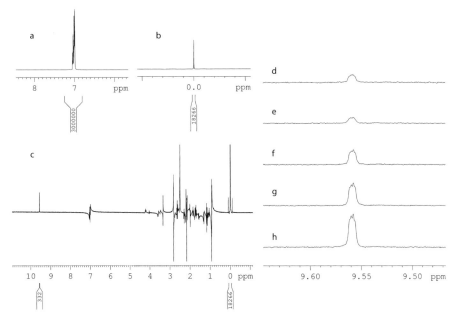

Figure 13.21   Proton spectra of 100 mg API(4) in d₆-DMSO (a and b) companion proton experiment with 150 ppm spike. (c) Selective pulse experiment with 150 ppm spike (d and e) duplicates with no spikes. Spiked with (f) 50 ppm aldehyde GI, (g) 100 ppm, (h) 150 ppm. Spectra run at 600 MHz at 300 K over 10 min of acquisition.

TABLE 13.5   Case Study 1: An Aldehyde Functionalized GI—Calculated ppm Levels and Recoveries from Selective Experiment on 600 MHz Instrument

	Level (ppm)	Recovery (%)
Duplicate 1	41	
Duplicate 2	45	
50 ppm spike	89	95
100 ppm spike	137	96
150 ppm spike	191	99

13.5.2   Case Study 2: Use of ¹⁹F NMR

Compound (6) is an intermediate in the development of a fluorinated API. At this intermediate stage of the synthesis, it was necessary to control the level of impurity (5), trifluoronitrobenzene (TFNB), down to 10 ppm.

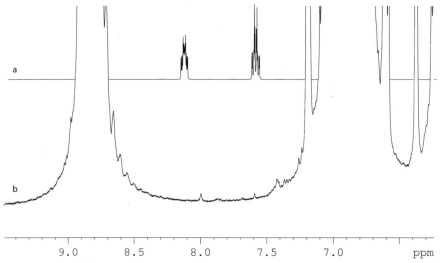

Figure 13.22 (a) ^1H NMR spectra of trifluoronitrobenzene and (b) 50 ppm spike of trifluoronitrobenzene in 500 mg/mL intermediate (6).

It was noted that the solubility of intermediate (6) was extremely high (>3 g/mL in d_6-DMSO), so both ^1H and ^{19}F experiments could conceivably give the necessary sensitivity. Initially, ^1H experiments were attempted, but although the GI signals were in a region of the spectrum distinct from signals from the intermediate other impurities and poor resolution prevented detection below 50 ppm despite experimental optimization, as shown in Figure 13.22.

However, ^{19}F with ^1H decoupling experiments were more successful. As can be seen in Figure 13.23, the three F signals from (5) are well resolved from the one in the intermediate (6). $^{19}F_1$ at −156 ppm was chosen for further study, as it had the simplest multiplet structure, and hence would give the highest sensitivity. To achieve the required sensitivity, the sample had to be prepared with 1 g of (6) in 300 μL d_6-DMSO. Due to the very high concentration and hence high viscosity, it was necessary to run the NMR spectra at 343 K to achieve sharp spectra. Under these conditions, the required level of detection was achieved on a 400 MHz instrument in 3.5 h of acquisition (see Fig. 13.24). Calculation of ppm levels was performed by simple integration, and recoveries from spiking experiments were comparable with those expected from other techniques for trace analysis, such as LC or GC. The data obtained is summarized in Table 13.6.

Using this method, a number of batches of material were screened, and it was quickly shown that none contained the TFNB impurity.

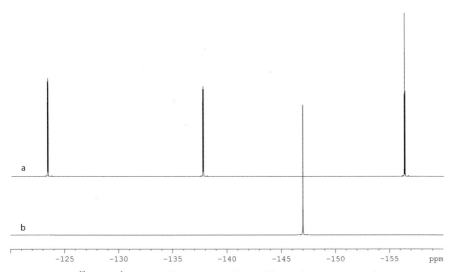

Figure 13.23 ^{19}F with ^{1}H decoupling spectra of (a) trifluoronitrobenzene and (b) intermediate (6).

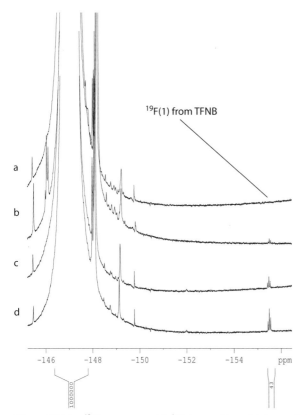

^{19}F(1) from TFNB

Figure 13.24 ^{19}F spectrum with ^{1}H decoupling of intermediate (6) at approximately 1 g in 300 mL d_6-DMSO, recorded on a 400 MHz instrument in 3.5 h at 343 K (a) not spiked. Spiked with (b) 9 ppm TFNB, (c) 23 ppm, and (d) 47 ppm.

TABLE 13.6 Case Study 2: Use of ^{19}F NMR—Recoveries

	Level (ppm)	Recovery (%)
Duplicate 1	Not detected	
9 ppm spike	10	111
23 ppm spike	22	97
47 ppm spike	45	96

TABLE 13.7 Case Study 3: Epoxide and Chlorohydrin GIs—Recoveries

	Epoxide (7) level (ppm)	Recovery (%)	Chlorohydrin (8) level (ppm)	Recovery (%)
3 ppm spike	4.1	137	2.6	87
10 ppm spike	10.0	100	8.8	88
30 ppm spike	27.6	92	31.9	106
100 ppm spike	78.9	79	102.3	102

13.5.3   Case Study 3: Epoxide and Chlorohydrin GIs

In another compound, two GIs were of concern, an epoxide (7) and a chlorohydrin (8), which were early synthetic intermediates of the API. Initially other techniques apart from NMR were considered. GC was not considered an alternative due to likely matrix interference, so first to be tried was HPLC-MS. However, it was quickly apparent that method development would not be straightforward.

Second, ion chromatography was attempted, and in the absence of the API, the GIs were readily retained and detected in aqueous media. However, in the presence of the API, there were interfering signals in addition to concerns around the solubility of the API in water. NMR was therefore considered as an alternative.

(7)   (8)

An initial comparison of ^{1}H spectra for the API, epoxide and chlorohydrin quickly suggested that resolution could be achieved, and hence the NMR methodology was pursued.

It was determined that the maximum API solubility that could be obtained was only approximately 60 mg/mL, and a level of detection of 10 ppm was required. Therefore, immediately, a 600 MHz system with a cryoprobe was utilized.

Spikes were performed of both epoxide (7) and chlorohydrin (8) at 1000, 100, 30, 10, and 3 ppm to confirm the method was specific and had sufficient sensitivity (Table 13.7).

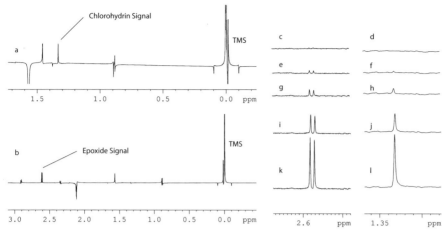

Figure 13.25   (a) Selective excitation experiment on spiked sample selecting chlorohydrin signal at 1.35 ppm and TMS at 0 ppm. (b) As (a) but selecting epoxide at 2.56 ppm and TMS. (c and d) Epoxide and chlorohydrin selective experiment respectively on sample with no spike. (e and f) With 3 ppm epoxide and chlorohydrin spike (g and h) 10 ppm spike (i and j) 30 ppm spike and (k and l) 100 ppm spike. All spectra recorded at 600 MHz.

To obtain maximum sensitivity, a companion proton and pair of selective experiments (one selecting the chlorohydrin and one the epoxide) were used.

As can be seen in Figure 13.25, both GIs were detected at the required level, and the recoveries obtained were acceptable.

A series of batches were screened, and it was shown that no batches contained the GIs. In this case, to achieve a greater level of confidence, each sample analyzed was subsequently spiked with 10 ppm epoxide and chlorohydrin. These samples were then rerun to prove 10 ppm could be detected.

13.5.4   Case Study 4: Sulphonate Esters

Sulphonate esters are a very common class of genotoxic impurities. Although they are easily detected using a range of other traditional techniques, it is also possible to detect them by NMR, as long as they are resolved from the substrate.

In this example, ethyl methanesulphonate, EMS (9) and methyl methanesulphonate, MMS (10) are detected in the presence of a certain API. Proton A in (9) is a quartet at 4.26 ppm, and proton B in (10) is a singlet at 3.87 ppm in d_6-DMSO.

(9)   (10)

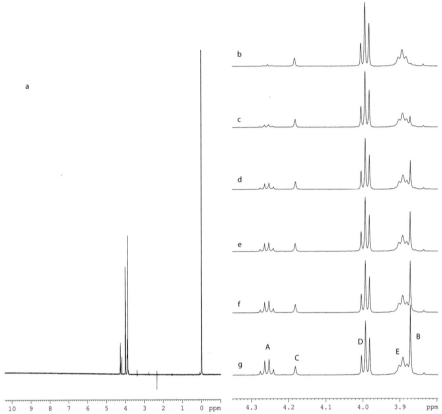

Figure 13.26 ^{1}H excitation sculpting with double gradient echo exciting the TMS signal at 0 ppm, the MMS singlet at 3.87 ppm (B), and the EMS quartet (A) at 4.26 ppm. Sample of API prepared at 100 mg/mL in d_6-DMSO, (a) showing the full expansion of a 20 ppm spike of EMS and MMS. No other signals are present in the spectra apart from those around the excited regions. Expansion of the region around the two GI signals are shown: (b) no spike, (c) 4 ppm spike of EMS and MMS, (d) 8 ppm, (e) 12 ppm, (f) 16 ppm, and (g) 20 ppm. C, D, and E are unknown impurities.

Both appear in an unoccupied region of the spectrum of the API in question. However, in contrast to previous examples, excitation sculpting has been used rather than a simple selective pulse. As described in Section 13.4.8.4, this allows the measurement of both impurities in the same experiment, and the removal of artifacts from the intense peaks at the expense of a small amount of sensitivity. This removal of artifacts is clearly seen when comparing Figure 13.26a with Figure 13.21c.

Figure 13.26b–g shows a series of spikes into the API present at a concentration of 100 mg/mL in d_6-DMSO. The NMR methodology is successful with a level of detection of approximately 4 ppm. This example highlights one difficulty with NMR. Down at ppm levels, there are often a large number of other unknown impurities present. If these happen to resonate at the same frequency as the GIs of interest, they can interfere. In this case, while the signals C-E shown in Figure 13.26, which are from unknown impurities, do not obscure the EMS and MMS signals, impurity E does make the integration of MMS (signal B) more difficult.

13.6   CONCLUSION

It has been demonstrated that NMR is a feasible technique for GI analysis that provides an excellent orthogonal technique to the more traditional methods.

It has a number of advantages over other techniques, such as:

1. Inherent quantitative nature.
2. Ease and speed of sample preparation.
3. Ability to provide a quick answer as to whether NMR is a feasible technique.
4. Ability to detect more than one GI into the same analysis and conceivably combine with other measurements, such as residual solvent analysis.

These advantages mean that NMR is a logical choice for problems, particularly in the earlier stages of pharmaceutical development when fit-for-purpose answers are required in a timely fashion. A suggested strategy is to think about NMR, investigating the spectra of both the substrate and GI independently, and do an assessment of whether any GI signals are likely to be resolved. In addition, perform some work to determine the likely solubility in a common NMR solvent, such as DMSO.

If there is resolution and a high solubility can be obtained, performing a spike at a high level, such as 1000 ppm, will quickly give an indication as to the success of the method. If such a spike is successfully, further work can continue at lower levels to determine whether NMR has sufficient sensitivity.

If the NMR work fails at this first attempt, further work can be done with different solvents or by the addition of additives to obtain resolution, or one can simply quickly move on and investigate different techniques.

There are, of course, a number of disadvantages of NMR that must be considered:

1. Inherent insensitivity.
2. Expense and available of some NMR equipment particularly higher fields and cryoprobe systems.
3. If resolution cannot be achieved between a substrate and GI, there is a limited amount that can be done compared with other chromatographic techniques, except a different solvent choice, use of additives, and possibly higher fields to give extra resolution.
4. Due to inherent sensitivity difficulties, it might be difficult to apply NMR to problems involving formulations.

In conclusion, NMR is a great orthogonal technique, and an extra tool that for certain problems can really speed up the tricky task that is trace analysis.

REFERENCES

1. Claridge T. 2008. *High Resolution NMR Technique in Organic Chemistry*. Wiley, Cambridge.
2. Cavanagh J, et al. 2006. *Protein NMR Spectroscopy: Principles and Practice*. Academic Press, San Diego, CA.
3. Ernst RR, Bodenhausen G, Wokaun A. 1990. *Principles of Nuclear Magnetic Resonance in One and Two Dimensions*. Clarendon Press, Oxford.
4. Levitt MH. 2008. *Spin Dynamics*, 2nd ed. WileyBlackwell, Chichester, UK.
5. Keeler J. 2006. *Understanding NMR Spectroscopy*. Wiley, Chichester, UK.
6. Williams DH, Fleming I. 2007. *Spectroscopic Methods in Organic Chemistry*, 6th ed. McGraw-Hill Higher Education, Maidenhead, UK.
7. Wawer I, Diehl B, Holzgrabe U. 2008. *NMR Spectroscopy in Pharmaceutical Analysis*. Elsevier Science, Amsterdam.
8. Kovacs H, Moskau D, Spraul M. 2005. Cryogenically cooled probes—a leap in NMR technology. *Progress in Nuclear Magnetic Resonance Spectroscopy* 46:131–155.
9. Hore PJ. 1989. Solvent suppression. *Methods in Enzymology* 176:64–77.
10. Guéron M, Plateau P, Decorps M. 1991. Solvent signal suppression in NMR. *Progrsss in NMR Spectroscopy* 23:135–209.
11. McKay RT. 2009. Recent advances in solvent suppression for solution NMR: a practical reference. *Annual Reports on NMR Spectroscopy* 66:33–76.
12. Bauer C, et al. 1984. Gaussian pulses. *Journal of Magnetic Resonance* 58:442–457.
13. Freeman R. 1998. Shaped radiofrequency pulses in high resolution NMR. *Journal of Progress in Nuclear Magnetic Resonance Spectroscopy* 32:59–106.
14. Vincent SJF, Zwahlen C. 1997. Selective pulses in NMR. In: *Methods for Structure Elucidation by High-Resolution NMR*, edited by G Batta, KE Kövér, C Szántay Jr. Elsevier Science, Amsterdam, pp. 1–19.
15. Hwang T-L, Shaka AJ. 1995. Water suppression that works. Excitation sculpting using arbitrary waveforms and pulsed field gradients. *Journal of Magnetic Resonance. Series A* 112:275–279.
16. Stott K, et al. 1995. Excitation sculpting in high-resolution nuclear magnetic resonance spectroscopy: Application selective NOE experiments. *Journal of the American Chemical Society* 117: 4199–4200.

CHAPTER 14

MECHANISM AND PROCESSING PARAMETERS AFFECTING THE FORMATION OF SULFONATE ESTERS: SUMMARY OF THE PRODUCT QUALITY RESEARCH INSTITUTE STUDIES

Andrew Teasdale

14.1 INTRODUCTION

Since the advent of the EMEA Guideline—Limits for Genotoxic Impurities (GIs)—the issue of genotoxic impurities has been the subject of significant regulatory scrutiny. Within the variety of classes of GIs, none have come under more scrutiny than sulfonate esters, the theoretical product of a reaction between a sulfonic acid and an alcohol. Indeed concerns over sulfonic acids and the potential to generate sulfonate esters when in contact with alcoholic solvents predate the advent of the guideline. The first clear reference to such concerns came with the publication within PharmEuropa in 2000[1] of a short article that drew attention to the potential risk of formation of sulfonate esters as a result of a combination of sulfonic acids in alcoholic solution as part of a salt formation process. At the time of publication, this was merely a call for "further information," it being an attempt to prompt the generation of data to understand better the extent of any of risk. This publication is now seen by many as one of the triggers eventually leading to the EMEA guideline. Thus, in many ways, the concern over sulfonate esters was itself the trigger for the drive for specific control over the broader range of GIs.

The specific reason for the concerns relating to sulfonate esters stems from the properties of the sulfonate group and its labile nature, that is the fact that it can readily displaced by a nucleophile, resulting in the alkylation of the nucleophile

Genotoxic Impurities: Strategies for Identification and Control, Edited by Andrew Teasdale
Copyright © 2010 by John Wiley & Sons, Inc.

concerned. This, of course, includes biological nucleophiles such as DNA. Indeed, studies conducted by Glowienke et al.[2] demonstrate that many such sulfonate esters are mutagenic.

During the period of time between 2000 and mid-2006, when the EMEA guideline was itself under development, sulfonate esters came under ever increasing scrutiny. This led to calls either to avoid the use of alcoholic solvents when handling sulfonic acids in salt formation processes, or, even more extreme, to eliminate their use altogether, that is not to develop sulfonic acids as counterions at all.

The potential loss of sulfonic acids as counterions was a major concern.[3] Doing so would have a significant impact. It would eliminate an entire class of pharmaceutically useful counterions, leading to the potential development of suboptimal API forms, for example hygroscopic. It could also impact on the synthesis of the API through restricting the use of reagents such as mesylates/tosylates. The frustration was compounded by the fact that both industry and regulators alike poorly understood the extent of the risk and even the mechanism involved in the formation of sulfonate esters.

Matters to some extent came to a head during a Drug Information Association (DIA) meeting held in Bethesda, Maryland in late 2005. During one of the sessions at this meeting, a debate took place between FDA officials and members of the audience from the pharmaceutical industry. FDA queried as to why were industry still using sulfonic acids as counterions. The response for a number of participants was to look to defend their use on the basis that many had examined the resultant APIs, for example mesylates, tosylates, and no one had found predicted esters such as ethyl methanesulfonate (EMS) at a level of concern in isolated materials. The debate continued after the session, with the FDA showing interest in the scientific understanding behind these results. What was clear was that although ester formation was controlled, exactly how was not fully understood. This directly set up the challenge for industry to develop a detailed understanding of the factors associated with the formation of sulfonate esters, and the work described in this chapter was born.

The Product Quality Research Institute (PQRI) is a nonprofit consortium of organizations involving the pharmaceutical industry and FDA's Centre for Drug Evaluation and Research (CDER) and Health Canada. Its mission is work together to generate and share relevant information that advances drug product quality and development. Given the nature of the problem with sulfonate esters and the FDA's interest, PQRI was seen as the ideal vehicle through which to conduct research into this area.

The keen interest in this initiative resulted in the formation of a multidisciplinary team with representatives from a significant number of major pharmaceutical companies. Individuals were selected to ensure that the team had the requisite skill set in the critical areas of analytical and physical organic chemistry/kinetics. Another critical decision taken at the onset of the project was to involve the Research Institute of Chromatography (RIC). The RIC, led by Professor Pat Sandra, is renowned for its expertise in the field of trace analysis, and thus was able to make a telling contribution from a technical perspective. Furthermore, by taking this approach, it was possible to ensure that the project had dedicated resource, which was a critical factor in conducting the work in the desired timeframe.

Soon after the work was initiated, the importance of the research became even clearer. In May–June 2007, it was widely reported in both the scientific and general press[4] that patients taking Viracept® (nelfinavir mesylate), an antiviral marketed by Hoffmann-La Roche (Basel, Switzerland), had complained of the tablets possessing a strong odor and of adverse reactions, such as nausea. It subsequently became clear that the tablets were contaminated with the sulfonate ester EMS, with levels of up to 2300 ppm eventually being reported. This led to the temporary withdrawal of Viracept and also further heightened concerns over sulfonic acid salts in general.[5,6]

14.2   REACTION MECHANISM

Sulfonic acids are widely used as counterions for APIs,[7] to modify and manipulate the physical properties of the API to develop an appropriate physical form. Low molecular weight alcohols such as methanol, ethanol, and isopropanol are widely used as solvents in processes used to produce such salts, and thus the risk is that the sulfonic acid can react with the alcohol during the manufacturing process, yielding the corresponding sulfonate ester.

The solvolytic behavior of sulfonate esters has been studied in great detail, particularly with respect to both kinetics of hydrolysis and the products from sulfonates of increasingly complex alcohols. Analytical methodologies based on spectroscopy or conductance used for some early kinetic studies assumed the solvolysis proceeded to completion, thereby implying no mechanism to form sulfonate esters in alcoholic solutions. Little consideration had been given to assessing any levels of residual ester, which might have characterized any propensity for the reverse reaction—the formation of esters. A *post facto* justification of the assumption of "complete" solvolysis can be found in the work described by Teasdale et al.,[8] as the low levels of ester reported would not been sufficient to have introduced noticeable errors in kinetic measurements.

At the advent of these studies into the potential reaction between sulfonic acids and alcohols, little was known about the mechanism of formation of sulfonic acid, with only one identified reference in the literature.[9] Within this paper, Snodin briefly commented on the possible mechanism and the low likelihood of reaction; however, there was no experimental data to provide proof of the postulated mechanism. That no data is available is unsurprising, as in synthetic terms, the reaction is of very little value. This is because there are far more effective means of generating sulfonate esters, usually employing the corresponding sulfonyl chloride.

As a result of the paucity of data, it was decided to look to study the reaction mechanism in order to be able to understand the factors that impact on the reaction, ultimately to be able to manipulate these to enable effective control during salt formation processes.

Ahead of the study, two mechanistic pathways were postulated, as shown in Figure 14.1, using the example of the reaction between methanesulfonic acid (MSA) and methanol.

Pathway "1" involves protonation of the alcohol by the sulfonic acid and subsequent nucleophilic attack of the resultant sulfonate anion on the protonated

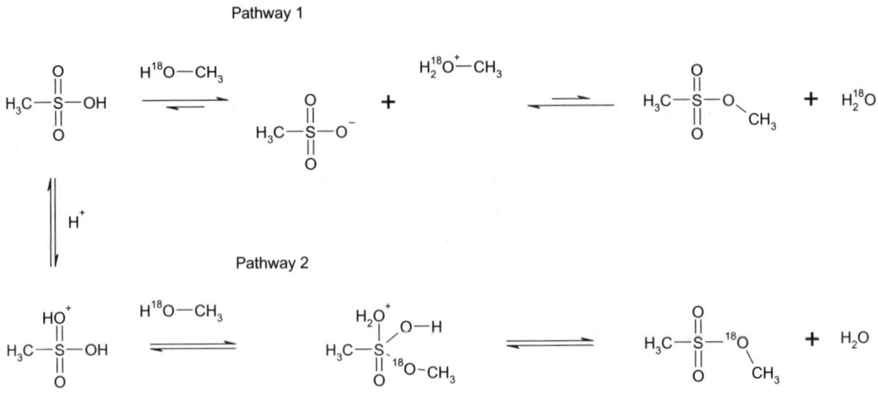

Pathway 1

Pathway 2

Figure 14.1 Potential mechanistic pathways for the formation of sulfonate esters.

alcohol, yielding the corresponding sulfonate ester. Pathway "2" is analogous to the $A_{AC}2$ mechanism associated with acid-catalysed esterification of carboxylic acids.

In order to elucidate the mechanism, a simple experiment was designed using ^{18}O-labeled methanol. Were the mechanism to follow pathway "1," then it would be expected that all of the ^{18}O label would be present in the water molecule. The reverse is true for pathway "2," where the label would expect to reside in the subsequent methyl methanesulfonate (MMS) molecule generated by the reaction.

Solutions of ^{18}O-methanol/MSA and unlabeled methanol/MSA were heated at reflux for a short period of time (2 h), and then the resultant solutions analyzed by direct injection GC-MS. Within the resultant chromatograms peaks corresponding to excess methanol, water and MMS were detected, the latter being positively identified based on it mass spectrum.

The level of conversion observed was low. Examining the mass spectrum of the MMS formed using isotope-labeled methanol showed only one molecular ion m/z 110. This was identical to that obtained from the corresponding reaction involving the unlabelled methanol. This clearly demonstrated that the ^{18}O was not incorporated into the MMS molecule, supporting pathway "1." Further evidence was provided through the extraction of ion chromatograms at m/z 18 (water) and 20 ($H_2^{18}O$). When these were overlaid, a peak at m/z 20 was only observed in the reaction involving the labeled methanol, confirming that the isotope label was incorporated into the water molecule. These findings were critical in not only clearly demonstrating the essential features of the mechanism, but also in proving that sulfonic acids are not analogous with their carboxylic acid counterparts as might have been postulated.

Another key observation is the proton dependency of the reaction. As will be illustrated later, this underpins all of the results seen in the kinetic studies.

In addition to pathways "1" and "2" describing reversible reactions, the well established *(vide supra)* solvolysis is a third competing reaction limiting net ester formation. This is shown in Figure 14.2 for the consumption of MMS. In the experiment, diethyl ether was detected, eluting just before methanol in the GC analysis.

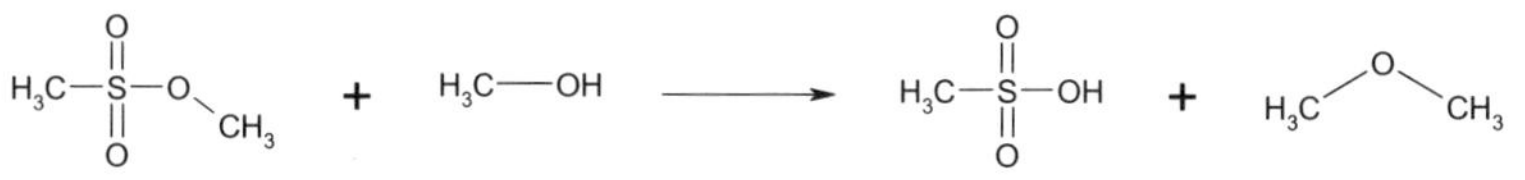

Figure 14.2   Solvolysis of sulfonate esters.

This was confirmed by analysis of the mass spectrum. In the case of the reaction involving the labeled methanol, the peak had shifted by two mass units showing that the ^{18}O label had been incorporated into the ether.

14.3   ANALYTICAL METHODOLOGY

At the onset of these studies, it was realized that in order to be able to profile and kinetically model any reaction between sulfonic acids and alcohols, it was critical that the data obtained from any reaction studies was accurate and precise. Within the PQRI working group, many of the individual companies represented had developed their own approaches to the analysis of sulfonate esters. Indeed, a comprehensive review of the literature[10] revealed a multiplicity of approaches. Included within the techniques employed were HPLC, direct GC analysis, liquid/liquid extraction, and derivatization techniques.

Direct analysis of alkyl esters of volatile methanesulfonates by gas chromatography (GC) is possible both in combination with mass spectrometric (MS) and flame ionization (FID) detection. Although ppm (μg/g) sensitivity can be achieved, matrix effects can be significant, resulting in contamination of the inlet and/or solute degradation. Furthermore, formation of sulfonate esters in heated inlet systems (through sample pyrolysis and flash reaction with solvents) has also been observed. The use of GC is also restricted to volatile sulfonate esters such as EMS and is not suitable for aryl sulfonate esters, for example ethyl tosylate. This was, however, briefly studied at the start of the studies, focused on EMS, but the level of precision was too poor for it to be of any practical value.

HPLC offered an alternative with the advantage being that decomposition of the API is less likely to occur, at least in solution. There are drawbacks to this approach, however, including concerns over the stability of sulfonate esters in aqueous solutions and mobile phases.

The issue of contamination/solute degradation can be avoided through extraction methods such as (micro-) liquid-liquid extraction, solid phase micro-extraction (SPME), and solid phase extraction (SPE); however, for the purposes of these studies, where rapid analysis of a high volume of samples was required, such techniques were ruled out as impractical.

In order to address the issue of analyte stability another alternative is derivatization. Two methods were described in the literature; Lee et al.[11] published a method where esters of methanesulfonic acid (MSA) were determined by GC after derivatization with sodium thiocyanate. The subsequent alkylthiocyanates and alkylisothiocyanates were analyzed by static headspace (SHS) coupled to GC-MS.

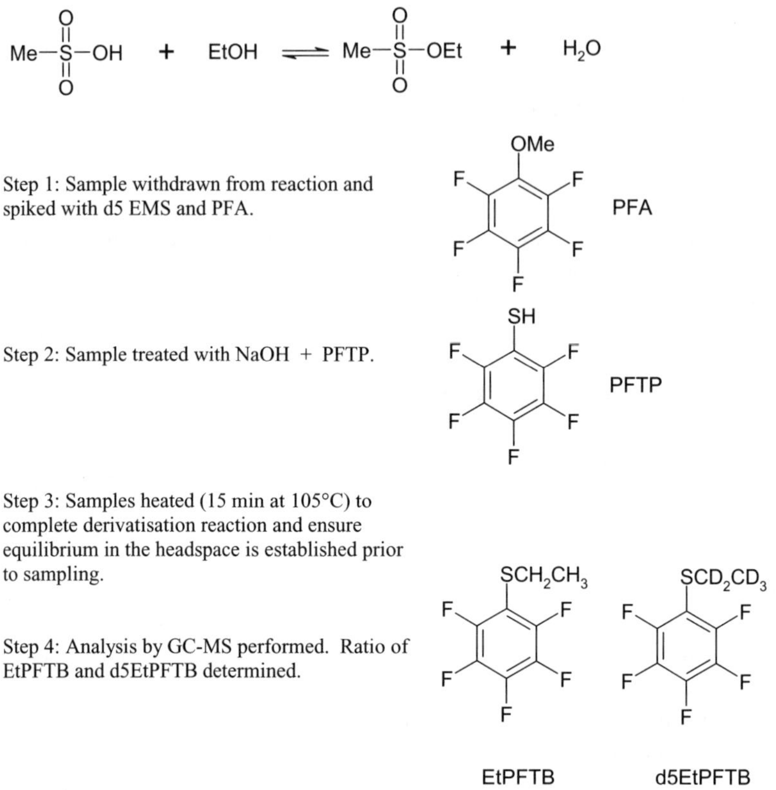

$$Me\!-\!\underset{\underset{O}{\|}}{\overset{\overset{O}{\|}}{S}}\!-\!OH \;+\; EtOH \;\rightleftharpoons\; Me\!-\!\underset{\underset{O}{\|}}{\overset{\overset{O}{\|}}{S}}\!-\!OEt \;+\; H_2O$$

Step 1: Sample withdrawn from reaction and spiked with d5 EMS and PFA.

PFA

Step 2: Sample treated with NaOH + PFTP.

PFTP

Step 3: Samples heated (15 min at 105°C) to complete derivatisation reaction and ensure equilibrium in the headspace is established prior to sampling.

Step 4: Analysis by GC-MS performed. Ratio of EtPFTB and d5EtPFTB determined.

EtPFTB   d5EtPFTB

Figure 14.3   Analytical procedure based on pentafluorothiophenol (PFTP) derivatization.

More recently, another derivatization method was published by Alzaga et al.[12] This had been used to determine the levels of methyl, ethyl, and isopropyl esters of sulfonic acids in API's at sub-ppm level. The method was developed in conjunction with the RIC and is based on derivatisation using pentafluorothiophenol (PFTP) to yield a stable volatile alkyl thio ether, which is subsequently analyzed by static headspace and GC-MS analysis.

Another critical aspect of this method was the utilization of an internal standard, significantly improving the method's precision and accuracy. The standards used were the deuterated form of the sulfonate ester; these were synthesized using deuterated alcohols.

The actual analytical procedure is illustrated in Figure 14.3, using the example of EMS.

This method was eventually selected as the basis for the studies described in the chapter.

However, the original method was focused on the determination of trace levels of sulfonate ester in API. In contrast, the present studies were focused on the formation of sulfonate ester in concentrated reaction mixtures. Thus, minor modifications (changes to the levels of derivatizing agent and NaOH added) were made to the method to ensure it demonstrated the requisite precision and reproducibility over the

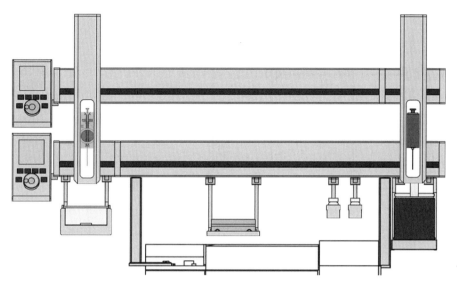

Figure 14.4   Schematic representation of the instrument used for the conduct of studies.

wide linear dynamic range required. One further modification was the incorporation of a second internal standard pentafluoroanisole (PFA). This internal standard, which has a chemical structure similar to the derivatized solutes (methyl ether instead of ethyl sulfide), was used to monitor instrument performance. A large deviation observed on the peak area of PFA would indicate an error in IS addition (liquid handling) and/or in static headspace analysis.

This derivatization-headspace GC-MS method was ultimately fully automated using a robotic system and applied to the analysis of multiple sulfonic acid/alcohol systems. A schematic representation of the system is provided in Figure 14.4. The key feature of this is the use of a dual rail system to allow both sampling of the reaction plus the derivatization process.

It should be noted that rather than performing one single reaction from which aliquots could be withdrawn, a series of identical reactions were established, these being placed in individual vials within the sample tray. Full details of the method are described in the paper published by Jacq et al.[13]

14.4   EXPERIMENTAL PROTOCOL

Having established the analytical methodology, the next step was to define the scope of the scope of the studies in terms of which sulfonic acid/alcohol systems to study and thereafter the design space for each system.

14.4.1   Sulfonic Acid/Alcohol Systems

Two extensive reviews by Berge et al.[14,15] have evaluated the relative frequency of usage of pharmaceutical salts. These show that of the sulfonic acids used, MSA is the most common, the next most prevalent being toluenesulfonic acid. On this basis,

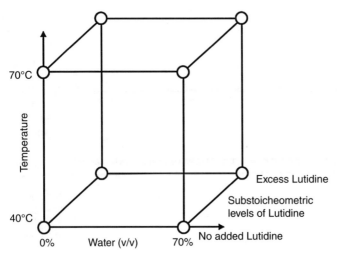

Figure 14.5   Reaction design space.

these two counterions were selected for study. By doing so, this also ensured that the studies exemplified the behavior of both alkyl and aryl sulfonic acids.

In terms of low molecular weight alcohols, methanol, ethanol, and isopropanol were selected, because they are the most commonly used alcohols. Their use also ensured that both primary and secondary alcohols were studied.

It should be noted, however, that the methodology described is flexible enough to also be applied to other systems, less common, systems.

14.4.2   Reaction Design Space

The scope of this was dictated by the desire to ensure that the conditions studied were directly relevant to typical process conditions associated with salt formation processes. This design -space can be visualized as cuboid, see Figure 14.5.

The front face of the cube addresses the strongly acidic alcohol/sulfonic acid system and the effect of temperature and water content, while the rest of the cuboid addresses salt-like systems, or measures of acidity.

All reactions were carried out in solution at concentrations appropriate to processes for salt formation processes.

The ethanol/MSA system was the starting point for these studies.

14.5   EXPERIMENTAL RESULTS

14.5.1   Experimental Results from Study of the EMS System

14.5.1.1   EMS Formation: Effect of Temperature   The effect of temperature on the level of EMS formed is graphically illustrated in Figure 14.6. This represents

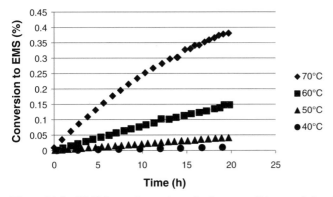

Figure 14.6   EMS formation under anhydrous conditions and the effect of temperature.

the molar conversion of sulfonate anion to ester in solution. Even at elevated temperature, 70°C, less than 0.4% conversion was observed after 20 h. After 80 h, reaction was approaching a pseudoequilibrium molar conversion at ca. 0.65%. This again illustrates the point made earlier that from a synthetic perspective, this is an extremely ineffective way to synthesize sulfonate esters, that is it is a chemically useless reaction.

From this, it can be clearly seen that controlling temperature can minimize the level of ester formed. It also illustrates the time taken to reach equilibrium, showing that minimizing the residence time of sulfonic acid in alcoholic solution can dramatically reduce the level of ester formed.

It is important to recognize that this study, focused on the simple binary (acid + alcohol) system, demonstrates the upper limit that may be formed in solution. In API manufacture, isolation processes would be expected to significantly reduce the levels, the majority remaining in the mother liquors. Thus, the level seen in solution represents an upper limit in terms of potential contamination and by comparing this to the level in isolated material it is possible to determine the efficiency of the salt formation process itself to purge any sulfonate ester present.

14.5.1.2 EMS Formation: Effect of Water
Reaction profiles in the presence of added water are shown in Figure 14.7. The water content in each reaction mixture was measured by Karl–Fisher titration at the start of the reaction, and expressed as % w/w. The presence of even moderate water at levels of 5% w/w reduced the levels of EMS by a factor of approximately one-third to below 1000 ppm molar conversion at 70°C after a reaction time of 18 h. This can be rationalized by both the stronger solvation of protons by water compared with ethanol reducing the forward reaction, and by the enhanced rate of hydrolysis of EMS compared with ethanolysis.

Where high levels of water are present in the system the level of conversion is very effectively suppressed.

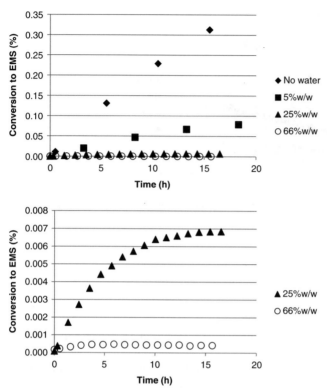

Figure 14.7 EMS formation—the effect of water on conversion; including Expansion of plots for 25 and 66% w/w reaction systems.

14.5.1.3 EMS Formation: The Impact of the Presence of Base

Low but appreciable sulfonate ester formation, as illustrated, does occur under strongly acidic conditions when combined with high temperature. However, salt formations using sulfonic acid counter ions often employ either stoichiometric amounts or at most small excesses of acid.

Experiments were therefore designed to have the sulfonate anion present at a comparable concentration to the binary system (acid + alcohol only), but with reduced proton availability. The formation of EMS under conditions of lower acidity was tested using the weak base 2,6-lutidine as a surrogate API. No measurable rate of EMS formation was observed (above background noise) when a slight excess of 2,6-lutidine was used, the "reaction" being studied over a time period in excess of 12 h at 70°C. (see Fig. 14.8).

When a 2% excess of MSA was present, a reaction did occur, however, at a very slow rate (approximately 0.004% conversion after 12 h at 70°C).

The lack of any reaction when an excess of base is present is entirely consistent with the reaction mechanism and the fact that the reaction is proton mediated. Without the transfer of the proton to the alcohol, no reaction can occur. The proton

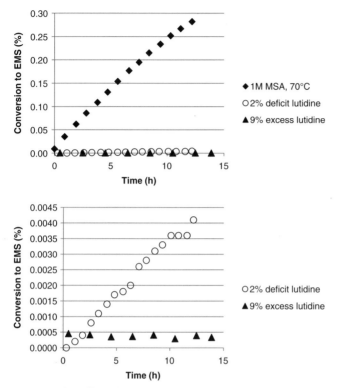

Figure 14.8   Effect of added base on EMS formation.

will react overwhelmingly with the strongest base present, in this case 2,6-lutidine, in preference to ethanol. This also illustrates that the conjugate acid of 2,6-lutidine is not strong enough to protonate ethanol.

This was tested further by conducting an experiment where a small excess of lutidine was used, to which was added a 10% excess of concentrated phosphoric acid, thus neutralizing the excess base. Even under these conditions, no reaction was observed, illustrating that an acid strength exceeding that of phosphoric acid is required in order for sulfonate ester formation to occur. The same experiment was conducted for all three alcohols studied, methanol, ethanol, and isopropanol, no reaction was observed in any of the systems.

14.5.2   Other MSA Systems

14.5.2.1   *Experimental Results from Study of the MMS System*   The above set of experiments was repeated studying the reaction between methane sulfonic acid and methanol. The results were consistent with those obtained for EMS. Figure 14.9 shows the results obtained for MMS, the plot showing the impact of both temperature and water content on the level of conversion.

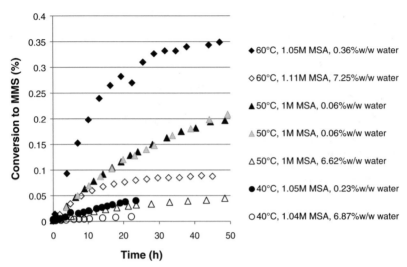

Figure 14.9   Combined plot showing the impact of both temperature and water content on conversion rates.

Most critically of all, no reaction was seen in the presence of a slight molar excess of 2,6-lutidine.

14.5.2.2 Experimental Results from Study of the Isopropyl Methanesulfonate (IMS) System   In terms of reaction profile, the results were very similar to those seen for the EMS and IMS systems. The level of conversion under anhydrous/high temperature conditions was higher at around 1% conversion in comparison with EMS/MMS, where levels were less than 0.5% over the same time period (Fig. 14.10).

Again, critically, no reaction was seen in the presence of a slight molar excess of Lutidine.

14.5.3   Experimental Results from Study of Toluenesulfonic (Tosic) Acid Systems

As well as studying the reaction between MSA and alcohols, an identical series of studies were performed for toluenesulfonic (tosic) acid, another common salt counterion. Studying this system also allowed us to determine what differences there were, if any, between an alkyl and aryl sulfonic acid, in particular whether there was any significant differences in terms of proton dependence and extent of reaction.

14.5.3.1 Experimental Results from Study of the Ethyl Tosylate (ETS) System   The reaction profile for formation of ethyl tosylate was directly comparable to that of the equivalent alkyl system (MSA + ethanol). Figure 14.11 shows

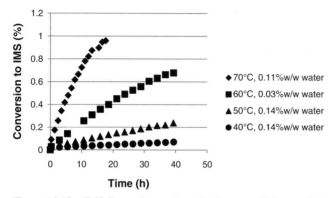

Figure 14.10   IMS Formation under anhydrous conditions and the effect of temperature.

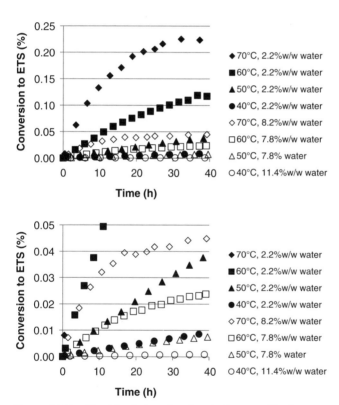

Figure 14.11   Combined plots showing the impact of both temperature and water content on conversion rates.

the impact of temperature and water on conversion rates. It is important to note that the studies described were performed using toluenesulfonic acid mono-hydrate; this was used, as the anhydrous form is not commercially available and therefore any production of a tosylate salt would involve the use of the mono-hydrate.

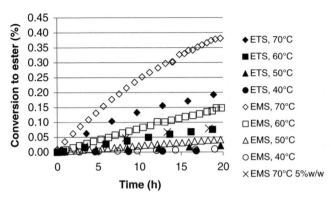

Figure 14.12 Comparison between conversions of MSA and TSA to ETS and EMS in ethanol.

A further critical result was the observation that for all of the tosylate systems studied (methanol, ethanol, and isopropanol), no observable reaction was observed where an excess of lutidine was present. This clearly demonstrates that the mechanism of reaction between sulfonic acid and alcohol (methanol, ethanol, and isopropanol) is common to both MSA and tosic acid. It would therefore seem reasonable to postulate that the reaction mechanism, elucidated through a study of MMS using isotope labeled ^{18}O methanol, is common to all sulfonic acid–alcohol reactions.

The data collected allows a direct comparison to be made between the EMS and ETS systems. This is illustrated in Figure 14.12. Visual comparison shows no substantive difference between representative alkyl and aryl sulfonic acids.

14.5.4 Solvolysis: The Impact of Alcohol, Water, Acid, and Base

As described earlier (see Figs. 14.1 and 14.2), as the reaction between acid and alcohol progresses a competing reaction, alcoholysis, starts to become increasingly prevalent as a build up sulfonate ester occurs. This, in combination with the reverse solvolysis reaction with water, eventually leads to the establishment of a pseudo-steady state condition within the reaction system.

The methodology developed for study of sulfonate ester formation was equally applicable to study of solvolytic reactions. This was simply done by starting at a predefined sulfonate ester concentration, and then studying the decline in level as a function of time.

The effect of acid and base and water on solvolysis rates was thus studied through the addition of 2,6-lutidine, MSA, and water. The observed rates of solvolysis were very similar (Fig. 14.13) in the presence of either MSA or 2,6-lutidine, but increased, as would be expected, with increasing water content. Hence, it was concluded that alcoholysis rates were not acid or base catalyzed.

Similar observations were made in the solvolysis of EMS. In addition, reactions were also performed with varying ratios of EMS to MSA. With a molar proportion of EMS higher than the pseudo-equilibrium ratio (7% vs. ca. 0.65%),

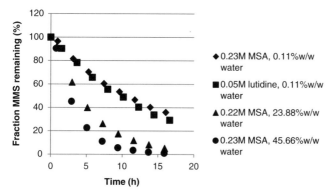

Figure 14.13   Solvolysis of MMS in aqueous methanol.

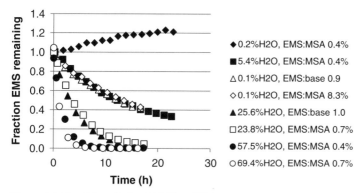

Figure 14.14   Ethanolysis of EMS at 70°C.

EMS was consumed *via* solvolysis, whereas with a lower proportion, EMS continued to be formed (Fig. 14.14).

14.5.5   Kinetic Modeling

At the onset of the work described within this chapter, the quality of the data collected through the experimental studies was recognized as critical were we to be able to achieve the stated aim of being able to generate a kinetic model of the system. As can be seen from the data illustrated above, the quality of the data is very high, clearly demonstrated by the smoothness of the reaction profiles. Indeed, the method used for the analysis, when validated, was found to achieve relative standard deviations of <5% across the full data range. To illustrate this point further, Figure 14.15 shows an overlay of two entirely separate experiments performed for MMS formation. As can be seen, they show excellent agreement.

Thus, with the assurance of the quality of data, it was possible to kinetically model each of the systems to determine rate constants and activation energies. Fitting data for the formation of sulfonate ester in "anhydrous" alcohols (no base present)

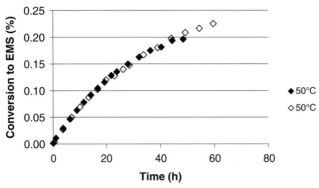

Figure 14.15   Comparison of data from two separate determinations of the conversion to MMS under anhydrous conditions at 50°C.

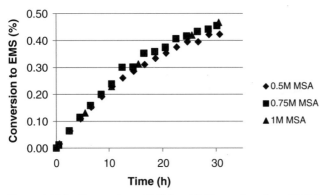

Figure 14.16   Conversion of MSA to EMS as a function of MSA concentration in "anhydrous" ethanol.

required a kinetic model which was first order in sulfonic acid. Plots of fractional conversion to ester showed (initial) rates independent of concentration of sulfonic acid (Fig. 14.16).

The kinetic modeling was performed using Dynochem® (DynoChem, Inc., Wilmington, DE). Rate constants for hydrolysis and alcoholysis were refined by including data from solvolysis reactions.

Table 14.1 illustrates the full kinetic data derived from the mesylate systems studied. Included are rate constants for formation, alcoholysis, and hydrolysis at reference temperatures, along with Activation energies.

Using these data, it becomes possible to predict sulfonate ester formation as a function of temperature.

Under anhydrous conditions, the observed kinetics, first order in terms of sulfonic acid, can be interpreted as a reaction of ion pairs (a "single" reacting species). However, this model does not describe the measured data in aqueous

TABLE 14.1 Kinetic Data

Sulfonate Ester	Forward rate (/sec)	Activation Energy (kJ/mol)	Hydrolysis rate[a] (L/ mol·sec)	Alcohol	Alcoholysis rate[a] (L/ mol·sec)	Activation energy (kJ/mol)[d]
MMS	7.10E-08 (60°C)	115[b]	3.03E-06	Methanol	8.50E-07	95
EMS	7.90E-08 (70°C)	114[c]	4.80E-06	Ethanol	6.0E-07	85
IMS	2.26E-07 (70°C)	123[c]	1.09E-5	Isopropanol	1.03E-06	105

[a] Rate constants were measured at the corresponding reference study temperature.

[b] Forward rate constants were measured at 60, 40, and 30°C and the activation energy calculated using Dynochem.

[c] Forward rate constants were measured at 70, 60, 50, and 40°C and the activation energy calculated using Dynochem.

[d] Estimate calculated from difference in equilibrium value projected at various temperatures.

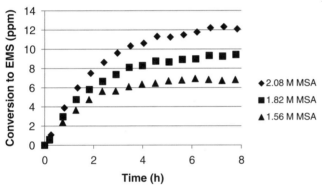

Figure 14.17   Conversion of MSA to EMS as a function of MSA concentration in 60% w/w water in ethanol.

alcoholic systems. Plots of fractional conversion to ester show formation rates are dependent on concentration of sulfonic acid, indicating non-first-order kinetics (Fig. 14.17).

Reactions of separated sulfonate anions and (solvated) protons might be expected to demonstrate second-order kinetics. The hydration of proton would favour ion separation in aqueous systems. However, clean second-order kinetics were not observed, even in solvent systems with high water content (where conversion to ester was very low), making good estimates of the second-order rate constant difficult to attain. Both mechanisms are operational in the presence of water. Fitting multiple data sets covering a range of water contents did not lead to satisfactory estimates of the second-order rate constant, as the partition between ion pairs and separated ions proved not to be a simple function of water content. Both kinetic models explain the requirement for acid to be present for the formation of sulfonate esters.

The conclusion from the available data was that the first-order model appears sound, and represents a "worst-case" model for predicting ester formation in systems where there is an excess of sulfonic acid present. In the presence of water, models are not yet sufficiently refined to be able to make accurate predictions, but the data-sets provide a series of "reference points," representing specific water contents, against which potential processes may be assessed.

14.5.6   Key Learnings and Their Implications for Process Design

What is clear from these studies is that under certain specific ranges of conditions, low levels of sulfonate esters can form. In particular, conditions favorable to the low-level formation of sulfonate ester include the presence of sulfonic acids under essentially anhydrous conditions in alcoholic solvents at elevated temperature, held there for prolonged periods. For example, levels of up to 0.3 mole% EMS are formed after MSA is held in solution in ethanol for 24 h at 70°C.

However, as would be expected of any kinetic process, the reaction rate can be modified through adjusting the reaction temperature, thus immediately offering a relatively simple way of affecting the rate of ester formation. Close examination of Figure 14.5 shows that the conversion can be reduced to well below 0.1% simply by reducing the temperature to below 40°C. This provides clear guidance to a process chemist to run the desired chemistry at the lowest practical temperature to minimize the ester formation.

Another key parameter affecting the extent of reaction is the level of water present. The presence of water has a twofold impact. First, formation rates are reduced due to the competition for protons between water and the alcohol molecules; reducing the number of alcoholic molecules protonated. Second, the accumulation of sulfonate ester is reduced by the back-reaction, that is hydrolysis. This, as demonstrated by the data in Table 14.1, is a significantly faster reaction than the analogous solvolytic pathway involving solvolysis through reaction between the sulfonate ester and alcohol. Close examination of Figure 14.7 shows the profound impact high water levels can have—under highly aqueous conditions—in excess of 50% w/w water: virtually no reaction occurs, at least in the timescales typically associated with a salt formation process. This again is a very simple precautionary step that can be taken should the process concerned be amenable to such high waters levels without having a negative impact, for example poor yields or a reduction in quality, that is higher levels of other impurities. Perhaps the simplest example of how this could be achieved is through the use of an MSA solution in water, as opposed to neat MSA. A 70% w/w aqueous solution of MSA is commercially available.

By far the most significant factor, though, in terms of control, is the manipulation of the level of acidity. Where a stoichiometric amount of base was present, no observable reaction was seen. This was the same within all of the systems studied. This observation is entirely consistent with the mechanism of the reaction, where it was elucidated that the first step in the reaction involved protonation of the alcohol. Where there is base present, there is competition for the proton between the base and the alcohol; however, given the relative basicity of the base in comparison with alcohols, the proton almost exclusively resides on the base. Use of a stoichiometric amount of base effectively removes the proton source that drives sulfonate ester formation. This is further explained by considering the relative rates associated with this proton transfer compared with the rates associated with sulfonate ester formation; proton transfer being many orders of magnitude faster.

All of the studies described here were carried out in solution; however, another important factor in control of sulfonate esters is their solubility. Levels of sulfonate ester are very likely to be substantially lower in isolated material, when the solubility of such species is considered, sulfonate esters effectively being freely soluble in alcohols. Certainly, the levels of ester formed are well below any practical limit in solubility terms. Thus, even in scenarios whereby esters are formed, these can be easily removed by effective/efficient deliquoring during work-up, thus providing yet more effective protection from the risk of sulfonate ester contamination of APIs.

14.5.7 Processing Rules

Taking the key points from these studies it is possible to devise a set of very simple rules that, where applied, mean that sulfonic acids can be used to form salts without risk of sulfonate ester contamination. These are:

Step 1: Use a stoichiometric amount or slight excess of free-base API when forming the salt, provided this does not significantly impact on the yield.

Step 2: If it is necessary to use a substoichiometric amount of base, try to introduce water into the process to inhibit sulfonate ester formation. This can be introduced, for example in the case of MSA through the use of an aqueous solution, a 70% w/w solution in water being commercially available.

Step 3: The greatest risk of sulfonate ester formation relates to where sulfonic acids are mixed with alcohols in the absence of base. In terms of salt formation, this is most likely to occur where a solution of the acid needs to be preprepared. Where this is necessary, try to use a partially aqueous solvent system, use the minimum temperature, and keep hold times to a minimum. Applying such controls should restrict levels of ester formed to a level that is inconsequential.

14.5.8 What About Viracept?

A common challenge to this work is the above question and the assertion that the events associated with Viracept conflict with these studies. The issues associated with Viracept were the result of prolonged contact between trace amounts of ethanol and MSA inadvertently present together within a head tank. Roche have disclosed the details of their investigation into the contamination.[16] This occurred due to a GMP failure. During the routine maintenance/cleaning of the plant, cleaning with ethanol was carried out. However, the tank was not dried, resulting in a small amount of ethanol remaining in the head tank. The tank was then charged with MSA, and over a period of time, several months, significant amounts of EMS were formed that, when introduced into the salt formation process, ultimately contaminated the isolated salt, levels of up to 2300 ppm being observed. Closer examination of this chain of events shows that rather than conflicting with the findings described above, they are in fact entirely consistent with them. Reflecting on the mechanism of sulfonate ester formation, as illustrated, this is proton mediated. In the Viracept incident, rather than the typical scenario, whereby acidity is limited, in that case, there was an unlimited source of acidity, MSA being effectively the solvent. Thus, it is entirely understandable that appreciable levels of EMS formed over the time period involved, the only limiting factor being that the "reaction" was held at room temperature.

14.5.9 What About Other Sources of Sulfonate Esters?

Another factor to take into consideration is the quality of raw materials, that is that of the sulfonic acid. The sulfonic acid itself can be contaminated with sulfonate esters or other reactive species, such as sulfonyl chlorides, that can readily form sulfonate esters on contact with alcohols. The level and nature of these is dependant upon the manufacturing process used. This is of particular significance in relation to MSA.

Traditionally, MSA has been manufactured through a two-step process involving the oxidative chlorination of methyl sulphide (methyl mercaptan) followed by hydrolysis of the resultant sulfonyl chloride (Fig. 14.18).

The resultant MSA can often contain several thousand ppm of residual methane sulfonyl chloride that if introduced into a salt formation involving an alcoholic solvent, will rapidly react with the alcohol to form a sulfonate ester. MSA produced via this route can also often contain both MMS and EMS, at variable, but appreciable, levels.

Relatively recently, an alternative process has been devised to manufacture MSA, this involving a two-step process. However, in this instance, the starting material is methanol.

The resultant MSA generated from this alternative process is significantly cleaner with virtually no sulfonyl chloride or EMS/MMS being present. MSA

Historical Process

$$CH_3SH + 3\,Cl_2 + 2\,H_2O \longrightarrow CH_3SO_2Cl + 5\,HCl$$

$$CH_3SO_2Cl + H_2O \longrightarrow CH_3SO_3H + HCl$$

Alternative MSA Manufacturing Process

$$H_2 + 2\,CH_3OH + 2\,S \longrightarrow CH_3\text{-S-S-}CH_3 + 2\,H_2O$$

$$CH_3\text{-S-S-}CH_3 + 5/2\,O_2 + H_2O \xrightarrow{\text{catalyst}} 2\,CH_3\text{-}SO_3H$$

Figure 14.18 Manufacture of MSA—Historical process + alternative process.

manufactured via this process is also available as an aqueous (70% w/w) solution, further eliminating any risk from a sulfonate ester perspective.

14.5.10   Potential for Ester Formation in the Solid Phase

A question that is often asked is: What is the potential risk of formation of sulfonate esters either during formulation processes such as wet granulation of a sulfonic acid salt in alcohols, or within the solid dosage form on storage?

Although no formal solid phase studies were performed as part of the PQRI research, many of the parties involved had themselves studied sulfonate ester formation both during formulation and subsequently on stability. No ester formation had ever been observed.

A recent paper relating to the chemical side of the Viracept incident[16] looked in detail at the level of EMS present in film-coated tablets and how this changed on storage. What they observed was that rather than any additional sulfonate ester forming on stability, the exact opposite occurred, that is the level was seen to reduce as a result of hydrolysis. This was seen under all storage conditions studied and is illustrated in Figure 14.19.

Using data from these studies, Roche reported hydrolysis rates of 0.3%/day at 25°C within Viracept 250 mg film-coated tablets.

These results and those informally reported by other organizations are not surprising when the postulated reaction is scrutinized. First, for any reaction to occur, there first has to be a proton source to initiate the reaction between the sulfonic acid

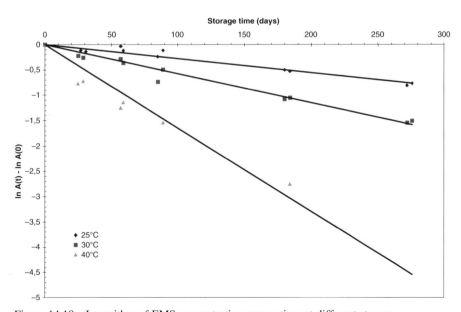

Figure 14.19   Logarithm of EMS concentration versus time at different storage temperatures. Reprinted from Gerber C, Toelle H-G. What happened: The chemistry side of the incident with EMS contamination in Viracept tablets. *Toxicology Letters* 190(3): 248–253. Copyright 2009, with permission from Elsevier.

and any alcohol. This would require the salt to disassociate. This in itself is very unlikely, as any such salt would have been selected on the basis of among several parameters, its stability. Furthermore, even if this was to occur, the likely kinetics of any reaction between sulfonic acid and residual levels of any alcohol present in the solid formulation (tablet) are likely to be extremely slow. Given the concentrations involved and the relatively low temperatures, levels formed are therefore likely to be miniscule. Far more likely, as demonstrated by the Roche data, is that any pre-formed ester present in formulated product will degrade through hydrolysis either as a result of water present directly in the formulation, or through moisture within the air picked up on storage.

14.6 CONCLUSIONS

At the onset of this work, many organizations had, through analysis of isolated sulfonic acid salts, demonstrated rudimentary control over levels of sulfonate esters. However, this was based on little or no understanding of the extent or nature of the reaction between sulfonic acids and alcohols.

These studies have delivered a clear understanding both of the reaction mechanism itself and of the key parameters that affect the kinetics of the reaction. This has made it possible to manipulate these key parameters in order to control sulfonate ester formation to such an extent as to render the risk it poses in terms of contamination of sulfonic acid salt inconsequential.

ACKNOWLEDGMENTS

I would particularly like to thank Dr Steve Eyley (AstraZeneca) for his help in constructing this chapter, especially in the help he has provided in the graphical representation of the data. I would also like to thank all those involved in PQRI working group (listed below). It has been a real pleasure working with such a committed team and finally I'd like to thank PQRI themselves for their support in undertaking the studies described.

PQRI Working Group
Steve Eyley/Andrew Teasdale (AstraZeneca)-Team Leader.
Andrew Lipcynski/Karen Taylor Worth (Pfizer).

- Kevin Facchine/Dave Elder (GSK)
- Van Reif (Schering Plough)
- Rolf Schulte-Oestrich (Roche)
- Ed Delaney (formerly BMS)—employed as a consultant to the project
- Simon Golec (Wyeth)

RIC
Karine Jacq/Frank David
FDA
Rick Lostritto

REFERENCES

1. European Directorate for the Quality of Medicines and Healthcare. 2000. Enquiry: alkyl mesilate (methane sulfonate) impurities in mesilate salts. *PharmEuropa* 12:27.
2. Glowienke S, Frieauff W, Allmendinger T. 2005. Structure-activity considerations and *in vitro* approaches to assess the genotoxicity of 19 methane-, benzene- and toluenesulfonic acid esters. *Mutation Research* 581:23–34.
3. Elder DP, Snodin DJ. 2009. Drug substances presented as sulfonic acid salts: overview of utility, safety and regulation. *Pharmacy and Pharmacology* 61:269–278.
4. EMEA press release, European Medicines Agency agrees on action plan following the recall of Viracept and recommends suspension of the Marketing Authorisation. Doc ref. EMEA/275367/2007.
5. Swissmedic Department for Control of the Medicinal Products Market. 2007. *Mesylate ester type impurities contained in medicinal products*. October 23, 2007.
6. Coordination Group for Mutual Recognition-Human Committee (CMDh). 2008. *Request to assess the risk of occurrence of contamination with mesilate esters and other related compounds in pharmaceutical*. EMEA/CMDh/ 98694/2008, London, February 27, 2008.
7. Elder DP, Teasdale A, Elyey S. 2010. The utility of sulfonate salts in drug development. *Journal of Pharmaceutical Sciences* 99(7):2948–2961.
8. Teasdale A, Eyley S, Delaney E, et al. 2009. Mechanism and processing parameters affecting the formation of methyl methanesulfonate from methanol and methanesulfonic acid: An illustrative example for sulfonate Ester impurity formation. *Organic Process Research and Development* 13:429–433.
9. Snodin DJ. 2006. Residues of Genotoxic alkyl mesylates in mesylate salt drug substances: Real or imaginary problems? *Regulatory Toxicology and Pharmacology* 45:7–90.
10. Elder DP, Teasdale A, Lipczynski A. 2008. Control and analysis of alkyl esters of alkyl and aryl sulfonic acids in novel active pharmaceutical ingredients (APIs). *Journal of Pharmaceutical and Biomedical Analysis* 46:1–8.
11. Lee CR, Guivarch F, Van Dau CN, et al. 2003. Determination of polar alkylating agents as thiocyanate/isothiocyanate derivatives by reaction headspace gas chromatography. *Analyst* 128:857–863.
12. Alzaga R, Ryan RW, Taylor-Worth K, et al. 2007. A generic approach for the determination of of residues of alkylating agents in active pharmaceutical ingredients by in situ derivatization-headspace –gas chromatography-mass spectrometr. *Journal of Pharmaceutical and Biomedical Analysis* 45:472–479.
13. Jacq K, Delaney E, Teasdale A, et al. 2008. Development and validation of an automated static headspace gas chromotography-mass spectrometry (SHS-GC-MS) method for monitoring the formation of ethyl methane sulfonate from ethanol and methane sulfonic acid. *Journal of Pharmaceutical and Biomedical Analysis* 48(5):1339.
14. Berge SM, Bighley LD, Monkhouse DC. 1977. Pharmaceutical salts. *Journal of Pharmaceutical Sciences* 66:1–19.
15. Bighley LD, Berge SM, Monkhouse DC. 1995. Preservation of pharmaceutical products to salt forms of drugs and absorption. In: *Encyclopodeia of Pharmaceutical Technology*, Vol. 13, edited by J Swarbrick, JC Boylan. Marcell-Decker, Inc., New York, pp. 453–499.
16. Gerber C, Toelle H-G. 2009. What happened: The chemistry side of the incident with EMS contamination in Viracept tablets. *Toxicology Letters* 190:248–253.

CHAPTER 15

ASPECTS TO CONSIDER WHEN LOW-LEVEL ACTIVE PHARMACEUTICAL INGREDIENT/DRUG PRODUCT DEGRADANTS HAVE THE POTENTIAL FOR GENOTOXICITY

Alan P. McKeown
Andrew Teasdale

15.1 INTRODUCTION

The safety of impurities present in active pharmaceutical ingredients (APIs) and drug products (DPs) is a concern for both pharmaceutical scientists and pharmaceutical regulatory agencies. The control of impurities (e.g. organic and inorganic impurities and residual solvents) is generally addressed by ICH guidelines covering both API and DP.[1-3] However, within the spectrum of impurities that need to be assessed, genotoxic impurities are a subclass that requires specific consideration. In recent times, European and American pharmaceutical regulatory expectations for genotoxic impurities have been described[4,5] to be used in conjunction with the ICH guidance. The scope of the specific guidance for genotoxic impurities includes synthesis-related impurities and those species resulting from degradation of the API or DP. Strategies for risk assessing genotoxic impurities arising from synthetic routes have been described previously,[6] and an example is explored within Chapter 9 of this book. Risk assessing a genotoxic degradant where the structure is known may follow similar principles to the process applied for synthesis-related genotoxic impurities. However, identified genotoxic degradants may require additional considerations or controls, as there is no opportunity for removal, and they need to be assessed over the shelf life of the API/DP. The more complex scenario (procedurally, technically) is devising an approach to understand the formation of degradants at low levels in the API/DP (e.g. sometimes at levels below ICH reporting thresholds), their identification, and, finally, determination of any genotoxic risk.

At present, there is no harmonized approach defining how to address such issues from an industry perspective, and little is known about the acceptance or otherwise of any approach from the perspective of regulatory authorities.

This book chapter therefore aims to discuss what may be important for the pharmaceutical scientist to consider when attempting to develop a strategy aimed at understanding the formation of low-level degradants and their potential for genotoxicity within a new medicine development program.

There are a number of factors to consider, and knowledge sources that may be useful to understand degradant formation and assess the potential for genotoxicity to reduce risk. It is highly likely, however, that any such evaluation and associated scholarship will include case specific elements. The following discussion aims to outline the main areas for consideration by the pharmaceutical scientist. The evaluation may be split into key areas:

- approaches to understanding low level degradant formation:
  - molecular assessments;
  - application of *in silico* tools;
  - stress studies; and
  - stability studies;
- compiling the different elements into a coherent and systematic approach.

15.2 APPROACHES TO UNDERSTANDING LOW-LEVEL DEGRADANT FORMATION

15.2.1 Molecular Assessments

Experience of molecule classes can be important during the development of new medicines. When a particular molecular framework has been identified as active in a disease area, it is not unusual for a sequence of new chemical entities to be progressed in parallel through the investigational phases of new medical product development. This can provide a useful broad knowledge of the physical and chemical attributes and behavior of the molecule class. Much of this information can be valuable for molecular class chemical degradation prediction, including the understanding of whether structural alerts for genotoxicity exist or may form. An evaluation of the parent molecule can establish whether any structural alerts exist and could be propagated to degradants, and whether functional groups within the parent molecule could yield structural alerting groups in a degradant. Finally, should a degradant form with an alerting group through a particular chemical degradation pathway/rearrangement, it is an important piece of knowledge when trying to understand degradation behavior for subsequent similar drug candidates, and the determination of such a species can be factored into experimental plans. The following general chemical degradation schemes provide examples to consider for the formation of degradants containing alerting groups, and may be useful in initial molecular assessments.

15.2.1.1   Examples of Nonalerting Molecules Yielding Structurally Alerting Degradants from Embedded Functional Groups

Amide Hydrolysis to Yield an Aniline/Hetero-Aromatic Amine

In this specific instance, due to the risk of hydrolysis of the amide bond, both through degradation and perhaps more significantly, metabolism, many organizations will now actively address this risk during the candidate drug selection phase, typically through evaluation of whether the bond remains intact, or through conduct of a bacterial reverse mutation assay, that is Ames test.

Formation of α,β-Unsaturated Carbonyl Groups through Oxidation

In this particular scheme, the alcohol group is converted to the corresponding carbonyl moiety. This reaction yields a α,β-unsaturated structure that flags as a structural alert with the potential for genotoxicity. This particular structure tends to be a minority product observed, with the major product being oxidation across the unsaturated bond. Nevertheless, this is a good example highlighting that even as a minor product of a chemical transformation, the α,β-unsaturated form may need to be considered due to its structural alerting status.

15.2.1.2   Examples of Nonalerting Molecules Yielding Structurally Alerting Degradants with Modification of Functional Groups

$$R-OH_2^+ + Cl^- \rightarrow R-Cl + OH_2$$

Formation of an Alkyl Halide through Nucleophilic Substitution of an Alcohol   The potential generation of alkyl halides through a reaction between alcoholic solvents and hydrochloric acid used in the process has recently been highlighted.[7] Such a risk potentially exists for drugs that possess an alcoholic functionality. This particular route of degradation has added significance when the potential of *in vivo* degradation is taken into account, that is degradation in the stomach. However, such a risk needs careful evaluation and should not be over interpreted and/or simplified. For instance, stomach pH varies considerably depending on whether or not food has been taken, ranging from pH2 (after overnight fasting) to pH5. Furthermore, when assessing any potential *in vivo* risk other factors, such as residence time in the stomach (for food between 3–5 h), dissolution rate of the DP and drug absorption kinetics through the stomach wall could well need to be considered. If there is evidence of acid instability derived from *in vitro* studies (i.e. stress studies), then specific targeted work under physiological conditions may be considered.

Oxidation of an Alcohol to Form an Aldehyde   Aldehydes provide a good example of the variance that can be seen in relation to a specific class. Although a small number of low molecular weight aldehydes present a concern from a genotoxic perspective, a significant number of other aldehydes are not genotoxic. It thus may be advisable that even if there is evidence of aldehyde formation, that the aldehyde in question be subject to further evaluation (e.g. Ames test) rather than simply assume it is genotoxic.

Aldehyde Formation through Radical Catalysis   A reaction that may be observed through photostability studies is a retro-aldol reaction. It may also be a key degradation pathway in radical catalyzed oxidation reactions.

15.2.1.3   Examples of Explicit Structural Alerts and Propagation to Degradants

In this example, a significant impurity, an alkyl halide, was found to be present in the API. In the actual example upon which this is based, the alkyl halide was found to be nongenotoxic. However, further degradation was observed; the labile amide bond hydrolyzed to split the molecule into two degradants: one, the carboxylic acid fragment, was of no concern; however, the other fragment retained the alkyl halide structural alert, flagging the degradant as having potential for genotoxicity.

It is important to note that degradants which share the same structural alerting group as the parent may be assessed using the mutagenicity data obtained for the parent.[4] However, in examples where the degradant is significantly different to the parent (e.g. molecular weight, functionality through degradation, reactivity), despite the fact the alert is common to both, it may be necessary to consider them separately, that is the degradant cannot be covered by the parent mutagenicity data (i.e. as a "Class 4" genotoxic alert[8]). Separate considerations/control strategies for the degradant may therefore be needed. Indeed, in this instance, the smaller, less sterically hindered alkyl halide was tested and found to be genotoxic.

15.2.2   Summarizing Molecular Assessments

Compiling the likely degradants list for a molecule can be a useful initial assessment to understand the genotoxic potential of degradants. If the pharmaceutical scientist is able to identify likely chemical reactions or functional group/molecule vulnerability (i.e. to acid, base, oxidant, etc.), then predicted degradants from the molecular assessment work can be verified/explored with subsequently well-designed stress studies.

15.2.3   Application of *In Silico* Tools for Predicting Degradation

The use of *in silico* tools could be a valuable, labor saving, and efficient approach to assessing drug degradation under a variety of conditions. The application of such tools may potentially save significant amounts of time while ensuring a consistent approach to the molecule assessment. This could be through the use of "rules" that have been programmed into the system to obey chemical transformations from organic chemistry knowledge, or even a neural network approach where a system could learn from previous examples/data and apply to future tasks. However, attempting to accurately simulate and predict chemical transformations under a variety of environments is a highly complex and specialized area. This may account for the relatively few tools available. At the time of writing, there are some software tools (commercial, proprietary, free and under development, which include CAMEO™ (Cemcomco, LLC P. O. Box 52 Madison, CT 06443 USA), DELPHI™ (Pfizer internal system), Pharma D3™ (CambridgeSoft Corporation, 100 CambridgePark Drive, Cambridge, MA 02140 USA), and Zeneth™ (Lhasa Limited | Registered office: 22-23 Blenheim Terrace, Woodhouse Lane, Leeds, LS2 9HD), respectively) available. The application of these tools to predict degradants, pathways, and behavior is not widespread. This is likely to be a major area for development over the next few years, with some companies developing products with pharmaceutical scientists for the pharmaceutical industry. This type of approach should provide the first specific *in silico* tool designed for degradation chemistry within the pharmaceutical industry. It is hoped that any software degradation tool is able to provide a comprehensive list of significant degradants for various conditions based upon chemical transformation rules and previous experience. Long lists of low probability degradants based on every theoretical degradation pathway (including multistep pathways) could be unhelpful, as the both ICH guidelines governing stability studies and the EMEA guideline covering genotoxic impurities themselves state that the focus for degradants (and impurities) should be on those species that might be reasonably expected. There is much hope that a well-designed software tool could provide significant strides forward for the pharmaceutical industry and regulatory agencies by providing an efficient means whereby a consistent and accurate understanding of degradant formation can be achieved.

Finally, it is important to sound a note of caution with regard to such systems, as they evolve and become more frequently applied within development programs in the industry. Any *in silico* prediction should ultimately be viewed as exactly that, a prediction, of note and interest, and not proof positive that a specific degradant will form. The approach prescribed by the EMEA guideline and its Q&A supplement both make it clear that for impurities (of which degradants are a subset), the focus should be on probable impurities (for which *in silico* tools can help the pharmaceutical scientist understand).

15.2.4 Stress Studies

One of the most difficult aspects in trying to understand the formation of degradants (in general, let alone if they possess a genotoxic risk) is how to assess their significance in relation to the anticipated long-term storage conditions of the product. In trying to define which degradants to focus on, it is useful to consider regulatory guidance. The ICH stability guideline Q1A(R) points out in the text on stress testing[9] that:

> Examining degradation products under stress conditions is useful in establishing degradation pathways and developing and validating suitable analytical procedures. However, it may not be necessary to examine specifically for certain degradation products if it has been demonstrated that they are not formed under accelerated or long term storage conditions.

Thus, stress studies (under conditions that may include heat, humidity, light, pH, oxidants) are a useful activity for understanding the range of degradants produced from API or DP under various conditions (as well as providing an insight to degradation pathways and samples to develop stability-indicating analytical methods). Studies crafted to encourage accelerated degradation (using appropriate energy/conditions) remain a useful activity to observe potentially relevant degradants. Most investigative degradation work inevitably applies stress conditions to induce degradation. From the resulting degradation profiles, it is usually straightforward to identify and understand principal degradation pathways. The assumption is made that principal degradants formed under suitable stress conditions (i.e. exaggerated storage conditions) will allow the pharmaceutical scientist to observe (or predict) the degradation profile that would result after a considerable time under long-term storage conditions of the product. This process serves well for the main degradants. (Specific guidance in terms of the conditions employed in such studies is covered in the work of Reynolds et al.[10] and Klick et al.[11])

Within such studies, the minor degradants are typically not identified, as it is proposed that if their presence after stress conditions is minor, then their likelihood of appearing at significant levels under the product's long-term storage conditions is a low risk. The challenge with genotoxic degradants is that control may be required at levels significantly below ICH thresholds (into ppm regions). To illustrate, the acceptable limit for any PGI (including PGI degradants) is calculated by dose as well as a variety of other factors. Therefore, a chronic use product with a 1000 mg/ day daily dose could result (based on a TTC of 1.5 mcg/day) in a maximum acceptable limit for the PGI degradant of 1.5 ppm. This in itself can be an analytical challenge. However, added to this is the knowledge that a lower limit (i.e. <TTC) will be required at product release, coupled with a thorough understanding of the genotoxic degradant formation kinetics to ensure the quality of the API/DP to the end of the designated shelf-life period. It is also highly likely that specific, validated analytical methods would be applied in such situations and such tests would be used for product release and stability monitoring purposes. It is clear from this example that the presence of a genotoxic degradant demands considerable additional efforts for the pharmaceutical scientist over and above nongenotoxic impurities to maintain a sufficient control strategy to assure quality and patient safety.

However, it is neither practical nor required to identify all ppm level species observed from all stress studies. Instead, there is potential to provide an insight to the low-level degradant formation, and extrapolate to real time under long-term storage conditions through the astute design of certain stress studies (i.e. elevated temperature/humidity), and this will be explored further. As already discussed, stress studies involve the exploration of degradation pathways induced by heat, humidity, a wide pH range in solution, oxidants, and light. Not all of these conditions may be directly relevant or useful for predicting degradants that will actually form during long-term storage of a particular API/DP. Exposing the API/DP to elevated temperature and humidity conditions could be the most appropriate approach to take, and should provide relevant, meaningful data (i.e. produce degradants more likely to be seen during long-term storage conditions). The other forced degradation conditions (pH, oxidant, light) are useful to build the complete understanding of the molecule degradation chemistry/pathways, but often may have little relevance in relation to the API/DP long-term storage. Such studies (i.e. pH, oxidant, light) are particularly useful in identifying a specific instability under certain conditions, as this can often trigger pharmaceutical development activities to minimize degradation, for example for oxidation, allowing the DP formulation to include an antioxidant, or, for light instability, ensuring storage of the API/DP in appropriately protective packaging.

Stability evaluations at elevated temperatures and humidities (the applicability and understanding provided by using modified Arrhenius equations that take account of the role of humidity in chemical degradation kinetics, along with Monte Carlo simulations to understand experimental variance[12–14]) have recently been successfully applied to longer-term stability predictions for API/DP. The approach effectively reduces stability study timelines to a matter of weeks (depending upon the protocol applied), and has been shown to give data that agree well with real-time studies.

Once these studies have been executed, the samples may be analyzed using a variety of orthogonal analytical tools to determine the nature of the degradants formed. A specific challenge faced when assessing data from stress studies is how to establish an identification threshold. This is only partially addressed through regulatory guidance from the recent formal EMEA Q&A response to submitted queries on the EMEA GTI document[15] states:

> In line with the ICH guideline, <u>no action is generally required for a new unidentified impurity found at levels below the ICH identification threshold.</u> When an impurity is found above the ICH identification threshold, but below the qualification threshold, and the structure gives rise to a structural alert, this can be negated by carrying out an Ames test on the active ingredient containing the impurity as long as the impurity is present at a minimum concentration of 250 µg/plate (estimated detection limit for most relevant mutagens in Ames test, see Kenyon et al., Reg Tox & Pharm, 2007, 75–86). <u>If the structure cannot be elucidated, then no action is generally required.</u> Above the ICH qualification threshold, then the ICH guidance should be followed. (Underline added for emphasis)

The problem, though, is how to relate this to degradation studies, especially where extensive degradation is observed. Such studies could well lead to the generation of degradation products that result from secondary degradation and even reactions between individual degradants, impurities that are very unlikely to form under "normal" storage conditions. Certain, empirical, approaches have been suggested: an identification threshold equivalent to 10% of the total degradation observed has been discussed informally between various pharmaceutical scientists in recent times, similarly for situations where the level of degradation is low (i.e. ≤1%); another approach suggested is to identify those degradants that consist of >30% of the total. While such approaches may provide pragmatic guidance, the appropriate identification threshold should be determined on a case-by-case basis, taking into account not only the extent of degradation, but also other factors, such disease area/dose/duration, etc. that impact on the permissible level for any GI.

15.2.5 Stability Studies

Long-term stability studies are typically performed to ICH conditions,[9] and are currently expected by regulatory agencies to demonstrate the quality and safety of products over the shelf-life period. The main degradants observed through stability studies are typically predictable from stress studies, and this is a useful correlation/corroboration of the main degradation behavior.

The long-term stability studies are also a pivotal source of samples to evaluate specific analytics to confirm or disprove the presence of suspected genotoxic degradants derived from the combined knowledge of the molecular assessment and stress studies work.

15.2.6 Combining These Different Elements into an Approach for Genotoxic Degradants

It should be possible for the pharmaceutical scientist to devise a framework to demonstrate that reasonable efforts have been applied, coupled with a strong science basis to investigate the presence of degradants that may be genotoxic by combining the "likely degradants" output from the molecular assessment, with the degradant profile observed from the elevated temperature/humidity studies and linking these data to the forced degradation work already performed. This would provide assurance for the pharmaceutical scientist and regulators of suitable due diligence.

This type of approach should ensure focused analytical attention on relevant degradants (i.e. prediction of major and significant minor species that may appear in long-term stability studies under standard storage conditions), and offers an alternative to developing a suite of highly sensitive, specialized methods that monitor down to low levels for potential and theoretical degradants that may not be present.

15.3   OTHER CONSIDERATIONS

15.3.1   Timing of Studies

The timing of the various evaluations described also needs to be considered. In general, it is advisable to have performed initial evaluations (molecular assessments and initial forced degradation studies) ahead of introducing the API/DP concerned into first-in-human clinical trials. It is, however, likely to be impractical to instigate detailed investigations as required for NDA/MAA submissions during the initial stages of development, as many factors that could affect stability will not be finalized. For instance the manufacturing process for the API will almost certainly not be finalized and could change significantly, this in turn could result in differences in the form of the API; which could itself affect stability. In addition, the initial formulated product is likely to be a probe formulation and thus significantly different to that of the final commercial product.

Such factors mean that any evaluation is therefore a continual process that builds on the initial assessments, constantly refining the knowledge through the input of specific scientific data from a variety of physical and chemical studies.

15.3.2   Safety Testing

In silico assessments for structural alerting motifs are performed using tools such as DEREK and/or MCase, and provide very useful indication of the potential genotoxicity of a compound. Such systems are deliberately designed to be sensitive to such a potential risk, and any output needs subject matter expert consideration and interrogation. Actual testing of degradants for mutagenicity in the form of a bacterial reverse mutation assay (Ames test) should also be considered as part of the risk assessment and control strategy deliberations.

15.3.3   Metabolites

There is, in some instances, a high degree of correlation between degradants and some metabolites; this can be particularly true of hydrolytic and oxidative degradants. It is therefore important that the results obtained from the *in vivo* or *in vitro* metabolite and parallel chemical stress studies are correlated. The topic of genotoxic metabolites and risk management approaches[16] is discussed in detail in Chapter 6 of this book.

15.4 CASE STUDY

The following case study has been compiled to highlight a number of the activities discussed in this chapter (including molecular assessment, stress study and stability data), and how they can be used for an assessment of genotoxic degradants. This case study also demonstrates the potential complexity of the genotoxic degradant topic.

NXY-059 was a candidate drug evaluated as a potential neuroprotectant. The synthetic route is described in Figure 15.1.

15.4.1 Molecular Assessment

NXY-059 was (like many experimental medicines) already in development at the point the EMEA guideline was being drafted, and hence a retrospective assessment of potential genotoxic impurities was performed. The NXY-059 molecule is relatively simple, and from a chemical degradation perspective, there would appear to be few potential products. The dissociation of the parent molecule to the subsequent benzaldehyde-2,4-disulfonic acid and, *tert*-butylhydroxylamine (tBHA) had already been identified as a degradation pathway.

15.4.2 Stress Studies

Further stress studies, however, illustrated the degradation profile to be more complex. A potentially genotoxic compound, azoxy-*tert*-butane (Fig. 15.2), was subsequently identified. This coincided with the development of the guideline, and thus investigations were initiated to understand the origin of this compound.

Azoxy-*tert*-butane had already been observed as a minor by-product (<0.02 area % by GC) in the final intermediate, *tert*-butylhydroxylamine acetate (tBHA-acetate, see Fig. 15.1). Subsequent analysis of the API showed azoxy-*tert*-butane levels to be approximately 10 ppm. However, NXY-059 was intended for continuous

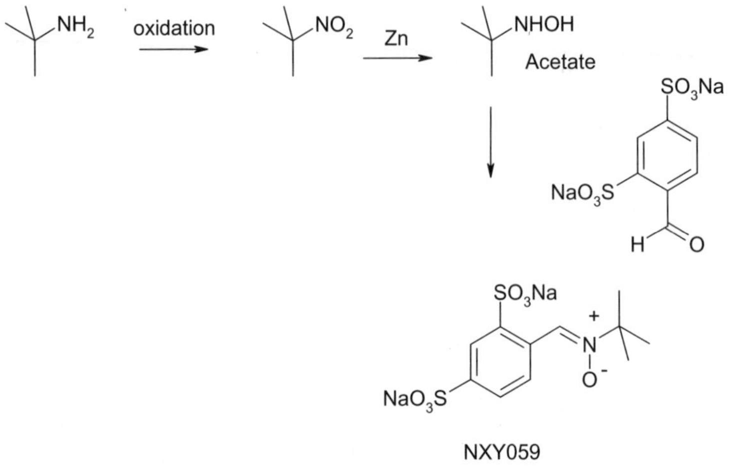

Figure 15.1 Synthetic route to NXY-059.

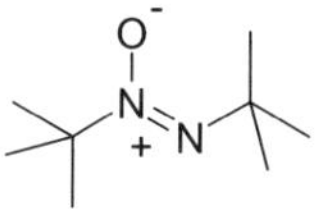

Figure 15.2   Structure of the potentially genotoxic compound azoxy-*tert*-butane.

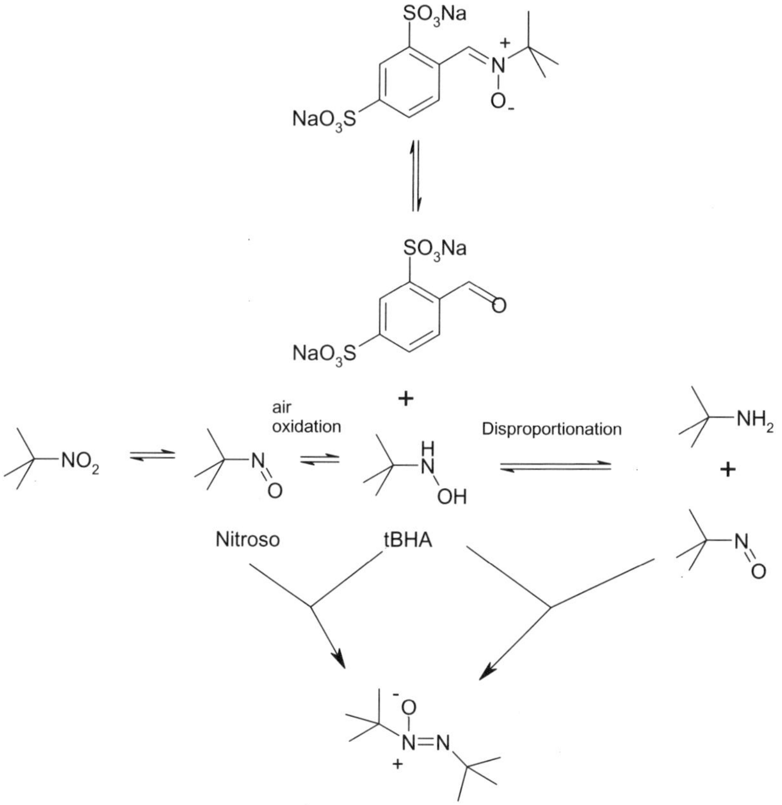

Figure 15.3   Potential pathways leading to the generation of azoxy-tert-butane.

infusion for a period of 72 h post, an ischemic event (stroke) with a total intended drug dose (73 g). At the time this was investigated, there was no formal acceptance of the staged TTC concept linking limits for GIs to duration of exposure. Thus, based on the standard TTC limit of 1.5 µg/day a very conservative target, a limit of ≤60 ppb was imposed.

Further investigations into the degradant through mapping activities revealed that azoxy-*tert*-butane was believed to form as a dimer of tBHA and the corresponding nitroso compound. Several proposed routes to the formation of azoxy-*tert*-butane were proposed (Fig. 15.3).

These included the evidence of trace levels of azoxy-*tert*-butane in tBHA-acetate originating from the tBHA-acetate synthesis and the formation from 2-methyl-2-nitropropane via the intermediate nitroso compound. The nitroso compound could also be formed by degradation or oxidation of tBHA in the API process

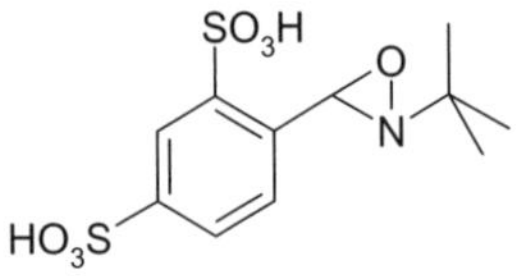

Figure 15.4   Oxaziridine.

(reaction, drying, etc.), or during storage of the API or during formulation to the IV DP and subsequent storage of the IV DP. Finally, NXY-059 was also found to partly dissociate into benzaldehyde-2,4-disulfonic acid and tBHA in solution, as initially predicted by the molecular assessment.

This story illustrates the complexity of degradation pathways and how stress studies are key to understanding degradation pathways.

Control over levels was eventually achieved through optimizing the API process by introducing a recrystallization step and drying the API at a low temperature (30°C as opposed to the original drying temperature of 80°C).

In parallel to the activities described above, preclinical safety studies were also being pursued. Despite being an azoxy type impurity (and hence part of a group of compounds considered to be of particular concern identified in the EMEA guideline), the azoxy-*tert*-butane was found to negative in a rat comet assay. This illustrates another very important point, and that is that there may always be value in performing preclinical safety studies.

In addition to azoxy-*tert*-butane, another degradant, an oxaziridine (Fig. 15.4), was also observed and identified from the stability studies. This was found to form predominantly within the final IV formulated product. Despite possessing no structural alert when screened both in DEREK and MCase, regulatory agencies requested Ames and mouse lymphoma (MLA) testing.

In parallel to the conduct of these safety tests, extensive investigations were conducted in order to control levels of this oxaziridine. It was discovered that light was the main contributing factor to the formation of this impurity, and thus control ultimately required the use of UV-resistant plastic tubing and infusion bags. Oxaziridine was ultimately found to be negative in both Ames and MLA tests, and was subsequently controlled to standard ICH thresholds.

This case study highlights a number of important points.

- Degradation processes are complex.
- Intermediates are often degradants, too, so linking the degradant investigations to the synthetic route PGI assessment is vital.
- The molecular assessment identified one of the three main degradants.
- Stress studies helped identify key degradants.
- Degradant/impurity mapping activities help build a complete understanding of the chemical behaviour of degradants/impurities in API/DP.
- Photostability studies identified a separate degradant not seen elsewhere, and influenced the product packaging requirements.

- The appropriateness of genotoxicity testing should always be considered, as it can help reduce potential risks (e.g. the oxaziridine).
- In the context of genotoxic impurities, this case study highlights that structural alerts alone do not necessarily always confer genotoxicity—there are only indicative of a potential risk (e.g. the azoxy-*tert*-butane).

15.5   OVERALL CONCLUSIONS

At present, there is a lot of discussion within the pharmaceutical industry in relation to which factors to include when trying to understand the risk that API/DP could produce genotoxic degradants. The discussions in this chapter outline the elements that could be considered for a data-driven, science basis for genotoxic degradant risk management. We have attempted to highlight topics for the pharmaceutical scientist to consider when trying to understand an API/DP degradant profile and risk manage potentially genotoxic degradants. The suggestions in this chapter try to build a picture to allow appropriate focus on those degradants of specific concern, that is those degradants relevant to the long-term storage of the API/DP. This is principally achieved by correlating molecular assessment knowledge with data derived from elevated temperature/humidity protocols and stress studies. Once efforts have been made to identify degradants, they can be evaluated for potential genotoxicity through the established process and the use of appropriate *in silico* tools. Should genotoxic degradants be confirmed, further considerations, which include formation kinetics and specification limits at product release and end of shelf life, need to be analyzed. Should no degradants with potential for genotoxicity be identified then, provided that a systematic, scientifically justifiable process such as that outlined in this chapter has been followed, it should be possible to argue that reasonable efforts have been to provide assurance to the pharmaceutical scientist and pharmaceutical regulatory agencies.

The case study highlights the application of elements discussed and described in this chapter used to compose information and data when attempting to understand degradant formation and the potential for genotoxicity. Combining the knowledge from molecular assessments and data from stress and stability studies with degradant/impurity mapping activities provided the breadth of information to compile a data-driven, scientific position. What is clear is that each candidate should be assessed individually to ensure an appropriate risk assessment, balancing safety and ensuring practical and real progression in the development of new medicines to maintain and improve patients' health.

REFERENCES

1. ICH. *ICH Q3A (R2), Impurities in new drug substances (revised). Step 4 version.* Available at http://www.ich.org (accessed September 2010).
2. ICH. *ICH Q3B (R2), Impurities in new drug products (revised). Step 4 version.* Available at http://www.ich.org (accessed September 2010).

3. ICH. *ICH Q3C (R4), Impurities: Guideline for residual solvents. Step 4 version.* Available at http://www.ich.org (accessed September 2010).
4. *Guideline on the limits of genotoxic impurities.* EMEA/CHMP/QWP/251344/2006, London, UK, effective January 1, 2007.
5. FDA. 2008. *Genotoxic and carcinogenic impurities in drug substances and products: Recommended approaches.* Draft Guidance for Industry, published December 2008. FDA, CDER, USA.
6. Dobo KL, Greene N, Cyr MO, et al. 2006. The application of structure-based assessment to support safety and chemistry diligence to manage genotoxic impurities in active pharmaceutical ingredients during drug development. *Regul. Toxicol. Pharmacol.* 44:282–293.
7. Yang Q, Haney BP, Vaux A. 2009. Controlling the Genotoxins Ethyl Chloride and Methyl Chloride Formed During the Preparation of Amine Hydrochloride Salts from Solutions of Ethanol and Methanol. *Org. Process Res. Dev.* 13:786–791.
8. Müller L, Mauthe RJ, Riley CM, et al. 2006. A rationale for determining, testing, and controlling specific impurities in pharmaceuticals that possess potential for genotoxicity. *Regul. Toxicol. Pharmacol.* 44(3):198–211.
9. ICH. *ICH Q1A (R2), Stability testing of new drug substances and product. Step 5 version 2003.* Available at http://www.ich.org (accessed September 2010).
10. Reynolds DW, Facchine KL, Mullaney JF, et al. 2002. Available guidance and best practices for conducting forced degradation studies. *Pharm. Technol.* 48–56.
11. Klick S, Muijselaar PG, Waterval J, et al. 2005. Towards a generic approach for stress testing of drug substances and drug products. *Pharm. Technol.* 48–64.
12. Waterman KC, Adami RC. 2005. Accelerated aging: prediction of chemical stability of pharmaceuticals. *Int. J. Pharm.* 293:101–125.
13. Waterman KC, Carella AJ, Gumkowski MJ, et al. 2007. Improved protocol and data analysis for accelerated shelf-life estimation of solid dosage forms. *Pharm. Res.* 24:780–790.
14. Waterman KC, Colgan ST. 2008. A science-based approach to setting expiry dating for solid drug products. *Regulatory Rapporteur* 5:9–14.
15. EMEA. 2009. *Question and answers on CHMP guideline on the limits of genotoxic impurities,* Revision 2. EMA/CHMP/SWP/431994/2007, London, UK, December 17, 2009.
16. Dobo KL, Obach RS, Luffer-Atlas D, Bercu JP. 2009. A strategy for the risk assessment of human genotoxic metabolites. *Chem. Res. Toxicol.* 22(2):348–356.

INDEX

Genotoxic Impurities: Strategies for Identification and Control, Edited by Andrew Teasdale
Copyright © 2010 by John Wiley & Sons, Inc.

423